Integrated Primary Care

The Future of Medical and
Mental Health Collaboration

Vance,

I'll always be grateful for your support + your ideas.

Sandy

Integrated Primary Care

The Future of Medical and
Mental Health Collaboration

Alexander Blount, Editor

W. W. NORTON & COMPANY
NEW YORK • LONDON

For information about permission to reproduce selections
from this book, write to
Permissions, W. W. Norton & Company, Inc., 500 Fifth Avenue,
New York, NY 10110.

Library of Congress Cataloging-in-Publication Data

Integrated primary care : the future of medical and mental health
  collaboration / Alexander Blount, editor.
     p.   cm.
  Includes bibliographical references and index.
  ISBN-0-393-70253-7
  1. Primary care (Medicine)   2. Mental health services.
  3. Integrated delivery of health care.   4. Medical cooperation.
  I. Bount, Alexander.
  R729.5.G4I58   1998
  362.1 – dc21   97-44806   CIP

W. W. Norton & Company, Inc., 500 Fifth Avenue, New York, N.Y. 10110
http://www.wwnorton.com
W. W. Norton & Company Ltd., 10 Coptic Street, London WC1A 1PU

1 2 3 4 5 6 7 8 9 0

In memory of
Dick Auerswald

Contents

Contributors

Edgar H. Auerswald, M.D., was, at the time of his death in November, 1997, Director, Applied Epistemology Project, Iona Foundation, Inc., San Francisco, California.

George R. Biltz, M.D., is Coordinator, Center for Exercise and Nutrition, HealthPartners, Minneapolis, Minnesota.

Richard J. Bischoff, Ph.D., is Assistant Professor, Marriage and Family Therapy Program, University of San Diego, San Diego, California.

Alexander Blount, Ed.D., is Associate Professor and Director of Behavioral Science, Department of Family and Community Medicine, University of Massachusetts Medical Center, Worcester, Massachusetts.

Thomson F. Davis, Ph.D., is Director of Research, Mental Health Department, HealthPartners, Minneapolis, Minnesota.

Alison Del Vento, R.N.C., is Geriatric Nurse Specialist, Group Health Cooperative of Puget Sound, Seattle, Washington.

Tillman Farley, M.D., Director of Medical Services, Salud Family Health Center, Fort Lupton, Colorado.

James L. Griffith, M.D., is Professor of Psychiatry, Director of Consultation-Liaison and Emergency Psychiatric Services, George Washington University Medical Center, Washington, D.C.

Richard L. Heinrich, M.D., is Assistant Medical Director for Behavioral Health, HealthPartners, Minneapolis, Minnesota.

Margaret Heldring, Ph.D., is Health Policy Advisor, Office of Senator Paul Wellstone, Washington, D.C.

Leita McIntosh-Koontz, M.A., is Intern in Marriage and Family Therapy, Sharp Health, San Diego, California.

JoEllen Patterson, Ph.D., is Associate Professor and Director, Marriage and Family Therapy Program, University of San Diego, San Diego, California.

C. J. Peek, Ph.D., is Consulting Psychologist for Medical Management Development, HealthPartners, Minneapolis, Minnesota.

Patricia Robinson, Ph.D., is Psychologist, Behavioral Health and Primary Care, Group Health Cooperative of Puget Sound, Seattle, Washington.

Robert E. Simpson, Jr., D.S.W., is Vice President for Behavioral Health, Baystate Health Systems, Springfield, Massachusetts.

Kirk Strosahl, Ph.D., is Staff Psychologist and Research Evaluation Coordinator, Group Health Cooperative of Puget Sound, Seattle, Washington.

Charles Wischman, M.D., is Primary Care Physician, Group Health Cooperative of Puget Sound, Seattle, Washington.

Introduction

INTEGRATED PRIMARY CARE is an idea that is quickly taking hold in the current market-driven reorganization of health care. The trend is toward primary care and away from specialty services; toward care managed by a primary care physician as gatekeeper and away from patients shopping to find the right specialist for each different ailment; and toward capitated relationships in which the gatekeeper is partly at risk for high utilization of specialty services and away from patients' unlimited access to care. For years, evidence has been accumulating that the separation of "emotional" and "physical" problems into separate "mental health" and "medical" treatment tracks is a poor reflection of how human problems are generated and how they are best resolved. For the first time, there is a growing economic incentive to initiate the most effective approaches to addressing these problems, even if they violate the structure of caregiving as it has previously existed.

By *integrated primary care* I mean both the service that unifies medical and mental health care in a primary health care setting and the practice of avoiding the dichotomy of "physical" or "mental" in defining the problems brought by a patient. This book focuses more on the former than the latter because there is a developmental relationship between them. First, it is necessary to set up the new integrated service. Practitioners who work in integrated settings, in my experience, tend to begin to understand the problems their patients present differently. When they develop a service that can meet the broad array of "pains" that are brought to the primary care door, they begin to find that the conceptual distinctions that went with the separate service systems begin to transmogrify. New concepts and classifications, different from the "mental" and "physical" etiologies of pain, become more sensible. This transformation of conceptual systems is the generative side of integrated primary care.

When this project was first conceived, integrated primary care was being considered by mental health providers and a few physicians in some of the more evolved markets for medical services, such as Minneapolis and San Diego. It was already being practiced in settings where the usual organization of medical services did not fit and people tended to just "do what works," such as in small rural settings, urban primary care health centers, or settings serving particular populations. Advocates were convincing physicians and administrators to locate mental health providers in the primary health care setting. It now appears that in the most evolved markets, integrated primary care is being implemented in whole health care systems. The fact that this is happening in these markets supports the contention that the practice is spreading across the nation.

It is my concern that colocation will become fashionable but then fail because administrators, physicians, and mental health providers do not understand the possibilities or the pitfalls of integrated primary care. Integrated primary care is built as much on organizational structures as on the enthusiasm of team members. It requires different approaches to space, scheduling, and data reporting than many settings are used to. It requires a shift in the thinking of both physicians and behavioral health providers about the work they do and how they do it. The benefits of integrated care include increased patient and provider satisfaction with the process of health care delivery, lower cost of services, especially for the highest utilizing patients, a different way of understanding medical and behavioral health practice, even a new way of conceiving the mind and the body. The pitfalls include creating inefficiencies and resentments that exacerbate the precise problems that colocation was meant to address. Examples of colocation that has gained little in reducing medical utilization or improving patient outcomes or satisfaction are legion. In one staff model HMO that wanted to begin to integrate services, the mental health providers and the primary care physicians were located in the same small community health center building. Both medical and mental health providers were intrigued by the possibility of collaborating on patient care. Yet, the physicians had to call an "800" number to arrange for a therapist colleague to walk down the hall and join a consultation with a patient. In this HMO, willingness and enthusiasm for collaboration between providers were never the problem; supportive organizational structures were what was needed.

Integrated Primary Care: The Future of Medical and Mental Health Collaboration was written out of this concern. The contributors describe current best practices in integrated primary care. We spend as much effort showing how to successfully develop and implement these programs in different settings as we spend arguing for their usefulness. The book is addressed to several different players in the evolving world of health care in mind: the decision makers in HMOs and other primary care settings who are responsible for overall quality of care, patient satisfaction, provider satisfaction and cost; the administrative and clinical leaders who make the actual care delivery systems work and who see firsthand the problems that develop when primary care does not address the psychosocial needs of patients adequately; and all the practitioners who want to be relevant (and employed) in the new world of industrialized health care, including primary care physicians, psychiatrists, psychologists, family therapists, medical social workers, nurse practitioners, and physician's assistants. It is also designed as a resource for the academics who are training the next generation of practitioners for an ever-changing health care marketplace.

Chapter 1 is an overview of the book's ideas and issues. Next, James Griffith provides a sampling of the research on the role of psychosocial factors in the etiology and course of physical illness. He makes the case for the need of a different way of thinking, not just a different way of *doing*. Edgar Auerswald describes a fully integrated primary care program from the 1970s. It is a striking example of how easily a new culture of medical care could be formed and how far it had to be removed from mainstream medical and mental health practices. The distance required between the way the program was organized and how most care was organized was part of why the program was not sustainable. Tillman Farley, in Chapter 4, offers another view of integrated care arising in an environment that is somewhat isolated from the mainstream of primary care. It is a simple, one-office implementation of integrated primary care in a rural practice. In Chapter 5, Robert Simpson tells the story of how a multioffice implementation of integrated care in a fairly rural setting became the basis for integrated primary care becoming the cornerstone of a comprehensive behavioral health service system in the largest health care system in western Massachusetts.

Kirk Strosahl, writing from the perspective of work in a very advanced and highly organized HMO setting in Seattle, then describes the changes in behavioral health practices when providers become integrated into a primary care environment. C. J. Peek and Richard Heinrich cover the same ground, but from the perspective of administrators who have nurtured the development of integrated care in a few settings in a large health system and must find a way to expand the program to the whole system.

The next three chapters portray specific programs that developed in primary care practices in large organized health systems. Patricia Robinson, Alison Del Vento, and Charles Wischman discuss care of the frail elderly in primary care; Thomson Davis and George Biltz focus on their program for obese children, and how their team developed; Margaret Heldring argues that only integrated care truly addresses the health care needs of women. Finally, JoEllen Patterson, Richard Bischoff, and Leita McIntosh-Koontz describe the development of an integrated training program that endeavors to prepare family therapists and family physicians for the future that we see arriving.

Making a unified book out of contributions from different authors in different parts of the country is difficult. In order to make the relationship of each chapter to the whole endeavor clearer and to make transitions smoother, I have placed a brief "connecting text" in front of each chapter after the first. These conntecting texts should not be taken as indications that a chapter is incomplete on its own.

The terminology for the process of integrated care can be quite confusing. Even the authors in this book use the terms in slightly different ways; this reflects the newness of the field and the lack of an accepted standardization of terminology. In general, "integrated" seems to be replacing "collaboration" as the descriptive term of choice. "Collaboration" originally referred to providers with separate sets of expertise and practice locations who brought their work closer together, resulting in a rich exchange of communication. Although mental health treatment was considered specialty treatment, mental health problems were seen as impacting upon physical problems; the reason for collaborating was to better coordinate treatments between the two. "Integration" implies one service consisting of various aspects. In an integrated setting, behavioral health service is seen as an aspect of primary care, rather than as a specialty service. The service may be offered to people with or without mental health diagnoses.

I believe that the changes in health care will be judged as one of the most important domestic stories of the late twentieth century in the United States. As the role of life experience in a patient's developing and overcoming physical disease becomes increasingly evident, the practice of integrated primary care seems to be "common sense" to more and more people. We offer here the nuts and bolts of that practice with the hope of enhancing its development and laying the foundation for a new synthesis, moving past the Cartesian dichotomy of mind and body, which has been the basis for medical science for the last two centuries.

Integrated Primary Care

The Future of Medical and
Mental Health Collaboration

1

Introduction to Integrated Primary Care

Alexander Blount

THIS CHAPTER WILL DEFINE integrated primary care (IPC) and describe it from the points of view of providers and patients. The chapter will also explain why IPC is better than referring patients to separate medical and mental health services, and why physicians alone should not be expected to meet all the mental health needs presented in primary care.* Then we will take a brief look at how IPC has developed and why many believe it will be much more broadly practiced in the future. We will look at models of how the service is structured and discuss the routines of practice that develop. Finally, we will discuss how to move from a small pilot project to a broader implementation across a health service system.

WHAT IS INTEGRATED PRIMARY CARE?

Integrated primary care is a service that combines medical and behavioral health services to more fully address the spectrum of problems that patients bring to their primary medical care providers. It allows patients to feel that, for almost any problem, they have come to the right place.

---

*The terms "mental health," "behavioral health," "psychological," "psychiatric," and "psychosocial" can be used almost interchangeably in this and other similar contexts throughout this chapter. Each has some utility and some drawbacks. I have tried to use the term that I thought would be most familiar to the most readers in a particular context.

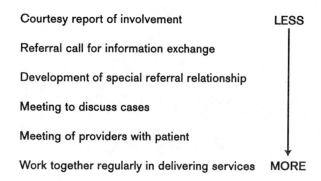

Figure 1.1. Collaborative care: The provider perspective.

It meets them "where they are" in their experience of problems or pain and does not require them to share the providers' understanding or language about etiology and treatment. By teaming mental health and medical providers, IPC is the structural realization of the biopsychosocial model (Engel, 1977) advocated so broadly in family medicine. It is the reunification in practice of mind and body usually represented in the separate worlds of medical and mental health treatment.

IPC is at one end of a continuum of ways medical and mental health practitioners collaborate. This continuum is perceived in different terms by providers of care and by patients. For providers, the continuum goes from the experience of working completely independently to working fully as part of a team.* For patients, the continuum goes from having two completely separate treatments to having one treatment plan with different providers carrying out different parts of the plan. We will first look at the continuum from the point of view of providers and then from the point of view of patients.

At the beginning of this continuum (Figure 1.1) is the courtesy contact that goes with a specialty-primary provider relationship. The mental health provider (MHP) notifies the primary care provider (PCP) that he or she is treating the patient. The primary care provider may well be the referring person. In any case, the PCP is the one other professional who is most likely to have an ongoing relationship with the patient. The notification of involvement allows the PCP to be reassured that there is some attention being given to the psychosocial aspects of the patient's care and invites further collaboration, should it be indicated.

---

*All of the collaboration described needs the consent of the patient. In many settings, the consent is built into the initial agreement between the patient and facility or between the patient and health plan.

Slightly more collaborative is a relationship in which the PCP and the MHP exchange information, usually over the telephone or in writing, at some point during the mental health treatment. Each may report aspects of the patient's situation that the other may not have had occasion to learn. There may even be coordination in areas such as medication that can be crucial for the patient's treatment. The exchange is done for the good of the patient, but does not reflect any regular working relationship between providers. The lack of working relationship between providers is often an impediment to this sort of exchange.

The next stage in collaboration is the development of a special referral relationship. Here the PCP and MHP are used to sharing the same patients. They are familiar with each other's work. They have informal but established protocols about referring back and forth. There is an opportunity to develop trust in the way patients are treated by the other provider, so that each one experiences the other as extending his or her treatment to some degree. Patients tend to notice how much faith each provider has in the work of the other.

At the next level providers meet face to face periodically to work together on treatment plans. This is most likely to happen when the providers are part of the same helping organization. This collaboration may occur because one or the other is having difficulty treating the patient. In this arrangement there may be an agreement on which aspect of the patient's situation to approach first and how each should behave to make that approach successful. Providers can also function as consultants to each other in working with the patient. The point of view of one provider can help to overcome a difficulty the other provider is having. The collaboration may be part of a regular reporting relationship between providers. Often the work of the MHP is presented to the patient as consultation to the PCP. Instead of referring the patient to the psychologist or therapist, the PCP tells the patient that there is a person who works in the practice who is very good at helping with "these sorts of problems." Work with the MHP can be "a trial" in the same way a person can have a trial of antibiotics. If a series of meetings with the MHP begins to ease the patient's anxiety or pain or helps the patient comply with medication, then that result is both information for the PCP and treatment for the patient. If it is not successful, that, too, is information for the PCP.

At the next level of collaboration the providers meet together with the patient. These meetings often include some members of the patient's family. This does not mean that in all IPC settings all patients meet with the PCP and MHP together. It means that the possibility of meeting with both providers and the patient exists in every case. In such meetings there is the chance not only to decide how to approach the patient's problem but also to define or redefine the patient's problem. A change in the definition of a problem can open up new options for solutions. Sometimes these meetings are called so that one provider can get help in his or her work with the patient. The consulting provider (usually the MHP) is addressing the relationship of the patient and the other provider (usually the PCP). In such meetings, both providers are likely to experience the patient and family as partners in developing the treatment plan.

Finally, there are situations in which each provider can represent a unified team responsible for treating the problem. In a population-based or vertically integrated approach, a multispecialty team that has developed protocols for treating a particular disorder or diagnosis, such as ADHD, obesity, or heart disease, may have worked together enough so that any one of the providers can represent the team in certain aspects of the treatment. This occurs at such times as intake or the explanation of the protocol for treatment to the patient. The team works together so regularly that over time each provider learns what the other does in certain situations. Each can fill in for the other in certain situations, even though multiple providers are necessary at other times and no provider will develop the expertise necessary to replace the other providers on the team.

In looking at this continuum from the patient's perspective (Figure 1.2) we must remember that it is not likely that he or she will be as concerned with how the contact between providers happens — by phone or face to face, regularly or on a case-by-case basis. He or she is likely to notice how much the providers agree or support each other's work. The patient experiences the degree to which either one or multiple treatments are occurring. In IPC, the more patients feel they have one treatment, the more they are likely to experience the treatment as fundamentally medical rather than psychological in nature. We will speak more about the importance of this later.

At the lowest level of collaboration, the experience of the patient is that the PCP and MHP each support the fact that the patient visits the other. The patient perceives that each provider believes that contact with the other is important and proper for the patient. At this level, the patient understands that neither the PCP nor the MHP knows many of the details of the patient's relationship with the other provider.

At the next level, the patient believes that each provider knows about and actively supports the specifics of the work being done with the other. For example, the MHP believes that the medication prescribed by the PCP is appropriate or that the PCP's doing further tests on the cause of the patient's headaches is sensible. The PCP believes that the MHP's

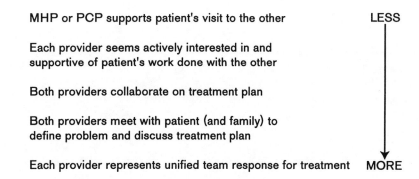

Figure 1.2. Collaborative care: The patient perspective.

engaging the whole family to work on a child's encopresis or headaches is sensible or that giving the parents specific guidance in behavioral management for their child with ADHD is useful.

At the next level patients know that the treatment plan followed by both providers was developed together, as when a physician and therapist agree that a patient with an eating disorder will be weighed every week and will be hospitalized if a certain weight threshold is crossed. Occasionally the treatment plan is generated by the MHP and PCP as equal collaborators. More often the MHP is seen as part of a team led by the PCP.

The next level is when providers meet with the patient (and sometimes the family) to develop the definition of the problem and the treatment plan. The patient sees the providers work together and understands why each of them addresses a particular aspect of the overall problem. Often in such meetings new definitions of the patient's situation are generated, creating new options for the work with each provider. Consequently, the patient and the family experience themselves as collaborative partners in the development of the treatment plan.

Finally, there are times when each provider represents a unified team responsible for treating the problem. In these settings, the patient is likely to perceive one treatment plan and a high degree of coordination between providers. Patients in these situations tend to expect and enjoy connection with other patients who are undergoing similar highly coordinated treatments for like conditions.

In practice, then, integrated primary care is the working together of medical and behavioral health providers so that the providers and the patient experience that there is one treatment plan, perhaps with several parts or steps, for the array of problems and diagnoses that the patient brings to the primary care setting.

WHY BOTHER TO INTEGRATE CARE?

For many reasons that will be discussed at the end of this chapter, it is not easy or convenient to advance along the continuum of collaborative relationships to integrated care. So why should anyone bother with the difficulties and expense that these changes represent? Here are nine reasons:

1. IPC reflects the way that the majority of patients present their distress in primary care. Their problems are not *either* biological *or* psychological; they are *both*, presenting in undifferentiated form.
2. For problems that are clearly psychological or psychiatric in nature, such as depression and anxiety, primary care medical settings are the predominant locus of treatment.
3. When the primary care service is a better fit for the way patients present, there is better adherence to treatment regimes, which leads to better outcomes.
4. Even when trained in psychiatry and counseling, primary care physicians cannot be expected to address the entire array of psychological/psychiatric problems that present in primary care, and referral out is often a poor alternative.
5. IPC is the best way of potentiating the skills of PCPs in dealing with the psychosocial aspects of primary care.
6. PCPs are happier with their work in integrated settings.
7. Patients are more satisfied with care in integrated settings.
8. It appears to be a break-even or cost-saving move in the long run.
9. Integrated primary care settings are the best laboratories for the further development and refinement of primary medical services.

Let's look at these reasons more closely.

1. *Patients come with undifferentiated problems.* Kroenke and Mangelsdorff (1989) report that less than 20% of patient visits to primary care physicians are for symptoms with discoverable organic causes and 10% are clearly only psychological in nature. That leaves the vast majority with no discoverable organic etiology in which organic factors and psychological distress are seen as mutually necessary from the physician's point of view to understand the purpose of the visit. The 14 most common presenting symptoms are: chest pain, fatigue, dizziness, headache, edema, back pain, dyspnea, insomnia, abdominal pain, numbness,

impotence, weight loss, cough, and constipation. The 10 most common complaints account for 40% of all visits, and for patients with these complaints, only 10–15% were determined, after a year of study, to have an organic diagnosis. These results are not unique (see Berkman & Breslow, 1983; Bridges & Goldberg, 1985).

Kroenke and Mangelsdorff's study sought to find the role of psychological factors in primary care visits by finding the magnitude of the role of solely biological factors. This is a welcome broadening of focus from earlier studies that looked for the magnitude of visits that were solely for psychiatric problems. These authors (e.g., Coleman, 1983; Glenn, Atkins, & Singer, 1984) tended to see the percent of primary care patients who need psychological treatment at between 15% and 20%.

By looking at the role of psychological factors in physical complaints, the picture changes dramatically: from 15–20%, which are felt to be psychiatric, to 75–80%, which are psychological in some way. As Katon (1995) put it, "I think mental health practitioners often believe that the somatizing patient is a rare phenomenon. In fact, to the primary care physician, the psychologizing patient is the rare phenomenon because people with psychological distress present the majority of the time with unexplained physical symptoms such as headaches or backaches" (p. 354).

Many people present the distress in their lives in the form of physical symptoms, but most primary medical settings are designed to treat people with biologically based problems. Physicians tend to focus on the biological and to shy away from the psychosocial side of what is presented. This tends to socialize the patient into believing that something is biologically wrong and that by looking harder he will eventually find a cure (Jenkins, 1996a). A pattern of misutilization develops for this group of patients. When the medical setting cannot relieve the problem the patient presents, he comes back repeatedly, wanting an answer and a treatment the PCP cannot provide. Katon's group (von Korff, Ormel, Katon, & Lin, 1992) found that the highest 10% of utilizers used more outpatient visits, as many prescriptions, and more specialty visits than the lowest 50% of utilizers. They also found that over half of the high utilizers were significantly psychologically distressed. Perhaps even more interesting, they found that physicians distinguish more than a third of high utilizers as frustrating to work with. These "frustrating" patients used more services than high utilizers who were equally distressed both physically and mentally. They were differentiated by the fact that their assessment of their distress was more serious than their physicians'. Compared with other high utilizers, their mental distress tended to be expressed more in somatizing and in anxiety (Lin et al., 1991).

Why not refer all these patients with nonbiologically based symptoms to a mental health professional? Patients come to the doctor because they see themselves as in need of medical services. Although a referral to mental health services may seem reasonable to the biomedical provider, it is a poor fit with patients' experience of their distress at the very least, and disrespectful or even insulting at the most. They came with what they believed to be a physical problem, and the doctor is telling them that they are fundamentally wrong about what is going on in their own body. No matter how nicely it is said, they hear that they are wasting the doctor's time. In addition, they often feel that they are losing the doctor if they accept the referral. Finally, they do not easily or lightly engage in the intimate exchange of information with a new provider, as they are accustomed to with their physician (Wolkenstein & Butler, 1993).

Bloch (1993) put it this way: "Referral of patients to mental health services (from primary care) needs rethinking. While it conforms to the biomedical model, it is often flawed and expensive. Patients and biomedical providers alike interpret referral as a sign of failure, rejection, and, often, pejorative labeling. Schematically, it signifies dysfunction at the provider/patient interface. These referrals often do not work out successfully: Either the patient does not arrive at the mental health provider's office, or, if he or she does, the contact is unproductive" (p. 4). Glenn (1987) reports that one of the reasons for establishing collaborative practice was that between 50% and 90% of the referrals to therapists "across town" did not result in a therapy.

Patients need to feel that they came to the right place. Even if they see another member of the team in that medical office, for many, the venue needs to be medical, not "mental," to fit their experience of their problems. They are much more likely to engage in psychological treatment that is housed in the same office. Katon (1995) reports that when patients who had been diagnosed as depressed by their primary physician were offered the opportunity to participate in a collaboratively structured approach to depression in the primary medical setting, 91% signed up. He reports that normally only about 50% of primary care patients who are referred to mental health practitioners actually show up for a first appointment.

2. *For problems that are clearly psychological or psychiatric in nature, such as depression and anxiety, primary care medical settings are the predominant locus of treatment.* Between 50% and 70% of patients with mental health problems in the United States are treated only in the primary medical care setting (Kessler, Burns, & Shapiro, 1987; Regier, Goldberg, & Taube, 1978; Reiger et al., 1993). This is a significant

portion of mental health treatment. These patients represent between 10% and 15% of the patients seen by PCPs. Depressive conditions, for example, take a larger toll than any of the chronic physical illnesses on patients' functioning (Katon & Schulberg, 1992; Wells & Burnam, 1991).

The actual magnitude of the problem seems to be much larger than these figures. Most studies of mental disorders that present in primary care settings have looked at groups of patients that meet criteria for specific diagnoses (major depressive disorder, anxiety disorder, somatization disorder) in the *DSM-IV* (American Psychiatric Association, 1994). There is evidence that many more patients who do not meet these criteria are still substantially disabled in their functioning due to depressive, anxiety, or somatization-type problems (Broadhead, Blazeer, George, & Tse, 1990; Katon et al., 1991; Katon, Hollifield, et al., 1995; Katon, von Korff, Lin, Bush, & Ormel, 1992; Zinbarg, 1994). Any improvement in the way that mental health problems are treated in primary care could have a dramatic impact on the functioning of a substantial portion of the population.

3. *When the primary care service is a better fit for the way patients present, there is better adherence to treatment regimes, which leads to better outcomes.* There is a significant discrepancy in primary care between physicians' prescription of and patients' adherence to treatment regimes. In one study (Katon, von Korff, Lin, Bush, & Ormel, 1992) only 45% of the "distressed high-utilizers" who were evaluated by a psychiatrist as needing antidepressant medication had been treated and only 11% had received "adequate dosage and duration of pharmacotherapy." The advent of HMOs with their own pharmacies has greatly increased the ability to track which patients at least obtain the medications prescribed by their physicians. Katon (1995) found that 44% of patients who were prescribed antidepressant medications had stopped filling prescriptions after three months. He maintains that physicians can be trained in specific techniques to make a difference in the adherence to antidepressant therapy. Physicians can also be offered psychiatric consultation to better fit prescriptions to protocols developed in specialty mental health services, but Katon's team found that the resulting improvements seem to be modest (Katon et al.).

Katon and his collaborators at the University of Washington have done some of the most exhaustive controlled research on interventions that can help primary care physicians manage mental disorders, particularly depression, more effectively. Katon conceives his studies, as well as similar ones by other researchers, as comprising three "generations." The first generation involved implementing screening procedures in primary care to more accurately identify depressed patients so that the physician could plan appropriate treatment. The second generation consisted of a diagnostic interview with a psychiatrist for patients who were identified as depressed; the psychiatrist consulted with the primary physician in developing a treatment plan for the patient. Patients were recruited to the study and then randomly assigned to the intervention or the control (usual care by their usual physician). In both generations, the diagnosis and sometimes the treatment of studied patients were more appropriate in the intervention cases than in the controls, but the outcomes in terms of patient functioning were not different (Katon, von Korff, et al., 1995; Katon, von Korff, Lin, Bush, Russo, 1992).

In the third generation studies (Katon, 1995; Katon, von Korff, et al., 1995), the intervention shifted from helping the physician (who did all the treatment) to integrating a mental health clinician into the treatment. A regular protocol of patient education about depression and brief treatment (two to four sessions) with a psychiatrist or psychologist was part of the treatment in the primary care setting. The visits with the biomedical provider alternated with the visits with the mental health provider. Outcomes began to change significantly. Table 1.1 is a summary of the study by Katon and his colleagues of an integrated approach to treating depression in primary care (Katon, von Korff, et al., 1995). The most powerful result was the difference in the patients with major depression who showed significant symptom reduction under the two conditions studied: 74% of the people with major depression in the integrated treatment plan showed significant symptom reduction while only 44% of the patients who had physician treatment and referral to mental health services at a separate site showed similar improvement.

Katon's summary of his team's findings was, "First, we know that a model of collaborative management with people with major depression dramatically improves adherence, satisfaction with treatment, and depressive outcomes" (1995, p. 364). Similar results have been reported in the United Kingdom. Balestrieri, Williams, and Wilkinson (1988) performed a meta-analysis of studies comparing treatment provided by mental health counselors in primary care and by general practitioners, and estimated that counselors achieve a 10% greater success rate.

4. *Even when trained in psychiatry and counseling, physicians cannot be expected to address the entire array of psychological/psychiatric problems that present in primary care, and referral out is often a poor alternative.* Why can't physicians do all of this themselves? After all, many primary care physicians, particularly those in family medicine, have had good training in psychosocial interventions and a few are qualified family or individual therapists. Here are just a few of the reasons:

TABLE 1.1
Impact of Integrated Approach on
Depression in Primary Care

INTERVENTION
- Patients recruited for a specific protocol to begin 4 to 6 weeks after depression first diagnosed.
- Visits 1 and 3 with physician; visits 2 and 4 (and 5 and 6 if needed) with a psychiatrist. The study was later replicated with similar results using psychologists.
- Patients were exposed to written and videotaped materials about depression and its treatment.
- Random assignment of recruited patients to treatment or control state. Control state involved regular treatment by physician with all usual opportunities for referral to specialty mental health services at a different site.

	TREATMENT	CONTROL
ADHERENCE TO MEDICATION		
major (n = 91)	75.5%	50.0%
minor (n = 126)	79.7%	40.3%
LIKED THE QUALITY OF CARE		
major	93.0%	75.0%
minor	94.4%	89.3%
RATED MEDICATION AS HELPING		
major	88.1%	63.3%
minor	81.8%	61.4%
SHOWED SIGNIFICANT SYMPTOM REDUCTION		
major	74.0%	43.8%
minor	approx. 60%	no. sig. difference

- The supply of physicians truly qualified to do family or individual therapy for the conditions found in primary care is limited (Barrett, Barrett, Oxman, & Gerber, 1988). Waiting for the supply to meet the need is futile.
- The economics of who supplies psychosocial treatment will always be against physicians as providers in cases that take more time.
- Fears of "opening a can of worms" tend to inhibit physicians' using their psychosocial training. In consulting to health centers looking to move toward integrated care, I have encountered many physicians who have substantial training in psychosocial assessment and intervention but who tend not to use that training. They fear asking a question and finding themselves with an answer that they either don't know how to address in the time allotted or are unable to address adequately, leading to a patient who feels abandoned.

This may be taken by some as a change from the general movement to help PCPs become better trained and more competent in treating mental disorders in primary care (Miranda, Hohmann, Attkisson, & Larson, 1994). It is not. It is only an acknowledgment that the physician cannot do it all and cannot reliably refer those she cannot treat to another office. As Shapiro and Talbot (1992) put it: "But one of the liabilities of Engel's 'comprehensive physician' model is that, no matter how diligently it is pursued, no one person can successfully master the totality of a wide range of desirable skills. This is especially true in the psychosocial domain in which physicians receive relatively limited training" (p. 249).

5. *It is the best way of potentiating the skills of PCPs in dealing with the psychosocial aspects of primary care.* When people of very different skill sets work together regularly in teams, there is a significant transfer of expertise among team members (Brulé & Blount, 1989). The transfer of expertise is attested to by people who have worked in integrated primary care settings. As one physician said to Mauksh and Leahy, "What is the best CME [continuing medical education] you get? It isn't taking a course, it isn't reading, it's dealing with a specific patient, learning about that patient in some way that helps you take care of that patient. Generally I will get something out of that, and so, to me, part of the collaborative relationship is an opportunity to see that as CME, as growth, as learning, not just about my personal self, but specifically about medical problems, social problems, and psychiatric problems" (Mauksch & Leahy, 1993, pp. 123–124). Katon (1995) agrees, "[Integrated models of care] provide a role for mental health practitioners, by potentiating the role of the primary care physician in treating depression rather than by supplanting him or her" (p. 364).

In integrated settings, the presence of the psychosocial provider not only keeps the skills of the biomedical providers honed, providing training through teamwork, it also allows biomedical providers to use their psychosocial expertise. If they get into a difficult situation, they know there is a colleague on site willing to help in reasonably short order.

Coleman and Patrick and their collaborators, who instituted the first large-scale integrated primary care service in an HMO in the United States (CHCP in New Haven), make the point that if the physician does not have to do all of the work of handling the emotional problems that present in primary care, she or he can actually be more effective in dealing with a wider range of these problems. "There is no reason to assume that primary physicians, on their own, without adequate mental health collaboration and support, can deal effectively with the entire range of emotional problems of their patients. The PCP needs more than a mental health referral or consultation resource; he needs the sustained, involved, daily collaboration of a mental health co-worker, with whom he can share his daily problems and concerns about emotionally disturbed patients. We find that with such collaboration, the PCP can deal with the great majority of psychiatric diagnostic categories, across the entire range of severity" (Coleman & Patrick, 1976, p. 895).

At CHCP, when mental health providers became part of the primary health team, there was a common pattern in the evolution of the way the primary care physicians related to them. At first, there was "dumping syndrome," where the PCPs tried to refer most of their patients with emotional problems to the MHP. As time went on, the rate of referral went down and the rate of consultation went up significantly. Physicians began to use the availability and expertise of the MHP to support their own management of mental health problems. Even with an MHP available and on the team, PCPs ultimately managed about 70% of the mental health problems with only consultative backup from MHPs (Coleman, Patrick, Eagle, & Hermalin, 1979).

6. *PCPs are happier with their work in integrated settings.* Being part of a team can be very helpful when providers confront the emotionally charged dilemmas presented by patients in primary care (Ross, Yudin, & Galluzzi, 1992). While a very high percentage of primary care physicians personally manage emotional problems of their patients, the percentage who feel prepared by their training to do this is much lower (Vazquez, Nath, & Murray, 1988). Dealing with many of these patients is extremely frustrating to physicians (Lin et al., 1991). The difference in job satisfaction in IPC has not been the focus of controlled studies that have been reported in the literature as yet. The anecdotal evidence seems to be that a few physicians find working in this sort of team uncomfortable, but

the great majority find it enhances their job satisfaction. In the study by Katon's group (Katon, von Korff, et al., 1995), 80% of the physicians who participated said that the collaboration with mental health professionals greatly increased their satisfaction in treating depression.

Corney (1986) assessed the already common practice of placing "marriage guidance counselors" into primary care practices in England. Besides the many positive comments from the counselors, the physicians felt that the practice made their workload lighter, there were fewer mental health referrals to outside agencies, and they prescribed fewer psychotropic drugs.

7. *Patients are more satisfied with care in integrated settings.* As in physician job satisfaction, the evidence for improved patient satisfaction is anecdotal as yet. Certainly patient satisfaction in the collaborative treatment of depression in primary care reported by Katon's group is very impressive (Katon, von Korff, et al., 1995), but it is only one study done in a limited number of settings. In general, patients tend to say they are happy with their physicians and their health care plans, which influences their staying with their health plan. This will be a telling factor in the future of IPC (this is discussed in more detail below, under item 8).

As the health care marketplace begins to be strongly affected by patient satisfaction measures, a recent study by Marshall, Hays, and Mazel (1996) may become important to those who design services. When they studied large groups of patients who had to cope with chronic illness and/or depression, they found no connection between the physical health status of patients and their satisfaction with their medical care; there was, however, a strong correlation between their mental health status and satisfaction with medical care. Although Marshall and colleages did not show that interventions to improve mental health status improves satisfaction with medical care, Katon, von Korff, et al. (1995) (see Table 1.1) have gone a long way toward demonstrating this.

8. *It appears to be a break-even or cost-saving move in the long run.* In evaluating the costs for integrated primary care, there are two competing trends to be considered. One is the trend toward lower medical cost in the presence of psychosocial intervention (Budman, Demby, & Feldstein, 1984; Cummings, Dorken, Pallack, & Henke, 1990; Jones & Vischi, 1979; Katon, 1995, Mumford, Schlesinger, & Glass, 1981; Mumford, Schlesinger, Glass, Patrick, & Cuerdon, 1984). The other is the trend toward wider utilization of mental health services when they are available in the primary care site. The literature on medical cost savings, especially in the presence of targeted, focused mental health services, is compelling. Cummings and his collaborators studied the Hawaii Medicaid Project

and found that when therapy was targeted toward the highest utilizers of medical care and focused on specific problem resolution, medical costs were reduced for all groups in the first year after the beginning of treatment, even when the cost of the mental health treatment was included. The cost reductions were 38% for Medicaid patients who were not chronically ill, 18% for Medicaid patients who were chronically ill, 35% for "employed" patients (i.e., patients on group health insurance through an employer) who were not chronically ill, 31% for employed patients who were chronically ill, and 15% for Medicaid patients who had substance abuse diagnoses.

These are typical results, yet all such studies contain one major problem when applied to IPC: They are studies of patients who, whether happily or reluctantly, accepted referral to mental health services. If we are right about the effectiveness of IPC in engaging patients who would not otherwise accept referral, then this group represents a significant number of new mental health treatment cases. Many are high utilizers of medical services and as such should show an impact in medical visits when their treatment more precisely fits their needs. On the other hand, many new cases are found as mental health treatment becomes more accessible and acceptable to patients. Not all of these will be people whose medical care will show a lot of change after mental health service.

Calculations about cost savings of locating mental health professionals in primary care in Britain are based on more experience with this model. In "fund holding" practices (capitated practices), a 36% reduction in referrals to specialist mental health services pays for the services of a full-time counselor in the practice (Jenkins, 1996b). Whether this is similar to the United States system or not, it is an interesting way of understanding the cost savings possibilities before we start to figure the medical cost savings of better treatment for the highest utilizers of services.

The claim that IPC appears to be a break-even or cost-saving proposition in the long run is based on a redefinition of the terms of the discussion as much as on evidence that is presently available. IPC represents a change in the most central venue of interaction between a health service system and its customers (patients). The improvement that IPC represents should be found in a number of different areas in the health system. In older cost-offset studies, much of the savings was in lower inpatient utilization. Much of that utilization is now believed to have been wrung out of the system in other ways, such as "drive-through deliveries" and outpatient mastectomies, that are much less effective than IPC at promoting patient and provider satisfaction or good public relations for the health plan.

If IPC makes patients more satisfied, there should be a lower rate of members leaving the health plan/health system in the presence of IPC. Macaran Baird, one of the pioneers of collaborative approaches in primary care, reported that in the health plan where he is Associate Medical Director for Primary Care, patients who say they have a good relationship with their PCP leave the plan at the rate of 3% per year and patients who report they do not have a good relationship with their PCP leave at the rate of 9% per year (M. Baird, personal communication, 1996). By improving fit of service to need, morale of providers, skill of PCPs and MHPs in caring for psychosocial problems, and clinical outcomes for some patients, IPC makes good relationships between PCPs and patients more likely.

Every new member recruited in a health plan in a mature health care market carries a cost. It may be in marketing or in lower charges to undercut the competition; in either case, it can be substantial. Interventions that increase patient satisfaction can lower those costs by limiting the number of members who leave the health plan and need to be replaced.

Another outcome that should be considered in calculating the cost offset of IPC is physician and other provider turnover. There is some evidence that providers are happier in the presence of IPC and are less likely to turn over, particularly if they had some choice about whether to participate in IPC. One local health plan (in New York and western Massachusetts) reports that it costs $13,150 to replace a physician and that the national figure for plans that do not have in-house recruiting departments is about double that; a nonphysician provider costs about half as much to replace as a physician (T. Benoit, personal communication, 1996).

Employers have much to gain from integrated care in both cost savings in health premiums and reduction of disability days (Broadhead et al., 1990). IPC appears to make the treating of psychiatric disorders in primary care more effective. The correlation between improvement in psychiatric disorders and improved functioning seems intuitively obvious. In fact, improved occupational functioning is one of the most immediate results of psychiatric improvement (Ormel et al., 1993). The effective treatment of depression, for instance, keeps people on the job. In one study, patients with severe depression who improved reduced their disability days by 36% and patients with moderate depression who improved reduced disability days by 72% (von Korff et al., 1992).

These savings have been documented in studies of behavioral health services offered by employers through employee assistance programs. A clear example was documented by the McDonnell-Douglas Corporation

(1989). An independent company conducted a comprehensive longitudinal analysis of approximately 20,000 employees who were identified as having alcohol and drug problems or emotional problems over a period of four years. Employees who used the EAP lowered their health care and dependent health care costs. The EAP users showed 34–44% decreases in absenteeism and had a 60–80% lower attrition rate. McDonnell-Douglas Corporation saved $4.00 in health costs, absenteeism, and attrition for every $1.00 spent on the EAP. But what about the employees who did not use the EAP? They were seen by their primary care physician. This is the other venue that needs to be incorporated into an overall approach to dealing with emotional and substance abuse problems in the workplace. Employers' direct dealing with health care systems and the evolution of EAP into the array of services provided by health systems now make this kind of overall approach feasible on a broad scale.

9. *Integrated primary care settings are the best laboratories for the further development and refinement of primary medical services.* Primary medical care is a special window on the human condition. It is the place where people bring the broadest array of their problems and pains. A team that integrates mental and physical health treatments creates the opportunity to think in different ways.

We are the products of what we do over time as well as what we think. *While we need to be able to think differently to act differently, we also need to be able to act differently to think differently.* The organization of social roles, the model by which we understand a particular set or domain of phenomena, and the regular routines of practice in that domain all interact recursively on each other. This interaction is discussed in more detail elsewhere (Blount & Bayona, 1994). By reorganizing social roles in a primary care medical service, new possibilities for understanding the phenomena presented there are created.

In Western medicine we have perpetuated the Cartesian dichotomy of mind and body in model (biomedical), organization (separate health and mental health systems), and practice, as well as in the basic structure of the language we use. Our linguistic and conceptual armamentarium is woefully lacking. There are no midway concepts between "mind" and "body," "psyche" and "soma," "physical" and "emotional" (or psychological) problems. The term "psychosomatic" is itself a dichotomy, implying that problems that belong in one dichotomized domain are found in the other. Somatizing patients are described as "patients who experience or express emotional discomfort and psychosocial distress as physical symptoms" (Kaplan, Lipkin, & Gordon, 1988, p. 177)—not a concept that transcends the dichotomy.

This dichotomous thinking can lead to explanations for physical problems for which we cannot find a biological cause that sometimes verge on the pathetic. We determine that patients are expressing psychological distress as physical symptoms because we cannot find a biological cause. It is a tautologic circle. The patients are somatizers because we cannot find a biological cause for their pain, and we cannot find a biological cause because they are somatizers. And how do we diagnose these patients when they do not show significant symptoms of psychological distress? We give them the diagnosis of "masked depression" (Lesse, 1968). Masked depression shows itself in unexplained physical symptoms *rather than in depressive symptoms*. So we have created a mental health diagnosis for patients who do not show mental health symptoms, but who must need a mental health diagnosis because we cannot find a physical diagnosis.

Though it is usual to describe biological or medical phenomena as different from emotional or psychiatric phenomena, this is a case of sloppy thinking in which we all engage. "Biological" and "emotional" describe different *worlds of explanation*, not different phenomena. The observer of the phenomena creates the difference by what he or she chooses to count as data. A smile is as biological as a cancer; it's just that the biological explanation of a smile is rarely needed to explain those aspects of the phenomenon that are important to us.

We have to be able to do better. But any attempt to do better that turns a blind eye to the practical applications of Western medicine or to the biological science that is behind these applications certainly fails to add to our expertise or our options.

Many of the studies of mental disorders in primary care (Barrett et al., 1988; Bridges & Goldberg, 1985; Kaplan et al., 1988; Katon et al., 1990; Kessler et al., 1987; Lesse, 1968) have documented the co-occurrence of mental and physical problems in patients, who are the highest utilizers of these services. This fact by itself can be seen as evidence of the unity of the mind and the body. The field of psychoimmunology or psychoneuroimmunology has made important strides in describing at the molecular level how this connection arises (e.g., Weiderman & Weiderman, 1988). Integrated primary care can organize professional roles and practice routines to provide a model that is much more detailed and integrated than the hierarchical systems of the biopsychosocial model (Engel, 1977). In this new model, "lower level systems" (biological), such as organ systems, could be part of the descriptions of "higher level systems" (psychosocial), such as families. The endocrinology of a mother whose son is not doing his homework can be as important in describing the system surrounding the problem as descriptions of the family communications or the family/ school system.

IF IPC IS AS USEFUL AS WE DESCRIBE, WHY HASN'T IT DEVELOPED MORE BROADLY?

Mauksch and Leahy (1993) list the barriers to collaboration as stigma, reimbursement rates, confidentialiy, territoriality, and fear of scrutiny by providers. "Other barriers include differing beliefs between mental health professionals and physicians about the process of behavioral change. Provider pace and the amount of time devoted to each patient varies from one discipline to another" (p. 122).

This is not to say that there haven't been large-scale attempts at IPC. The community health center movement that began in the 1970s tended to promote outreach to low-income patients by health care teams. The teams were made up of physicians, nurses, and nurse practitioners, and sometimes social workers or members of the community to be liaisons between the patients and the health team. Auerswald (see Chapter 3) gives an account of one of the most fully realized examples of this movement. The hope was that by reaching into the community, rather than having all health services in large hospital-based clinics, under-served populations with high vulnerability for preventable health problems could be better engaged in prevention and early treatment. These teams constituted a way of organizing medical services that were integrated within the team, but the whole approach was never integrated into the dominant forms of service delivery and funding. They operated on funds from the "war on poverty" and a few committed foundations. The whole effort tended to shrink as the pool of public money for serving low-income people shrank, though many of the community health centers it spawned still remain and serve a vital function.

WHY DOES IPC SEEM TO BE CATCHING ON NOW?

Evolution in the relative importance of primary care and in the funding structure of medical services have made IPC possible on a much broader scale than ever before. The development of family practice as a specialty in medicine created a new kind of collaboration. Family practice residencies required a behavioral science faculty member. When family medicine decided that expertise in the family should be one of the skills of its practitioners, family therapists (who were sometimes also psychologists or social workers) began to be as common as faculty in residencies. This made family practice the only medical specialty in which one of the central areas of expertise (the family) is best known by nonphysicians. Physicians trained in these residencies have the experience of seeing physicians as experts in matters of biomedicine and nonphysicians as experts in psychosocial matters. This creates a flexible hierarchy of expertise, which is the basis of the type of collaboration called for by so many authors.

The final and most important condition in the development of integrated primary care has occurred because of the development of the health care marketplace. As the marketplace has matured in areas like San Diego, Seattle, and Minneapolis, cost has become much less of a focus in the competition for market share. In mature markets most of the excess costs that can be wrung out of the system have long since been dispatched. Now the competition is based on quality as measured by things like customer satisfaction, rates of retention of members in the plan, and clinical outcomes (Luciano, 1996).

In this environment, where capitation dictates that the most efficient and satisfactory service will survive, the practice of locating mental health professionals in primary care is growing exponentially. As integrated primary care becomes familiar and accepted by physicians, mental health providers, administrators, and patients, it becomes possible to return to the model in which all referrals, even mental health referrals, go through the primary care physician's office. In this case the behavioral health provider often manages these referrals, treating some and passing others to the credentialed network of specialty providers or to the in-house specialty mental health services unit, which is much smaller and more focused on certain more impaired populations than was previously the case. When the referral is done by a behavioral health clinician who has the capacity to treat, it becomes sensible to patients that it go though the primary care office. The role of "gatekeeper," which has been part of the primary care service, changes to "case manager."

In such an organization, it becomes much easier to develop targeted behavioral health services for medical populations, including prevention/lifestyle training, mindfulness/relaxation/biofeedback training, and groups for patients and families coping with chronic illness, ADHD, neurological disorders, cardiac disease, eating disorders, juvenile diabetes, and chronic pain.

In organizations that have moved beyond cost cutting as their primary focus, the discourse of providers is moving beyond the discourse of loss that has dominated publications and conferences since the advent of managed care. People start to talk about what can be done and new possibilities in working together, rather than about the autonomy that has been taken away.

WHAT DOES IT TAKE TO BUILD A SUCCESSFUL TEAM?

Ten years ago, finding mental health clinicians to work in primary care might have been difficult. This is no longer true. The prediction that there will be fewer specialists needed in the future of health care is quite common (McDaniel, Campbell, & Seaburn, 1995). One analysis estimated a future need for only one-third of the current number of psychiatrists (Weiner, 1994). In the case of mental health professionals, these estimates have given everyone in the field reason to wonder about his or her future employability. It is no wonder, then, that many mental health practitioners see primary care as a place where they, or their trainees, might find employment.

As the training in the mental health disciplines is presently structured, each of the disciplines is potentially a good training setting for work in primary care and no discipline does the whole job of training its members for this work. Trainees from each discipline have a good deal to unlearn in order to work effectively in primary care.

Dym and Berman (1986) propose the role of "primary care therapist." This is a person who is trained in individual and family therapy with expertise in behavioral medicine (therapies aimed at changing health behavior and the body's reaction to stress). Primary care therapists need to be sufficiently familiar with anatomy, physiology, disease processes, and pharmacology to participate fully in meetings in a medical practice. If they can participate only in psychosocial discussions, they contribute to maintaining the dichotomy in roles and approaches. In the long run, they will not have to make diagnoses or prescribe treatments, but they will need to be able to function to some degree as the eyes and ears of the physician while they do their work. They need to be a consultative resource to medical staff on diagnosis and the need for psychopharmacology, though consultation with a psychiatrist needs to be readily available. Primary care therapists should have group therapy and psychoeducation skills so they can bring targeted programs to specific groups of patients and be comfortable with the role of patient educator in the areas of their expertise. They should also be comfortable in the role of case manager, following how a patient fares in relation to other agencies and providers.

A primary care therapist must be comfortable with variable amounts of time in a session, depending on what is being done. A first interview might take 30–40 minutes, a family interview could be 45–50 minutes, and an ongoing session with someone who is following a treatment plan could be 15–20 minutes. This kind of schedule meets the increased patient flow needs of primary care and the need for the MHP to be available for consultation with the PCP. This also means that session starting times, like other appointments in primary care, are approximate. The flow of urgent and routine situations in an office dictates how time will be used as much as the schedule.

Giving up the 50-minute hour means giving up many of the approaches to therapy that go with that hour. Therapy will need to be focused, goal oriented, and sometimes instructive. There will be a drift toward cognitive/behavioral and Ericksonian (strategic or hypnotic) techniques to make use of the shorter time. These techniques tend to use the time between visits for homework and use the visit for assessing progress. Some sessions will need to involve the patient's family, because many health-related problems involve family members as caretakers or holders of stress in the environment. All of these approaches fit easily with the solution-focused and systems approaches.

Mauksch and Leahy (1993) recommend the solution-focused approach of the Brief Family Therapy Center of Milwaukee as being particularly adaptable to mental health work in primary care (Berg, 1994; Berg & Miller, 1992; de Shazer, 1985, 1998; de Shazer et al., 1986; Furman & Ahola, 1992). McDaniel and colleagues (1995) assert that a family systems approach provides the best chance of healing the mind-body split in conceptual worlds and that it is the best model for therapists seeking to build what we are calling integrated primary care. This is also the advice of Coleman (1983), who is convinced that the mental health provider needs to be someone who operates with "the client in a family and social context" as a basic frame of reference (p. 116). Glenn (1987) concurs.

There are certain characteristics that emerge in the clinical models that are used in successful settings.

1. The model and language of mental health workers make sense to medical providers if medical providers are given a thorough introduction and have not already been trained in a different model.
2. There are aspects of the mental health treatment approach that can be utilized in a medical interview. In this way mental health work that must be done by physicians and nurses does not require a change of contract for service with the patient from "medical care" to "counseling" in order to be effective.

3. The approach tends to heighten hopefulness on the part of providers and ease of collaboration with patients. It fits comfortably into the range of roles and responses that patients expect in primary care.

Skills that Can Be Taught to MHPs and PCPs to Help Make IPC Work

Speaking in Front of the Patient

Often there are brief meetings between the PCP and MHP in which the patient's situation has to be introduced to the MHP and the request for the MHPs input has to be detailed. If these meetings take place away from the patient, it literally doubles the time that the consultation requires. Instead of the PCP and MHP meeting first in the hall and then in the examining room or physician's office with the patient, the whole event can occur once with the patient present. Time is used much more efficiently and the patient is part of a collaborative process rather than a staged presentation.

Conferring in front of a patient is a skill that is new to most PCPs and MHPs. It requires the ability to ask for help openly from a colleague. Symptoms must be accurately described in such a way that the patient does not feel blamed. It also requires the use of lay terminology or explanations of terms for which there is no lay person's word. This is a teachable set of skills, not, as is sometimes thought, a reflection of the personalities of providers. It is not a skill that is taught widely nor commonly identified as needed.

Working as a Team Member

Coleman and others (1979) describe the culture clash between physicians who are socialized to operate in hierarchical treatment settings and social workers or psychologists who are not. Early attempts at collaboration sometimes fell apart because of this conflict (Banta & Fox, 1972). The socialization of physicians to hierarchy does not mean that the physician always needs to be in charge just to have someone in charge. Robert Singer, a family physician, told therapists in his office to be ready to take the lead in difficult psychosocial cases and "Tell me what to do. . . . Instruct me, use me the way you think I'd be most effective. Do you what me to encourage a particular person to be independent? Do you want me to help a daughter get closer to her father, and less dependent on her mother? Tell me" (Glenn, 1987, p. 116).

Often collaboration requires a flexible hierarchy. In one situation the PCP is clearly taking the lead and in another the leadership is provided by the MHP. The MHP must be comfortable with the ultimate responsibility of the PCP, because primary care is (for the present, at least) ultimately defined as a medical service. Over time, the experience of all team members is likely to be that the medical versus psychological distinction is less necessary.

In the area of teamwork, both PCPs and MHPs should learn how to maintain a stance of *curiosity* in complex, non-life-threatening situations. Curiosity is the practice of noninterventive discovery, the attempt to understand a person's situation and experience without inevitably needing to change it. Such an approach enfranchises a team member to be active, even if he is not directing the treatment of a patient. It involves being interested in how a situation is maintained and what understandings influence the players without the requirement that any question be related to some potential action in the situation. This practice often opens up opportunities for change that cannot be found when the provider has to have a specific diagnosis and offer a treatment related to that diagnosis in the limited time available. Curiosity creates collaboration just as having to "get it right and fix it" invokes a hierarchical relationship.

If curiosity is part of the regular clinical practice of the team, it gradually influences the relating within the team. Curiosity makes it much easier to learn the language of the other culture represented on the primary care team. To be effective, MHPs must be reasonably fluent in speaking "medicalese" and PCPs need to be at least rudimentarily conversant in "psychologese." The practice of curiosity makes acquiring these languages natural and interesting rather than a compromise of the "true" language one learned in training. Teams that work together for an extended period of time tend to develop a common language. We do not yet know what commonalties of language will emerge in integrated primary care settings.

Interviewing Family Members

In describing the relief that physicians feel when MHPs are part of the practice, Glenn (1987) quotes one physician who says he did not go to medical school to wind up "in a room with three screaming adults and a teenager with a drug problem" (p. 354). He would rather find himself up at night worrying about fetal heart tones. It probably doesn't make sense to have the physician doing the therapy in such a case, but if the only thing standing between the physician and working in such a case is the screaming, that is fairly easy to deal with. The skill of conducting a family interview, keeping a focus, eliciting information, and maintaining comfortable decorum is teachable. It does not require several courses in family therapy. It can be taught by a family therapist who is experienced in the primary care setting to the advantage of PCPs and MHPs alike (Crouch & Roberts, 1987). It is a different skill from that of practicing family therapy (Doherty & Baird, 1983).

Bringing a family together to talk about their stress and ambivalence in trying to plan for a parent whose health is deteriorating is a service that should be offered in primary care, not referred to a mental health specialty service. There is no mental health diagnosis necessarily present. Similarly, both PCPs and MHPs need to be able to discover that a particular man's refusal to comply with his medical regimen is an expression of his maintaining his independence by refusing to comply with his wife's wishes. She tells him to follow his doctor's advice and he refuses to show that he is "his own man." Being able to make this assessment is a skill that can save time and frustration on the part of providers and can lead to better health outcomes if the situation can be successfully addressed in primary care.

Practicing Solution-Focused Interviewing

Solution-focused interviewing is a way of building on what patients are doing "right" rather than spending all of the time focusing on what they do "wrong." It involves *studying with patients* what is working for them rather than telling them what they need to do next or congratulating them when they cooperate with their medical regimes. It is built on the finding that the more the patient talks about the solution to the problem, as opposed to talking about the problem and what causes it, the more likely they are to report later that the problem is solved (Gingrich, de Shazer, & Weiner-Davis, 1988). I believe it is a skill to which every provider in primary care should have access, whether or not they ever do "therapy."

Perhaps a reverse example would be helpful. A resident at chart rounds once described the interview with a patient. The patient was a middle-aged woman who was overweight and had high blood pressure and heart trouble. The resident reported that since the last visit the patient had stopped smoking and lost 20 pounds. Since these two health behaviors were better, the resident spent most of the visit pushing the woman to lower her salt intake. The patient seemed very disappointed with the visit. She was heavier when she returned for her next visit.

A solution-focused interview would have asked the woman how she was able to accomplish the changes she did, what ideas helped, whose advice or support helped, even how the doctor might use what the patient had learned to help other patients. Only at that point might the patient be asked what her next goal was in her process of taking charge of her health or how she could apply these learnings to her salt intake. By eliciting the patient's story of herself as a person committed to improving her health, the likelihood of her taking the next step in that direction is increased. This is a very different relationship than one in which the patient feels she practices health behaviors to please her physician who is never satisfied.

Utilizing Brief Cognitive/Behavioral Interventions

While cognitive/behavioral techniques have proved to be effective and easily adaptable for use by MHPs in a primary care setting (see chapter 6), Patrician Robinson and her collaborators (1995) have found that they are also used effectively by PCPs as part of the regular office visit. They found that very simple techniques like talking to depressed patients about planning pleasurable activities or activities that enhanced their confidence correlated with patients subsequently using these techniques, showing higher than usual levels of compliance with any prescribed medication, and having good outcomes in terms of reductions of depressive symptoms (see also Cranwath & Miller, 1986).

When Should the Mental Health Provider be Involved?

Dym and Berman (1986) describe a relationship in integrated practice in which the physician and therapist always jointly interview a new patient at the first meeting. This joint meeting helps to elicit a full biopsychosocial view of the patient and the problems he or she brings. It allows them to determine a treatment plan in which the patient continues with one or both members of the team, rather than being referred within the office to someone other than the first interviewer. This protocol also allows for future involvement of the team member who did not carry out the initial treatment plan without having a new person brought in.

Dym and Berman illustrate this with the treatment of a man with a 16-year history of intractable headaches who had always refused a referral to a therapist because it was a sign of weakness to him. "But in our mode of practice, the primary care therapist had been in the room from the start. Gradually an alliance was built and a contract was made to deal with the tremendous tension which this very rigid man maintained for himself. Little by little, the family physician was phased out, and by the fourth meeting, he came in only to answer some questions about allergy testing" (p. 18).

Most practices will not elect to do a collaborative interview for all new patients, but the role of these interviews in the practice is no less important. If collaborative consultative interviews are common, whether they occur in all cases or a selected group, it is reasonable to expect that over time the physician will gain expertise at psychosocial interviewing and begin to handle problems alone that previously needed the psychosocial provider. If, however, the regular practice in an office involves referral and separate interviews, it is reasonable to expect physicians to get more expert only at case finding and referral. Joint interviews can be done at any point the MHP is brought into a case by the PCP or vice versa.

Glenn (1987) has articulated criteria for a physician's decision to involve a psychosocial provider:

- The patient's symptoms are unexplained by medical findings.
- The problem appears to involve other family members.
- Noncompliance of any kind is developing.
- The physician feels over his or her head with some emotional or relational problem presented by the patient.
- The physician feels hopelessly triangulated between family members.
- The physician feels chronically in conflict with the patient over diagnostic or treatment issues.
- The patient's problem appears to significantly coincide with a stage in the family's developmental cycle.
- The patient's problem involves the discovery of cancer, sudden change in physical health, or is terminal.
- A cloak of secrecy seems cast over some critical family member.
- Obvious emotional difficulties are presented by the patient in the course of treatment.

If the MHP was not involved in the initial interview with a patient, some sort of introduction is necessary when the PCP wants to involve him or her in a case. Different settings have developed different ways of handling this moment. There can be no best way of doing this because of differences in the personal styles of PCP, MHP, and patient. Following are three examples. It is important to keep experimenting to see which way of describing the MHP's involvement leads to the most comfortable and effective entry.

Glenn (1987) describes a way of making the patient a "consultant" to the MHP, at least in the first few months of the MHP's service in the practice. "I have a new therapist in the practice who is learning about how physical illnesses impact people's lives. Would you be willing to meet with him and tell him about your illness and how it has affected your life?" (p. 146) This request helps the patient to start talking about his or her social/emotional life without the implication that it needs fixing. There is no charge for this meeting since it is for the use of the provider. When the patient discovers that the MHP is knowledgeable and understanding, often a request for help is forthcoming. If this happens, subsequent meetings are billed. If not, the process is, in fact, exactly what the PCP described and may constitute an introduction that could make the involvement of the MHP easier in the future.

A second way is for the MHP to be seen as a consultant to the physician on what the physician might need to learn in working with the patient, rather than what the patient needs to learn. Physicians are usually willing to use this script because they want very much to find a way to get the MHP involved. They typically say something like, "The last few visits haven't resulted in as much relief for you as I would like, but I want to keep trying. I'd like to bring in Dr. Johnson. She is a psychologist working with me in our office. Her job is to help the physicians understand their patients better so that they can find better ways to help their patients." This introduction leads to a meeting or meetings in which the MHP discovers the contexts of the patient's life, possibly with family members. It makes perfect sense for the physician to attend, since the purpose is to aid her understanding. If both the PCP and MHP are skilled at speaking in front of patients, a portion of the first meeting can be an interview of the physician about her understanding of the patient's situation.

A third way involves a script for bringing in the MHP that is especially effective at keeping a medical definition of the process. It can be used in almost any situation without regard to whether the physical symptoms are explained by findings. The physician says, "Your pain is obviously very real. I need to assess whether stress has a role in making it worse. I want to bring in Ms. Jones, the staff member in our office who is most expert on stress." The patient waits until Ms. Jones can join the meeting. At that point the physician says to Ms. Jones in front of the patient, "I want you to make an assessment of whether stress has a role in making Mr. Smith's pain worse. Meet with him and with anyone else you need to in order to see if a reduction of stress could give him even a little relief. Report back to me with Mr. Smith within a month." An interview of the physician in front of the patient can then orient the MHP for working with the patient while the patient hears and can comment on the physician's findings and concerns. By reporting back together, the patient and MHP are defined as a team working together for the patient's good, rather than as a patient who is being treated by a new provider. They are a "subcommittee" of the medical treatment. The physician stays in charge. If the report indicates that some reduction of stress may reduce pain, then the physician can prescribe a "trial" course of treatment to reduce stress. This can lead to any of the psychosocial treatment options available within or outside the office. In all likelihood, there will have already been some relief during the "assessment" period and the MHP will simply need to finish what was begun.

HOW IS IPC ORGANIZED WITHIN THE OFFICE?

Mauksch and Phillips (Glenn, 1985) report that a receptionist who serves both the MHP's and PCP's practices seems to facilitate patients' using the counselor. Patients, at the suggestion of the physician, can go back to the same receptionist and schedule a time with the therapist.

The more integrated the practice, the more proximity is crucial. Mental health providers must be located in the primary care site. There must be overlapping time as well as shared space between the MHP and PCP. Coleman and his collaborators (Coleman et al., 1979) found that 92% of consultations between PCPs and MHPs in their setting were brief and unscheduled. Almost none of these would have happened if they were not located in the same space.

Scheduling can facilitate integrated practice. Some practices have designated times when the MHP and PCP work together. Each can schedule patients into these times knowing that the other is available. At other times, if the MHP usually sees patients for a half-hour, there are two times each hour when they can be brought in for a brief meeting with another patient or buttonholed for a consultation by a PCP.

Every practice will also need regular meetings (most choose one hour per week) to talk together about difficult cases and to work on the problems that IPC raises. Agendas should be set for these meetings, or they tend to learn more toward complaining than problem solving. Some practices reserve part of the time for difficult cases and ask that providers sign up in advance to use the time. The rest of the time is used either for administrative matters or to discuss articles or present subjects of interest to all providers. The more providers work together and learn about each other's language and work, the broader the range of topics that are of interest to all. Providers become comfortable discussing a wider range of topics. As they work together, this skill becomes important for the maintenance of the team.

Levine (1983) points out a phenomenon that has been much more thoroughly discussed in the family therapy literature (Selvini-Palazzoli, Boscolo, Checchin, & Prata, 1978). The interaction between team members will inevitably reflect the tensions and paradoxes of the particular patients and families with whom they are involved. Team problems are diagnostic tools for discovering unacknowledged patient problems. It takes a fairly sophisticated, well-joined team to observe these patterns and not take them personally. Professionals who become comfortable with the questioning of their approaches and experience it as inevitable on a regularly collaborating team will, in all likelihood, become more comfortable with the questions of patients about their methods. They will engage more easily in collaboration with their patients and the patients' families.

Special treatments can be undertaken in the primary care setting that would be less likely to occur through a referral to a specialty mental health setting. As providers meet and discuss regularly, patterns in the population being served tend to emerge, leading to special targeted services for groups within the practice. Groups or other treatments for patients with chronic illness, heart disease, depression, or obesity, for example, can be developed to meet the immediate needs presented in the practice. This makes treatment much more responsive than is the case when a PCP has to find appropriate specialized treatment outside the practice.

Confidentiality is a very important topic that must be addressed in the meetings of providers in the practice. Medical providers usually understand confidentiality to mean that information is not shared beyond the medical team providing care. This team can include physicians, nurses, other providers in the office, and relevant specialists outside the office. Mental health providers usually believe that confidentiality means that information is not shared without permission beyond the people who attend the session. In some settings, the likelihood that office staff might see personal therapy records has led to the therapists maintaining separate records and writing in the medical chart only as necessary. In other settings, patients sign releases as part of the initial paperwork of joining the practice for all providers to be able to share information; these settings usually keep all records in one chart.

I have found I can use the same skills required to talk in front of the patient, described earlier, to compose a treatment note. I routinely read the last note in the chart to patients at the start of the next meeting. This means they have no anxiety about what is written about them in the chart, and the notes are written in a way that is clear to other providers. It also helps with continuity and with highlighting progress in treatment.

STARTING A PILOT PROGRAM AND MOVING TO BROADER IMPLEMENTATION

Mauksch and Leahy (1993) have a set of recommendations for implementing integrated primary care plan-wide in an HMO. (Recommendations are quoted, elaborations are paraphrased.)

1. "Improve physical proximity." Locate mental health practices in primary care when possible, and when space does not allow this, have a mental health practitioner on site at least one day per week.
2. "Keep a joint medical record."
3. "Improve coordination of care." In difficult cases with many providers involved, designate a case coordinator and have the functions of the role understood by all.
4. "Focus on primary care providers as important customers for mental health providers." Mental health providers need to be comfortable and effective in the role of consultant in many cases, since the majority of mental health treatment will continue to be done by the primary care physicians and nurses, even in integrated settings.
5. "Explore new practice styles that may be effective in a managed care setting." Mental health practitioners need to try more episodic models of care, shorter treatment sessions, etc.
6. "Create coverage policies that avoid an adversarial relationship between providers and patients" (and between providers).
7. "Avoid double standards (between mental health and medical) when designing coverage policies."
8. "Include mental health consultation earlier in the course of a patient's evaluation in order to minimize unnecessary expenses."
9. "View patients as people [the organization] is committed to working with over time, rather than as people presenting a series of isolated treatment episodes."

This list is a good example of the scope of the potential impact of IPC: It begins with suggestions about the location of providers and moves to basic assumptions about coverage, service structures, and mission.

Integrated primary care needs to be offered as a remedy to perceived problems, rather than as a good idea to be pursued for its own sake. In any primary care site there will be some problems presented by patients that are particularly bothersome to the staff of that unit, whether these patients are noncompliant, overutilizing, somatizing, depressed, substance abusing, or have a particular medical diagnosis. Focusing on those problems makes it most likely that staff will support the endeavor. It should not be hard to find some mental health providers and some biomedical providers who are interested in this kind of work. A pilot project tends to generate enthusiasm on the part of its members. Nevertheless, the enthusiasm of a limited group will not be enough to sustain the project.

I conceive of this process of developing IPC and implementing it across a primary care providing entity as precipitating four distinct crises in the organization. By "crisis" I mean to invoke both of the meanings of the word as it is represented in Chinese, by a combination of the characters for "danger" and "opportunity." If the dangers can be forseen and met creatively, the opportunities become the most salient aspect of the crisis. If only the opportunities are forseen, the dangers tend to dominate everyone's experience. The organizational crises are:

1. the undertaking of a new type of project (the project to create IPC)
2. the creation of new ways of understanding and working with the problems patients present
3. the creation of a new cohesive team within the organization
4. the impact on people who were not in on the development of these ways of understanding and working when a broader implementation is attempted

How each these crises will ultimately be experienced depends in great measure on how they are understood and addressed by the managers of the IPC process.

Crisis 1: Undertaking a New Type of Project

Any new project impacts the members of the project and the various staff members whose work support the project.* In the case of IPC, there will be different levels of anticipation and acceptance among project members. As an MHP joins the primary care team, everyone's role will undergo some change. This will impact nurse practitioners, physicians' assistants, nurses, medical assistants, as well as physicians. In addition, support staff will have to change their work as they deal with new scheduling, billing, and patient communication problems.

The hierarchical structure of medical care delivery can make it tempting to assume that if the physician or physicians in a setting are in favor, the project can simply be announced and begun. In most settings this would be a mistake. The clinical team plus the office manager should sit together to talk about how the psychosocial aspects of care are currently handled, to remind themselves of some of the more difficult cases in which they all wanted someone there to help, to strategize about how an MHP could be useful immediately, and how to bring a person onto the team in a way that will get him or her oriented and functioning the fastest. There may well need to be a series of meetings to accomplish this

---

*For a much more detailed analysis of the reciprocal impact between a specialized project and the host organization, see Brulé and Blount (1989), chapter 14.

discussion fully. Later, this group plus the MHP will need to assemble periodically to address problems as they come up and to make recommendations concerning such central practices as how to handle the medical record. This group will also form the vehicle for allowing the larger organization to connect with the process of IPC and to make a broader implementation possible. This is discussed below.

The office manager will need to assemble the support staff to talk about how having an MHP will help the practice and to assign the necessary tasks to prepare for the MHP's arrival. These include researching the regulations of payers related to psychiatric billing codes and planning for scheduling and space utilization changes.

The more people feel that their concerns about IPC are being addressed, the more they will be able to understand and participate in the opportunities IPC presents.

Crisis 2: The Creation of New Ways of Understanding and Working with Problems Patients Present

New ways of working, even if they are clearly improvements, can be very upsetting to people. It can make them feel they have been doing things wrong. This can be destabilizing, particularly in medical care, where providers often feel they are supposed to have the answer and get it right the first time.

A powerful example comes from a primary care setting where family therapists and physicians began collaborating in the examining room with very little orientation or other preparation. The family therapists did not know how to contribute or what was expected of them, so for the first few weeks they were mostly quiet. The physicians did not know what to do with them, so for a while they acted as if the therapists were not there. As they became more familiar with each other, the physicians began urging their guests to participate. The family therapists began joining in on the interview of the patient, inevitably asking questions that the physicians would never have thought to ask. Occasionally they would "get lucky," opening up areas of the patient's relational context, which shed a very different light on the patient's problem. One physician's comment to his therapist collaborator may have represented how many of them felt, "After what happened today, I think you should be seeing 80% of my patients instead of me." Shortly thereafter, problems developed in the health center that made it impossible to continue the project. The physicians were no longer available.

To avoid such an outcome, a "learning environment" needs to be supported, in addition to the preparation for IPC described above. This means that making learning a value for all staff is crucial for the kind of organizational culture in which change can be accepted. The weekly meeting of internal continuing education, even if it is only an hour over breakfast or lunch, is essential. If learning is a group norm, then discovering something new is an opportunity for exchange rather than an indictment of previous practices.

To help providers learn IPC, it is useful to offer training in skills that everyone needs and that no one discipline is expected to have already mastered. The list above (speaking in front of the patient, working as a team member, interviewing family members, practicing solution-focused interviewing, and utilizing brief cognitive/behavioral interventions) can form the nucleus of a training program that all can join. Sometimes the initial stages of the program can be framed as "discovering the problems of IPC." Then a series of two or three meetings can be assembled with the purpose of sharing the problems, forming work groups to propose solutions, and devising trial procedures to be evaluated in the next meeting. In this way, everyone has a part in the process of change and the possibility of people feeling left out or blamed is greatly reduced.

Crisis 3: The Creation of a New Cohesive Team within the Organization

IPC may be implemented as a pilot program in a larger organization consisting of several primary care settings or in a practice with a small number of providers. In either case, as the project goes forward, the surrounding organization will notice. Unless proper steps are taken, the more successful the project is, the higher the morale and excitement of the project staff and the more they become successful at handling cases that before would have languished (with patients and providers frustrated and unsatisfied), the more the organization around the project may punish the project.

This is a common pattern in all organizations, not just those in the medical world. A cohesive team that has a high morale and is developing its own way of working inevitably excludes people who are not part of the team. People who feel "left out" are often disparaging of whatever it is they are "out" of. In a large organization, the staff members of other health centers or middle and upper managers who are not directly involved in the implementation of IPC may be disparaging. In a small practice, colleagues in the specialties or representatives of payors or regulatory agencies may look askance on the team's work. This is heightened by the fourth crisis.

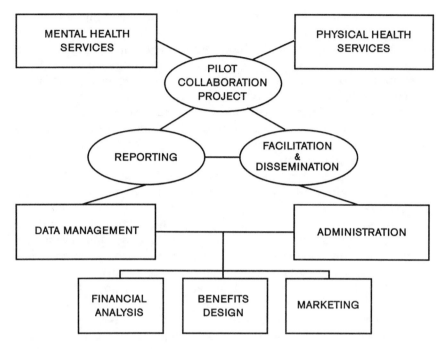

Figure 1.3. Getting from the pilot program to full implementation.

Crisis 4: The Impact of a Broader Implementation

The same problems described in crisis 2 are back at this point, but this time they can be widespread and less manageable. People who were not in on developing IPC in the organization are asked to change some of the ways they practice because of the project. It is common for people in this situation to feel that they are being told that there is something wrong with the way they have been practicing and to avoid assenting to this idea by avoiding the new way of practicing.

Figure 1.3 illustrates the series of conversations that can be convened and maintained as the pilot project develops in order to make the move to full implementation possible when the pilot stage is over. In order to mitigate crises 3 and 4, is important to turn the people who might be in a position to make things difficult for IPC into "stakeholders" in IPC. In a large organization, all of the managers and providers who might be asked to implement IPC later on should be in on this process. This is done by communicating with them early in the process, before they would hear about the project some other way. A memo or announcement or newsletter should be written, explaining why IPC is being started in one setting, what sort of difficulties it is designed to address, and that it is an experiment. It helps if there is some documenting of the need for a different approach in terms that other staff can understand. One HMO did an internal study (which remains proprietary) in which they simply looked at all members and their families who were prescribed any sort of psychotropic medication. The average overall medical cost for this group was three times the plan average. This is the kind of tantalizing finding that can energize an experiment.

After making the announcement that IPC is being tried on a pilot basis, hold regular facilitation and dissemination meetings to update the group on the progress of the "experiment." It is important that key staff who are not involved in the pilot feel that they are in on the ground floor. Communication should be frequent enough so that the project does not develop new ideas or procedures without the stakeholders understanding where they came from and how they work. The updates should be candid, describing the blind alleys that the project staff tried as well as the successes. In this way, stakeholders learn what the project staff learns without having to make all the same mistakes later. It gives them the sense that they are in on the development of the project. The updates should tell stories and not just talk in programmatic language. They should describe the problem a patient presented, how it would have been dealt with in the past, what was tried differently this time, what happened, and what the providers learned. It is the stories that people remember and that make them feel they are part of what is happening.

The facilitation and dissemination group is made up of the project providers, the office manager, and the manager representing administration. It can be the source for the communication of material to the larger organization. This probably should be done by the manager in the larger organization who will be responsible for the broader implementation. By meeting regularly with this group, with the goal of eliciting and publishing the story of their development, the manager makes the broader implementation possible.

Regular discussion between the project group and the data management staff needs to occur as the process develops. This "reporting" group designs the data reports that make the pilot project able to be more effective and to run smoother. IPC tends to require different reporting than the usual primary care service simply because new problems need to be addressed that once did not need to be identified. The field of data management for integrated primary care is very new and there is little agreement about what should be tracked or reported. In a few centers routine reports about patients for medical and mental health providers has been developed, but the specifics of those reports tend to be proprietary. The categories to be tracked must arise from a conversation about the ongoing development of the pilot(s). The manager who is going to be in charge of broader implementation will want to shepherd this process.

The following is an example of the kind of data that would allow a medical provider to assess when to take a more psychosocial approach to treatment or to look for the input of the MHP:

- number of visits
- percentile in utilization
- number of visits by family members
- problem list (long- and short-term)
- pharmacy list, including refills
- most recent health status and lab data
- date of last health maintenance exam
- nurse triage calls
- visits to other providers in the system
- any alerts by other providers concerning drug seeking, suspected depression, etc.

This is a report that could come off the computer and be available on the encounter form or in the chart at each patient visit. This is not easy to produce in most primary care practices. It takes constant discussion between providers and information management personnel to develop such reporting as a regular feature of the primary care interaction.

Integrated primary care involves levels of communication between medical and behavioral health providers that are new to most settings. Implementing IPC across a large health system requires new levels of communication in all of the domains described above. This is the kind of communication that is required for total quality management initiatives or other sorts of organizational reengineering. In this case, the reengineering starts out addressing the immediate problems brought by a large number of the highest utilizers of care. It goes on to offer opportunities for renewel in the routines of practice, the organization of social roles, and ultimately the explanatory model behind the expertise that is provided (Blount & Bayona, 1994).

There is reason to take very seriously the potential impact of IPC on health care as we know it. On the other hand, no one has had much success selling fundamental fixes for health care in the recent past. The fate of the Clinton health plan is an example of what can happen to even the most powerfully supported attempts at fundamental change. Integrated primary care offers far-reaching possibilities for expanding the way primary medical care is delivered and for facilitating the development of new ways of conceptualizing and approaching human pain. Whether these possibilities will be realized will be seen in the next decade or so as IPC becomes more common and better developed across the United States. It will become more common, however, because it offers the possibility of solving very real problems that primary care providers face every day.

BIBLIOGRAPHY

Akamatsu, T. J., Parris-Stephens, M. A., Hobfoll, S. E., & Crowther, J. H. (Eds.). (1992). *Family health psychology*. Washington, DC: Hemisphere.

Amercian Psychiatric Association. (1994). *Diagnostic and statistical manual of mental disorders* (4th ed.). Washington, DC: Author.

Backett, E. M., Mabin, R. P., & Dudgeon, Y. (1957). Medicosocial work in general practice. *Lancet, i*, 37–40.

Badger, L. W. (1994). Patient presentation, interview content, and the detection of depression by primary care physicians. *Psychosomatic Medicine, 56*, 128–135.

Balestrieri, M., Williams, P., & Wilkinson, G. (1988). Specialist mental health treatment in general practice: A meta-analysis. *Psychological Medicine, 18*, 711–717.

Ballenger, J. (1987). Unrecognized prevalence of panic disorder in primary care, internal medicine and cardiology. *American Journal of Cardiology, 60*, 39J–47J.

Banta H. D., & Fox, R. C. (1972). Role strains of a health care team in a poverty community. *Social Science and Medicine, 6*, 698–722.

Barrett, J., Barrett, J., Oxman, T., & Gerber, P. (1988). The prevalence of psychiatric disorders in a primary care practice. *Archives of General Psychiatry, 45*, 1100–1106.

Belar, C. D., Deardorff, W. W., & Kelly. L. E. (1987). *The practice of clinical health psychology*. New York: Pergamon.

Berg, I. K. (1994). *Family-based services: A solution-focused approach*. New York: Norton.

Berg, I. K., & Miller, S. (1992). *Working with the problem drinker: A solution-focused approach*. New York: Norton.

Bergsma, J., & Thomasma, D. C. (1982). *Health care: Its psychosocial dimensions*. Pittsburgh: Duquesne University.

Berkman, L. F., & Breslow, L. (1983). *Health and ways of living: The Alameda County study*. New York: Oxford University.

Bernard, L. C., & Kaupat, E. (1994). *Health psychology: Biopsychosocial factors in health and illness*. Orlando: Harcourt Brace.

Bhagat, M., Lewis, A. P., & Shillitoe, R. W. (1979). The clinical psychologist and the primary health care team. *Update, 18*, 479–484.

Bloch, D. A. (1988). The partnership of Dr. Biomedicine and Dr. Psychosocial. *Family Systems Medicine, 6*, 2–4.

Bloch, D. A. (1993). The "full service" model: An immodest proposal. *Family Systems Medicine, 11*, 1–7.

Blount, A. (1985). Toward a "systemically" organized mental health center. In D. Campbell, & R. Draper (Eds.), *Applications of systemic therapy*. Orlando: Grune & Stratton.

Blount, A., & Bayona, J. (1994). Toward a system of integrated primary care. *Family Systems Medicine, 12*, 171–182.

Bridges, K. W., & Goldberg, D. P. (1985). Somatic presentation of DSM-III psychiatric disorders in primary care. *Journal of Psychosomatic Research, 29*, 563–569.

Broadhead, W., Blazeer, D., George, L., & Tse, C. (1990). Depression, disability days and days lost from work in a prospective epidemiologic study. *JAMA, 264*, 2524–2528.

Broskowski, A., Marks, E., & Budman, S. (1981). *Linking health and mental health.* Beverly Hills: Sage.

Brulé, J. F., & Blount, A. (1989). *Knowledge acquisition.* New York: McGraw-Hill.

Budman, S. H., Demby, A. B., & Feldstein, M. L. (1984). A controlled study of the impact of mental health treatment on medical care utilization. *Medical Care, 22*, 216–222.

Canino, G., Bird, H., Shrout, P., Rubio-Stipec, M., Bravo, M., Martinez, R., & Sesman, M. (1987). The prevalence of specific psychiatric disorders in Puerto Rico. *Archives of General Psychiatry, 44*, 727–735.

Christie-Seely, J. (Ed.). (1984). *Working with the family in primary care: A systems approach to health and illness.* New York: Praeger.

Cleary, P., Miller, M., Bush, B., Warburg, M., Delbanco, T., & Aronson, M. (1988). Prevalence and recognition of alcohol abuse in a primary care population. *American Journal of Medicine, 85*, 466–471.

Coleman, J. V. (1983). Interdisciplinary implication of primary medical care. In R. S. Miller (Ed.), *Primary health care: More than medicine.* Englewood Cliffs, NJ: Prentice-Hall.

Coleman, J. V., & Patrick, D. L. (1976). Integrating mental health services into primary medical care. *Medical Care, 14*, 654–661.

Coleman, J. V., Patrick, D. L., Eagle, J., & Hermalin, J. A. (1979). Collaboration, consultation and referral in an integrated health-mental health program at an HMO. *Social Work in Health Care, 5*, 833–896.

Corney, R. H. (1986). Marriage guidance counseling in general practice. *Journal of the Royal College of General Practitioners, 36*, 424–426.

Coulehan, J., Zettler-Segal, M., Block, M., McClelland, M., & Schulberg, H. (1987). Recognition of alcoholism and substance abuse in primary care patients. *Archives of Internal Medicine, 147*, 349–352.

Crane, D. D. (1986). The family therapist, the primary care physician, and the health maintenance organization: Pitfalls and possibilities. *Family Systems Medicine, 4*, 22–30.

Cranwath, T., & Miller, D. (1986). *Behavioral psychotherapy in primary care: A practice manual.* Orlando: Academic.

Crouch, M. A., & Roberts, L. (Eds.). (1987). *The family in medical practice: A family systems primer.* New York: Springer-Verlag.

Cummings, N. A., Dorken, H., Pallak, M. S., & Henke, C. (1990). *The impact of pshchological intervention on healthcare utilization and costs.* South San Francisco: The Biodyne Institute.

de Shazer, S. (1985). *Keys to solution in brief therapy.* New York: Norton.

de Shazer, S. (1988). *Clues: Investigating solutions in brief therapy.* New York: Norton.

de Shazer, S., Berg, I. K., Lipchik, E., Nunnally, E., Molnar, A., Gingerich, W., & Weiner-Davis, M. (1986). Brief therapy: Focused solution development. *Family Process, 25*, 207–221.

Doherty, W. J., & Baird, M. A. (1983). *Family therapy and family medicine: Toward the primary care of families.* New York: Guilford.

Doherty, W. J., & Campbell, T. L. (1988). *Families and health.* Thousand Oaks, CA: Sage.

Dym, B., & Berman, S. (1986). The primary health care team: Family physician and family therapist in joint practice. *Family Systems Medicine, 4*, 9–21.

Ell, K. O., & Northen, H. (1990). *Families and health care: Psychosocial practice.* New York: Aldine de Gruyter.

Engel, G. L. (1977). The need for a new medical model: A challenge to biomedicine. *Science, 196*, 129–136.

Engel, G. L. (1980). The clinical application of the biopsychosocial model. *American Journal of Psychiatry, 137*, 535–544.

Engel, G. L. (1982). The biopsychosocial model and medical education: Who are the teachers? *New England Journal of Medicine, 306*, 802–805.

Froom, J., Culpepper, L., Kirkwood, R. C., Boisseau, V., & Mangone, D. (1977). An integrated medical record and data system for primary care, Part 4: Family information. *Journal of Family Practice, 5*, 265–270.

Furman, B., & Ahola, T. (1992). *Solution talk.* New York: Norton.

Gingrich, W. J., de Shazer, S., & Weiner-Davis, M. (1988). Constructing change: A research view of interviewing. In E. Lipchick (Ed.), *Interviewing* (pp. 21–32). Rockville, MD: Aspen.

Glenn, M. L. (1985). Interview: William Phillips, MD, MPH, and Larry Mauksch, M.Ed. *Family Systems Medicine, 3*, 344–355.

Glenn, M. L. (1987). *Collaborative health care: A family oriented approach.* New York: Praeger.

Glenn, M. L., Atkins, L., & Singer, R. (1884). Integrating a family therapist into a family medical practice. *Family Systems Medicine, 2*, 137–145.

Helsing, K. J., Szklo, M., & Comstock, G. W. (1981). Factors associated with mortality after widowhood. *American Journal of Public Health, 71*, 802–809.

Henao, S., & Grose, N. P. (Eds.). (1985). *Principles of family systems in family medicine.* New York: Brunner/Mazel.

Hoyt, M., & Austad, C. (1992). Psychotherapy in staff model health maintenance organizations: Providing and assuring quality care in the future. *Psychotherapy, 29*, 119–129.

Huygen, F. (1981) *Family medicine: The medical life histories of families.* New York: Brunner/Mazel.

Ingram, W. J. (1981). *Clinical psychiatry in primary care.* Menlo Park, CA: Addison-Wesley.

Jenkins, G. C. (1996a). Psychological aspects of chronic illness: The challenge to the family doctor. *Section of Psychotherapy pages.* Staines, UK: Conselling in Primary Care Trust. *http://psyctc.sghms.ac.uk/cpct/chronic.htm*

Jenkins, G. C. (1996b). Cost implications of counselling services in primary medical care. *Section of Psychotherapy pages.* Staines, UK: Conselling in Primary Care Trust. *http://psyctc.sghms.ac.uk/cpct/cost.htm*

Jones, K. R., & Vischi, T. R. (1979). Impact of alcohol, drug abuse and mental health treatment on medical care utilization: A review of the literature. *Medical Care, 17*, 1–82.

Kaplan, C. L., Lipkin, M., & Gordon, G. (1988). Somatization in primary care: Patients with unexplained and vexing medical problems. *Journal of General Internal Medicine, 3*, 177–190.

Katon, W. (1995). Collaborative care: Patient satisfaction, outcomes and medical cost-offset. *Family Systems Medicine, 13*, 351–365.

Katon, W., Berg, A. O., Robins, A. J., & Risse, S. (1986). Depression, medical utilization and somatization. *Western Journal of Medicine, 144*, 564–568.

Katon, W., & Gonzales, J. (1994). A review of randomized trials of psychiatric consultation-liaison studies in primary care. *Psychosomatics, 35*, 268–278.

Katon, W., Hollifield, M., Chapman, T., Mannuzza, S., Ballenger, J., & Fyer, A. (1995). Infrequent panic attacks: Psychiatric comorbidity, personality characteristics and functional disability. *Journal of Psychiatric Research, 29*, 121–131.

Katon, W., Lin, E., von Korff, M., Russo, J., Lipscomb, P., & Bush, T. (1991). Somatization: A spectrum of severity. *American Journal of Psychiatry, 148*, 34–40.

Katon, W., & Roy-Byrne, P. (1991). Mixed anxiety and depression. *Journal of Abnormal Psychology, 100*, 337–345.

Katon, W., & Schulberg, H. (1992). Epidemiology of depression in primary care. *General Hospital Psychiatry, 14*, 237-247.

Katon, W., von Korff, M., Lin, E., Bush, T., & Ormel, J. (1992). Adequacy and duration of antidepressant treatment in primary care. *Medical Care, 30*, 67-76.

Katon, W., von Korff, M., Lin, E., Bush, T., Russo, J., Lipscomb, P., & Wagner, E. (1992). A randomized trial of psychiatric consultation with distressed high utilizers. *General Hospital Psychiatry, 14*, 86-98.

Katon, W., von Korff, M., Lin, E., Lipscomb, P., Russo, J., Wagner, E., & Polk, E. (1990). Distressed high utilizers of medical care: DSM-III R diagnosis and treatment needs. *General Hospital Psychiatry, 12*, 355-362.

Katon, W., von Korff, M., Lin, E., Walker, E., Simon, G., Bush, T., Robinson, P., & Russo, J. (1995). Collaborative management to achieve treatment guidelines: Impact on depression in primary care. *JAMA, 273*, 1026-1031.

Kessler, L., Burns, B., & Shapiro, S. (1987). Psychiatric diagnoses of medical service users: Evidence from the epidemiologic catchment area program. *American Journal of Public Health, 77*, 18-24.

King, M. (1986). Brief communication: At risk drinking among general practice attenders: Validation of the CAGE questionnaire. *Psychological Medicine, 16*, 123-127.

Knesper, D. (1982). A study of referral failures for potentially suicidal patients: A method of medical care evaluation. *Hospital and Community Psychiatry, 33*, 45-52.

Kroenke, K., & Mangelsdorff, A. D. (1989). Common symptoms in ambulatory care: Incidence, evaluation, therapy and outcome. *American Journal of Medicine, 86*, 262-266.

Lareau, M. W., & Nelson, E. S. (1994). The physician and licensed mental health professional team: Prevalence and feasibility. *Family Systems Medicine, 12*, 37-45.

Lesse, S. (1968). Masked depression: A diagnostic and therapeutic problem. *Diseases of the Nervous System, 29*, 169-173.

Levine, S. (1983). Interprofessional implications in primary care. In R. S. Miller (Ed.), *Primary health care: More than medicine*. Englewood Cliffs, NJ: Prentice-Hall.

Lin, E., Katon, W., von Korff, M., Bush, T., Lipscomb, P., Russo, J., & Wagner, E. (1991). Frustrating patients: Physician and patient perspectives among distressed high users of medical services. *Journal of General Internal Medicine, 6*, 241-246.

Lin, E., von Korff, M., Katon, W., Bush T., Simon, G., Walker, E., & Robinson, P. (1995). The role of the primary care physician in patients' adherence to antidepressant therapy. *Medical Care, 33*, 67-74.

Luciano, L. (1996). Developments in managed care. *Business and Health, 14*, 45.

Marshall, G. N., Hays, R. D., & Mazel, R. (1996). Health status and satisfaction with health care: Results from the Medical Outcomes Study. *Journal of Consulting and Clinical Psychology, 64*, 380-390.

Mauksch, L. B., & Leahy, D. (1993). Collaboration between primary care medicine and mental health in an HMO. *Family Systems Medicine, 11*, 121-135.

Mayfield, D., McLeod, G., & Hall, P. (1974). The CAGE questionnaire: Validation of a new alcoholism screening instrument. *American Journal of Psychiatry, 131*, 1121-1123.

McDaniel, S. H., & Campbell, T. L. (1985). Physicians and family therapists: The risks of collaboration. *Family Systems Medicine, 4*, 4-8.

McDaniel, S. H., Campbell, T. L., & Seaburn, D. B. (1990). *Family-oriented primary care: A manual for medical providers*. New York: Springer-Verlag.

McDaniel, S. H., Campbell, T. L., & Seaburn, D. B. (1995). Principles for collaboration between health and mental health providers in primary care. *Family Systems Medicine, 13*, 283-298.

McDaniel, S. H., Hepworth, J., & Doherty, W. J. (1992). *Medical family therapy: A biopsychosocial approach to families with health problems*. New York: Basic.

McDonnell-Douglas Corporation. (1989). *Employee Assistance Program Financial Offset Study: 1985-1988*. Long Beach, CA: Author.

Miranda, J., Hohmann, A., Attkisson, C., Larson, D. (Eds.). (1994). *Mental disorders in primary care*. San Francisco: Jossey-Bass.

Miranda, J., & Munoz, R. Intervention for minor depression in primary care patients. *Psychosomatic Medicine, 56*, 136–142.

Mumford, E., Schlesinger, H. J., & Glass, G. V. (1981). Reducing medical costs through mental health treatment. In A. Broskowski, E. Marks, & S. H. Budman (Eds.), *Linking health and mental health*. Beverly Hills, CA: Sage.

Mumford, E., Schlesinger, H. J., Glass, G. V., Patrick, C., & Cuerdon, T. (1984). A new look at evidence about reduced cost of medical utilization following mental health treatment. *American Journal of Psychiatry, 14*, 1145–1158.

Novack, D. H. (1987). Therapeutic aspects of the clinical encounter. *General Internal Medicine, 2*, 346–355.

Ormel, J., von Korff, M., Van den Brink, W., Katon, W., Brilman, E., & Oldehinkel, T. (1993). Depression, anxiety, and social disability show synchrony of change in primary care patients. *American Journal of Public Health, 83*, 385–390.

Patrick, D. L., Eagle, J., & Coleman, J. V. (1978). Primary care treatment of emotional problems in an HMO. *Medical Care, 16*, 47–60.

Peek, C. J., & Heinrich, R. L. (1995). Building a collaborative healthcare organization: From Idea to invention to innovation. *Family Systems Medicine, 13*, 327–342.

Regier, D., Goldberg, I., & Taube, C. (1978). The de facto mental health services system. *Archives of General Psychiatry, 35*, 685–693.

Regier, D., Narrow, W., Rae, D., Manderscheid, R., Locke, B., & Goodwin, F. (1993). The de facto mental health and addictive disorders service system. *Archives of General Psychiatry, 50*, 85–94.

Robinson, P., Bush, T., von Korff, M., Katon, W., Lin, E., Simon, G., & Walker, E. (1995). Primary care physician use of cognitive behavioral techniques with depressed patients. *Journal of Family Practice, 40*, 352–357.

Rosen, G. M., Geyman, J. P., & Layton, R. H. (Eds.). (1980). *Behavioral science in family practice*. New York: Appleton-Century-Crofts.

Ross, J. L., Yudin, R., & Galluzzi, K. (1992). The geriartic assessment team: A case report. *Family Systems Medicine, 10*, 213–218.

Rowland, N., & Irving, G. (1984). Towards a rationalization of counseling in general practice. *Journal of the Royal College of General Practioners, 34*, 685–687.

Sammons, M., Belar, C., & Bally, R. (1996). Integrated health deliver systems: Psychology's potential role. *Professional Psychology: Research and Practice, 27*, 107–108.

Saultz, J. (1995). Collaborative care of Medicaid patients: Lessons from the Oregon Health Plan. *Family Systems Medicine, 13*, 343–349.

Schulberg, H. C., & Pajer, K. A. (1994). Treatment of depression in primary care. In J. Miranda, A. Hohmann, C. Attkisson, & D. Larson (Eds.), *Mental disorders in primary care*. San Francisco: Jossey-Bass.

Seaburn, D., Gawinski, B., Harp J., McDaniel, S., Waxman, D., & Shields, C. (1993). Family systems therapy in a primary care medical setting: The Rochester experience. *Journal of Marital and Family Therapy, 19*, 177–190.

Seaburn, D. B., Lorenz, A. D., Gunn, W. B., Gawinski, B. A., & Mauksch, L. B. (1996). *Models of collaboration: A guide for mental health professionals working with health care practitioners*. New York: Basic.

Selvini-Palazzoli, M., Boscolo, L., Checchin, G., & Prata, G. (1978). *Paradox and counter-paradox*. New York: Jason Aronson.

Shapiro, J., & Talbot, Y. (1992). Is there a future for behavioral scientists in academic family medicine? *Family Systems Medicine, 10*, 247–256.

Shemo, J. P. (1984). Primary care management of mental illness: Medication as a tool. *Southern Medical Journal, 77*, 1010–1014, 1019.

Smith, R. C., & Hoppe, R. B. (1991). The patient's story: Integrating the patient- and physician-centered approaches to interviewing. *Annals of Internal Medicine, 115*, 470–477.

Stuart, M. R., & Lieberman, J. A. (1986). *The fifteen minute hour: Applied psychotherapy for the primary care physician*. New York: Praeger.

Suchman, A. L., & Matthews, D. A. (1988). What makes the patient-doctor relationship therapeutic? Exploring the connexional dimension of medical care. *Annals of Internal Medicine, 108*, 125–130.

Sullivan, M., Katon, W., Russo, J., Dobie, R., & Sakai, C. (1994). Coping and marital support as correlates of tinnitus disability. *General Hospital Psychiatry, 16*, 259–266.

Sweet, J. J., Rozensky, R. H., & Tovian, S. M. (1991). *Handbook of clinical psychology in medical settings*. New York: Plenum.

Usdin, G., & Lewis, J. M. (1979). *Psychiatry in general medical practice*. New York: McGraw-Hill.

Vacarinno, J. M. (1977). Malpractice-the problem in perspective. *JAMA, 238*, 681–683.

Vazquez, A. M., Nath, C. L., & Murray, S. P. (1988). Counseling by family physicians: Report of a survey and curriculum modification in West Virginia. *Family Systems Medicine, 6*, 463–469.

von Korff, M., Ormel, J., Katon, W., & Lin, E. (1992). Disability and depression among high utilizers of health care. A longitudinal analysis. *Archives of General Psychiatry, 49*, 91–100.

Weiner, J. P. (1994). Forecasting the effects of health reform on U.S. physician workforce requirements. *JAMA, 272*, 222–230.

Weissman, M., Klerman, G., Markowitz, J., & Ouellette, R. (1989). Suicidal ideation and suicide attempts in panic disorder and attacks. *New England Journal of Medicine, 321*, 1209–1214.

Wells, K., & Burnam, A. (1991). Caring for depression in America: Lessons learned from early findings of the medical outcomes study. *Psychiatric Medicine, 9*, 503–519.

West, N. D. (1979). *Psychiatry in primary care medicine*. Chicago: Year Book.

Wiederman, C. J., & Wiederman, M. (1988). Psychoimmunology: Systems medicine at the molecular level. *Family Systems Medicine, 6*, 94–106.

Wise, H. (1972). The primary-care health team. *Archives of Internal Medicine, 130*, 438–444.

Wittchen, H. (1986). Epidemiology of panic attacks and panic disorders. In I. Hand, & H. Wittchen (Eds.), *Panic and phobias*. New York: Springer-Verlag.

Wolkenstein, A., & Butler, D. (1993). Teaching the stages of mental health referral to family practice residents. *Family Systems Medicine, 11*, 397–406.

Zinbarg, E. (1994). The DSM-IV field trial for mixed anxiety-depression. *American Journal of Psychiatry, 151*, 1153–1162.

ACKNOWLEDGMENTS

I want to thank Anthony Giuliano and Laura Rome for reading drafts and providing important feedback.

2

The Importance of
Nondichotomized Thinking

James L. Griffith

Any book about integrated primary care should include a discussion of the relationship between psychosocial experience and biomedical disease. The field of psychosomatic medicine has a long and distinguished history, but until recently was given comparatively little attention. In the last 10 to 15 years, the amount of research being done in a number of different specialties on the interaction of psychosocial and biomedical factors in the etiology and treatment of disease has mushroomed dramatically. Because this research is one of the foundations of the argument for integrated primary care, it is important that a careful review of this literature be made early in this book.

As Director of Consultation-Liaison Psychiatry at George Washington University, a psychiatric service that serves people who are hospitalized for medical reasons, James Griffith is uniquely qualified and positioned to offer this review. His book, *The Body Speaks*, written with Melissa Elliott Griffith (Griffith & Griffith, 1994), is a detailed and sensitive discussion of how life's pain and troubles can become expressed in bodily distress and the kinds of conversations that can lead to the relief of this distress. In the present chapter, he lays the groundwork for a shift in thinking about the mind and the body. His review makes the case for the inadequacy of our usual dichotomized mode of thinking about the phenomena that are emerging in biobehavioral research. The dichotomy between mind and body, between psychosocial and biomedical factors, needs to be transcended.

The organization of Griffith's chapter by disease entities provides a way for practitioners working with specific populations of patients to find an entry into the biobehavioral literature that is most relevant to them. For those who are not focused on a particular population, Dr. Griffith provides a panoramic view of the world of biobehavioral etiology and treatment. It is a structure the reader can use to assess the importance of each new study within the continual stream of research reports in which we are all immersed.

In one sense, this is the chapter in the volume that is most doomed to obsolescence; in the time between writing and publication there will be new research reported that should have been included. In another sense, this is a chapter that is fundamental and unchanging. The particular programs in other chapters will evolve over time and health care itself will change dramatically in the next few years. The need to get beyond the dichotomous way we have thought about human problems and the separate service structures (medical and mental health) we have set up to address these dichotomized problems will continue for as far into the future as anyone can foresee.

As MEDICINE PROGRESSED through the twentieth century, two trends in the delivery of health services helped create a system that treated mental disorders and medical disorders as if neither had much to do with the other. First, medical science made major advances by viewing the human being as if it were a physical machine. Medicine's success in using this biomedical perspective to develop antibiotics, cancer chemotherapy, microsurgical techniques, and computerized imaging technologies pushed into the background any awareness of psychosocial influences in the generation of disease, including insights of which previous generations of physicians had been cognizant. Second, psychiatry, dominated until the last decade by psychoanalysis, treated patients as though problems of thought, emotions, and behavior could be fully explained in psychological terms, ignoring roles played by disordered brain physiology.

This splitting of mind from body had detrimental consequences that became more and more evident as the century neared its end. One strand of evidence came from the realization by clinicians that medical research could not advance further in treating a number of chronic medical disorders, among them hypertension, heart disease, end-stage renal disease, and diabetes, unless salutary changes occurred first in patients' health habits, lifestyle, and mental health. A second strand of evidence came from clinical studies showing that certain neurological, nutritional, and endocrinological diseases gave rise to psychiatric disorders, even in the absence of poor parenting or life stresses. Finally, somatization emerged as a major public health problem that not only generated suffering for patients and families, but also cost the health care system billions of dollars annually. It was evident that only clinical approaches that brought an integrated understanding of mind and body would have useful solutions to offer for problems of somatization. The following overview illustrates how complex, reciprocal relationships between psychosocial problems and diseases shape the form and course of medical illnesses. Our health care system must find ways to utilize the possibilities for healing that lie within these reciprocal relationships.

HOW PSYCHOSOCIAL DISTRESS AND MEDICAL DISEASES INTERACT

It is now generally accepted that psychological, social, and physiological processes interact and modulate one another in both health and illness. A useful framework for conceptualizing the treatment of medical diseases is to imagine a *biobehavioral continuum* along which every disease can be placed according to the relative influence that psychosocial factors or physiological factors hold over its course of illness (Wood, 1993, 1994). Such diseases as Alzheimer's disease or Duchenne's muscular dystrophy, little influenced in their progression by psychosocial factors, are at one end of the spectrum. Disorders such as irritable bowel syndrome or anorexia nervosa, strongly influenced by psychosocial factors, are at the other end. In the middle region of this continuum, usually positioned more toward one end or the other, are most other diseases and medical disorders, including asthma, cancer, coronary artery disease, or migraine headaches. A clinician can maximize healing possibilities by assessing the unique pattern for each illness through which psychosocial or physiological interventions can influence its outcome and composing a treatment plan that employs what each can offer. Surveying a variety of illnesses will illustrate the range of patterns through which psychosocial factors share influence with physiological ones along the biobehavioral continuum.

CARDIOVASCULAR DISEASES: PSYCHOSOCIAL FACTORS CREATE DISEASE RISK

The impact that a patient's personality style can have on disease progression has been best demonstrated by research linking type A behavior to the onset and progression of cardiac disease (Friedman, 1969). Type A behavior is characterized by aggressiveness, time urgency, competitiveness, body tension, and a hostile, "in your face" style of communication with others. Epidemiologic evidence suggests that type A behavior, especially its component of hostility, is a risk factor for the development of coronary artery disease (Dembroski, MacDougall, Costa, & Grandits, 1989; Siegman, Dembroski, & Ringel, 1987). These adverse consequences appear to be mediated through its effect in keeping the endocrine systems and the autonomic nervous system of the body in a state of perpetual alarm and mobilization (Goldstein & Niaura, 1995; Krantz & Durel, 1983; Manuck & Krantz, 1986).

Fortunately, psychological treatments have been developed that enable change in type A behavioral patterns. Programs have been developed that teach about the risks of type A behavioral patterns and help patients eliminate type A-associated patterns of thinking. Such programs have been successful in reducing hostility, impatience, and anger behaviors, while strengthening a patient's social networks and self-esteem. Outcome studies have shown a statistically significant 50% reduction in coronary events after a 3-year follow-up (Nunes, Frank, & Kornfeld, 1987).

In addition to type A behavior, important relationships have also been delineated between heart disease and other psychosocial factors, including depression, sudden emotional distress, and stress in the workplace. These factors make both direct and indirect contributions to the risk for heart disease by fostering poor dietary habits, neglect of exercise, excessive alcohol consumption, and smoking (Niaura & Goldstein, 1995).

The co-occurrence of major depressive disorder with heart disease increases the risk for sudden death. Carney and colleagues (1988) found the presence of a major depressive episode to be a stronger predictor of serious cardiac disease during the year following coronary artery catheterization than any other variable in their study, whether physiological variables, such as severity of coronary artery disease or diminished left ventricular ejection fraction, or other risk factors, such as smoking. Why should depression be such a high risk factor for heart disease? There are multiple answers. At a behavioral level, depressed persons tend not to attend to the care of their health through diet, exercise, and avoiding cigarettes, alcohol, and other harmful substances. At a metabolic level, processes are triggered that may compromise health. Although depression outwardly may appear to be a state of behavioral withdrawal and immobility, inwardly the emotional systems of a person's brain are locked in a state of excessive arousal, as if responding to a continuous signaling of alarm. We are beginning to understand how the secondary processes that are then triggered—excess secretion of stress hormones, compromise of the immune system—impair physical health (Esler et al., 1982; Esterling, Kiecolt-Glaser, Bodnar, & Glaser, 1994). Some of these processes appear to directly harm the heart and cardiovascular system.

In contrast to depression, it is not clear that generalized anxiety—worry, apprehension, fearfulness—contributes significantly to the progression of heart disease (Booth-Kewley & Friedman, 1987). When anxiety comes as an acute shock—severe, sudden, and unexpected—it appears to be more dangerous, however. The onset of malignant ventricular arrhythmias was associated with an identifiable emotional trigger in 21% of patients referred for antiarhythmic management in one study (Reich, DeSilva, Lown, & Murawski, 1981).

In the workplace, work overload, excessive job responsibility, and job dissatisfaction are social factors that have all been shown to increase risk of cardiac disease. High job strain, defined as the combination of highly demanding work together with few opportunities to control the job situation, may increase the risk of coronary heart disease morbidity by as much as 50%. Low social support and social isolation have a multiplicative effect on this risk, with a worker who, even though working alongside others, feels isolated and alone while trying to cope with stressful work (Niaura & Goldstein, 1995).

CANCER: PSYCHOSOCIAL FACTORS AFFECT DISEASE PROGRESSION

Although alternative medicine claims that life stress can heighten the risk of developing cancer, there is little solid evidence to support that claim. However, there is controvertible evidence that cancer, once initiated, progresses more rapidly where adverse psychosocial factors are present, particularly depression, inadequate social and family supports, and a coping style described as type C personality style (Spiegel & Kato, 1996).

Type C personality describes a person who tends to respond to stress with acquiescence, hopelessness, and helplessness. Patients with a "fighting spirit," on the other hand, tend to live longer (Greer, Morris, & Pettingale, 1979). Some recent research has suggested that such factors as type C personality and "fighting spirit" are not simply characteristics of the individual patient, but are actively shaped by the patient's couple and family relationships (Weihs, 1996; Weihs, Enright, Simmens, & Reiss, 1997). As an example, one woman suffering from breast cancer acknowledged during marital therapy that she had been struggling alone with a decision whether to have additional surgery, not having let her husband know the surgery had been recommended: "[My husband] can't handle it if he sees me upset. He doesn't know how sick I am." Another breast cancer patient, who had spent her adult life caring attentively for her husband's and their three children's needs, resisted her doctor's recommendations that she discuss with them a shifting of roles, with their assuming more responsibility for meals and household duties so she could rest: "If it's me, it doesn't matter. I want my family to have the same wife and mother they have always known for as long as I am with them." (Griffith & Griffith, 1997). Such cases suggest that the state of well-being of a patient's couple and family relationships may be important for survival from cancer.

Depression and relational distress have both been shown in psychoimmunological studies to compromise the effectiveness of the immune systems, presumably the mechanism by which they adversely impact resistance to cancer (Andersen, Kiecolt-Glaser, & Glaser, 1994). These findings suggest that psychosocial therapies that can change how persons interact in family relationships and early recognition and treatment of depression both may contribute to resilience against cancer.

Already two psychosocial intervention studies, one with breast cancer and the other with malignant melanoma patients, have shown a specific form of group therapy to extend significantly the life expectancy of cancer patients (Fawzy et al., 1993; Spiegel, Kraemer, Bloom, & Gottheil, 1989). This group therapy was designed to facilitate among group members the sharing of personal experiences, collaborative problem-solving, and learning such pain-control methods as self-hypnosis and relaxation techniques. Patients in the treatment groups significantly extended their life expectancies compared to those in the control groups without treatment.

PULMONARY DISEASES: PSYCHOSOCIAL FACTORS CHANGE A PHYSIOLOGICAL SENSITIVITY INTO A DISEASE

Asthma is generally considered to be a psychophysiological disorder. A psychophysiological disorder arises when the meaning attributed to events in a person's life triggers a reaction from the autonomic, endocrine, or immune systems of the body that then cascade into a state of disease. This seems to occur when one or more of these systems normally shows a heightened responsiveness to emotional stimuli but without symptoms, then is recruited by new life events into responses so excessive as to produce symptoms of disease.

In asthma, this psychophysiological process ends in bronchospasm and increased mucous secretion. As with other psychophysiological disorders, precipitants for attacks of asthma can be either physical or emotional stimuli. Research studies have identified infections, allergens, and emotional stressors as the three most common precipitants of an attack of asthma (Moran, 1995).

For example, 9-year-old Jill was referred to our pediatric hospital due to asthma that had become increasingly severe during recent months, despite efforts by physicians in her community to treat her symptoms. During the hospitalization, her pulmonologist determined an optimal regimen for her inhalers and a plan for occasional use of steroids when she had upper respiratory infections. However, a family evaluation also suggested that a high level of emotional tension in the home from financial difficulties and fighting between Jill's parents may also be contributing to her worsening illness. Family therapy was initiated that included marital therapy for the parents and a family-wide project to help Jill learn how to use each of her inhalers properly and to free the home from house dust and other allergens that might be contributing to her illness. As with other psychophysiological disorders, a comprehensive plan of treatment required interventions that addressed both physical and emotional precipitants of her illness.

GASTROINTESTINAL DISORDERS: SIMILAR SYMPTOMS REQUIRE DIFFERENT PSYCHOSOCIAL THERAPIES

The gastrointestinal disorders that have as their symptoms abdominal pain, diarrhea, and constipation illustrate how a similar constellation of symptoms among different diseases require quite different approaches for psychosocial aspects of their treatment. Ulcerative colitis and Crohn's disease (regional enteritis) are both inflammatory bowel diseases that are serious and potentially life-threatening. Irritable bowel syndrome, with similar symptoms of pain, diarrhea, and constipation, accounts for 50% of ambulatory cases seen by gastroenterologists but is not associated with physiological disease that can be demonstrated by lab tests or physical examination (Folks & Kinney, 1995).

Ulcerative colitis is associated with a high risk of colon cancer, surgery, and colostomy. As such, it produces similar stress symptoms and psychosocial problems as do other medical diseases that share a chronic course of exacerbations, remissions, and an uncertain prognosis. Patients with ulcerative colitis, however, are no more likely to have associated depressive, anxiety, or somatization disorders than are most other medically ill patients (Helzer, Stillings, Chammas, Norland, & Alpers, 1982). Hence, psychosocial therapy for ulcerative colitis can be helpful by focusing on coping with stigma and practical strategies for "living alongside" a disabling chronic illness. However, there is no expectation that changing habits of thinking, emotional coping, or lowering life stress will alter onset or progression of the disease.

By contrast, patients with Crohn's disease show a higher prevalence of depression than most medically ill patients, as well as temporal associations between exacerbations of pain and diarrhea and stressful life circumstances. Psychosocial therapy focuses on recognition and treatment of depression and on coping strategies for life stresses that exacerbate symptoms (Andrews, Barczak, & Allan, 1987; Zisook & DeVaul, 1977). In order to sustain remission of symptoms, such psychosocial therapies are often needed in addition to medications that diminish the inflammation in the intestines.

Irritable bowel syndrome, unlike the inflammatory bowel diseases, results from a sensitivity to psychological factors by intestinal muscles, much like the sensitivity of bronchiolar muscles of the lungs in asthma (Folks & Kinney, 1995). An estimated 70% of patients with irritable bowel syndrome have other associated psychological, behavioral, or psychiatric disorders. Psychosocial therapy for irritable bowel syndrome combines diagnosis and treatment of associated depressive or anxiety disorders, often using psychotropic medications, with therapy for resolving personal and relationship conflicts that may be contributing to exacerbations of symptoms (Crouch, 1988; Wise, Cooper, & Ahmed, 1982). Even though a patient may not be showing mood symptoms, gastrointestinal symptoms can diminish with the administration of antidepressant or antianxiety medications (Folks & Kinney).

NEUROLOGICAL AND ENDOCRINE CONDITIONS: WHEN THE NEUROPHYSIOLOGICAL REGULATION OF MOOD OR COGNITION IS IMPAIRED, DISABILITY AND SUFFERING ARE MULTIPLIED

Neurological and endocrine disorders are unique in that the brain, as the target of physiological disease in these disorders, is also the organ most responsible for regulating how a person thinks, feels, and behaves. Neurological and endocrine diseases can destabilize these capacities in a direct manner not seen in other kinds of disease. When the neurophysiological regulation of mood or cognition is impaired, disability and suffering are multiplied.

Patients with strokes or tumors in the left hemisphere of the brain tend to develop a depressed mood, whereas lesions in the right hemisphere are associated with mood elevation and mania. Each pattern is attributable to different roles that each of the two hemispheres play in mood regulation (Robinson, Star, & Price, 1984). Due to the important roles that hormones play in mood regulation, disorders affecting the pituitary, adrenal, thyroid, and parathyroid glands also tend to destabilize moods (Kathol, 1996).

For example, Mrs. Jones was admitted to the hospital for diagnostic evaluation of probable Cushing's disease. In addition to gaining weight and becoming lethargic, Mrs. Jones had also become socially withdrawn during recent weeks and full of despair over lifestyle choices her children had made. Hospitalized on a fifth-floor medical unit, she jumped from an open window to her death. At least two-thirds of patients with Cushing's disease develop severe depressive symptoms, with an accompanying increase in incidence of suicide, due to brain effects from high levels of steroid hormones that are secreted by the adrenal glands. Had this risk been recognized earlier, her depression might have been anticipated and her suicide perhaps prevented.

In multiple sclerosis, depression has been shown to occur among 42% of patients, compared to 5% of persons in a normal population (Joffe, Lippert, Gray, Sawa, & Horvath, 1987). While one might suppose that these depressive symptoms are due to the psychological impact of a disabling illness, there has been found no correlation between degree of functional disability and severity of depression, suggesting that direct damage to brain systems that regulate mood accounts for much of the mood instability (Schiffer, Caine, Bamford, & Levy, 1983).

In epilepsy, a neurological disease affecting about 1% of the population, depression can be diagnosed in about half of patients. Patients with epilepsy have a suicide rate at least five times that of the general population (Mathews & Barbas, 1981). The patterns of relationship between epilepsy and mood are multiple and complex, but damage within brain systems that regulate perception and expression of emotion appears to mediate much of this high prevalence of mood disorders. Epilepsy is also a disease in which its severity correlates directly with a patient's reliability in taking daily anticonvulsants, appearing for regular office visits, and obtaining regular blood tests (McNamara, 1995). For this reason, unrecognized or untreated depression is a more serious hazard than with some medical conditions.

Mood symptoms frequently accompany degenerative diseases affecting subcortical systems of the brain, such as Parkinson's disease and Huntington's disease. In Parkinson's disease, about half of patients can be diagnosed with a depressive disorder (McNamara, 1995). A similar frequency of depression occurs in Huntington's disease, along with a several-fold increased incidence of suicide (Maricle, 1993). Since other diseases with comparable disability and suffering do not show these high rates of mood disorder or suicide, these effects appear to be mediated largely by damage to brain systems regulating mood, rather than a psychological response to difficult life circumstances (McNamara).

Patients who suffer strokes are doubly impaired when, in addition to their neurological deficits, they also suffer loss of the ability to concentrate, remember, and think abstractly. Depressed patients who suffer strokes have been found to show more cognitive impairment than would be expected solely from the brain damage. In one study (Robinson, Bolla-Wilson, Kaplan, Lipsey, & Price, 1986) all patients with major depression showed cognitive impairment, whereas only 40% of nondepressed patients were similarly impaired. Moreover, although nondepressed patients demonstrated some cognitive improvement six months after their stroke, the depressed patients showed no such improvement. When depression was appropriately treated, the patients' cognitive capabilities also improved.

RHEUMATOLOGICAL DISORDERS: A MULTIPLEX OF MIND-BODY PATTERNS SPREAD ACROSS THE BIOBEHAVIORAL CONTINUUM

Rheumatological disorders arise when the immune system of the body erroneously targets one's own body tissues for destruction. Depending upon the specific disease, particular regions of the body, such as the kidneys or the lungs, or particular types of body tissue, such as the skin or bone marrow, are selectively damaged. When the inflammation involves small arterioles, the blood vessels occlude, destroying whatever tissue had relied upon the vessels for nutrients and oxygen. Rheumatological diseases thus produce complex patterns of tissue damage and, as a consequence, the superposition of multiple patterns through which symptoms are generated.

About 25% of exacerbations of systemic lupus erythematosus are associated with acute psychiatric symptoms (Greenberg, 1996). Among these, symptoms of delirium, psychosis, or mood disorders occur and for widely different reasons. Symptoms often result from vasculitis that injures or destroys brain regions that regulate mood or cognition. In other cases, antibodies directly attack brain neurons. In others, high-dose steroids used to treat the disease precipitate psychosis, depression, or mania. In still others, mental confusion occurs due to metabolic abnormalities from damage to the kidneys or other body organs. In still others, a patient and his or her family members become demoralized and depressed from the uncertainty of a disease characterized by a chronic pattern of unpredictable, dramatic relapses that quickly become life-threatening. Finally, many patients with lupus suffer chronic pain, disfigurement, and neurological symptoms that bring demoralization and stigma. A program of psychosocial therapy must tease apart each of these strands, tailoring a specific component of therapy for each that can be integrated with medical treatment of the disease.

For example, William, a 19-year-old young man with lupus, was referred for treatment of depression. William now had a new renal transplant. He had lost his kidneys because he had refused during his early teenage years to take his immunosuppressive drugs reliably. Embarrassed by changes in his appearance — weight gain and hair loss — he had secretly discarded his medications on frequent occasions, a choice that eventually resulted in loss of his kidneys. A multidimensional assessment, involving interviews with William, alone and with his family members, consultations with his nephrologist, and a review of his medical records, suggested that two major patterns contributed to his current depressed mood: First, William lived with his mother who worked full time, with William staying home alone most of the day. Most of his access to a broader social world was provided through weekend visits in his older brother's home. However, the older brother would soon be transferred by the Army to Europe, and both William and his mother worried about their future without him. Second, there was a reliable pattern in which he had become depressed on each occasion that his steroid dose was increased to protect the transplanted kidney. In addition to these two major patterns, William's self-blame for losing his kidneys, his demoralization from not being able to visualize a hopeful future, and his social isolation from peers were adding other elements to his depressed mood. Therapy for William included a plan to pretreat his body with lithium carbonate prior to future increases in steroid doses in order to prevent the mood-destabilizing side effects; family meetings with William, his mother, and his brother to plan together how to compensate for the brother's absence; and individual meetings with William devoted to envisioning a future worth living even though lupus would also be part of it.

Fibromyalgia is a commonly diagnosed but poorly delineated rheumatological syndrome. Its diagnosis relies on the syndromal association of muscle aches and pains, disturbed sleep, daytime fatigue, and pain trigger points. Laboratory tests are normal, and there is no dire prognosis as is often the case with lupus. Nearly all patients meet diagnostic criteria for a depressive disorder, but it has never been clear whether the depression is a source or a consequence of the somatic symptoms. For example, Mrs. Morgan had suffered from multiple aches and pains for three years, during which she had undergone multiple medical evaluations and had taken a multitude of medications with no beneficial effects. A comprehensive, multidimensional evaluation led to the diagnosis of fibromyalgia and the prescribing of trimipramine, a sedating antidepressant, to deepen certain stages of her sleep, and clonazepam to stabilize symptoms of panic disorder. Physical therapy was instituted since aspects of her muscle and tendon pains appeared due to disuse atrophy from the minimal amount of physical activity in which she engaged. Marital therapy was begun to repair the alienation that had developed between Mrs. Morgan and her husband, who had wearied of medical bills and her frequent talk about physical complaints. Both spouses were provided extensive information about the syndrome so that discussions could focus on designing strategies to minimize the impact of fibromyalgia on their marriage.

END-STAGE RENAL DISEASE: DISEASE AND DEPRESSION CAN LOOK THE SAME

Depression is commonly associated with end-stage renal disease. When present, its identification and treatment are important. Multiple studies have found depression to be a better predictor of mortality and frequent hospitalizations than either age or physiological variables (Burton, Kline, Lindsay, & Heidenheim, 1986; Richmond, Lindsay, Burton, Conley, & Wai, 1982; Schulman, Price, & Spinelli, 1989; Wai, Richmond, Burton, & Lindsey, 1981). Also, reliability in adhering to the medical treatment protocol, of greater concern in end-stage renal disease than in most other diseases, is influenced by such psychosocial factors as patients' beliefs about health behaviors, self-efficacy, family problems, and social support.

Despite its importance, it is difficult to determine presence and severity of depression in end-stage renal disease because the physiological symptoms of uremia (poor appetite, disturbed sleep, poor energy, poor concentration) are nearly identical to those of depression. Moreover, such commonly used medications as steroids, metabolic abnormalities from underlying systemic illnesses, imbalances of blood electrolytes, and anemia can superimpose effects that further confuse assessment of mood.

For example, Mr. Jenkins was a 50-year-old man treated for end-stage renal disease with peritoneal dialysis. He was referred for a psychiatric evaluation when the staff of his dialysis unit noted that increasingly he showed little energy, was more withdrawn, showed little interest in the affairs of his children, and was irritable with his wife. On a Hamilton Depression Scale, he scored 15, which is an elevated score but below the usual range for a major depressive disorder. When he failed to improve after administration of the antidepressant Wellbutrin, greater attention was focused on his peritoneal dialysis, which left him with erratic shifts in his metabolic status. Eventually, a decision was made to replace the peritoneal dialysis with hemodialysis. With hemodialysis, his energy returned and his mood and thinking promptly cleared as his renal status improved. He had already discontinued treatment with the antidepressant.

SOMATIZATION: A BODILY IDIOM OF DISTRESS?

Patients with problems of somatization often suffer life-long torment from physical symptoms for which there is no evidence that a medical disease exists to account for them. These patients experience such symptoms as headaches, stomach aches, seizures, chest pains, vomiting, shortness of breath, diarrhea, dizziness, or a sense of body disfigurement, only to be told on visits to physicians that there is nothing wrong with their bodies. For patients and their families this is frightening, and for physicians it is frustrating. For health care systems, money spent in futile medical treatments of somatization is a serious drain on resources (Griffith & Griffith, 1994; Katon, 1996; Smith, Rost, & Kashner, 1995).

Among medical and psychiatric disorders, treatment of somatization has been uniquely difficult. First, many patients feel embarrassed that their bodily symptoms are labeled as psychiatric and feel abandoned when their medical doctors refer them to mental health clinicians. Second, mental health clinicians traditionally have avoided patients with somatized symptoms, considering them to be poor candidates for psychological therapies (Griffith & Griffith, 1994).

Cross-cultural research on somatization has opened a perspective for understanding somatization that appears to hold more treatment options than those suggested by traditional psychiatric theories. The work of Arthur Kleinman (Kleinman & Kleinman, 1985) and Laurence Kirmayer (1989) suggest that somatization is a bodily idiom of distress that becomes dominant when verbal avenues for expressing distress are suppressed. Kirmayer further noted that it is normative across cultures for a person in distress to express distress both through talk and through symptoms of the body — chest pains, loss of appetite, dizziness, fatigue. Only in Western culture, however, are persons expected to psychologize distress, speaking only about feelings.

If it is normal for human beings to express distress both through their words and through their bodies, why then do so many patients come to physicians' offices seeking treatment for bodily complaints that appear to have no associated disease? Griffith and Griffith (1994) noted that commonly somatization is accompanied by the presence of an *unspeakable dilemma*. An unspeakable dilemma is a bind with no good options for escape and whose existence must be kept hidden from other persons involved in the situation. Unspeakable dilemmas are typically characterized by feeling trapped, isolated, unable to let others know that a problem even exists.

For example, a 9-year-old child witnessed her father having an affair with another woman. Afraid to betray him, yet also unable to keep this secret from her mother, she began having blackout spells. After a series of fruitless neurological examinations, EEGs, and brain scans, the family began meeting with a therapist. She was able to speak the secret during a session, whereupon the spells stopped. Such symptoms commonly improve or disappear when the patient is able to speak openly to those involved in the problem, as did this little girl, even though the dilemma itself may remain unresolved.

Often, unspeakable dilemmas are associated with realistic threats of physical harm, as with a child who might have been physically harmed or abandoned had she revealed that she was being sexually abused by her stepfather. In other cases, it is the lingering effects of a story from the past that suppress expression, as with a woman whose memories of her parents' unhappy marriage had led her to stay silent, rather than to voice to her husband her distress in her marriage (Griffith, 1995).

Both severe depression and panic attacks hinder a person from resolving distressed relationships due to the sense of entrapment and isolation they foster. In addition, they sustain a focus of attention on the body's state of being. For such patients, treatment of somatization may succeed best when a therapy focused on distressed relationships is coupled with antidepressant treatment for depression or panic disorder symptoms (Griffith & Griffith, 1994; Katon, 1996).

IT IS DIFFICULT TO TAKE A BOTH/AND PERSPECTIVE

As these examples show, there is a compelling argument for integrating psychosocial and biomedical perspectives in medical treatments. Nearly every medical illness can be placed somewhere along a biobehavioral continuum, where both psychosocial and biomedical interventions can influence different aspects of disease. However, relationships that hold between the body and the psychosocial world, and through which therapeutic effects of psychosocial interventions must be mediated, are not only different for different diseases, but also sometimes multiple for a single disease or changing form over the course of an illness.

As in many of the above examples, a depressed mood can be not only a source of emotional distress, but also a risk factor for onset of heart disease, or a factor that exacerbates the progression of cancer, or an amplifier of the severity of dementia in stroke patients. In such examples, depression engenders illness.

However, a depressed mood also can be the consequence of disease. About a third of hospitalized patients across all medical diagnoses meet criteria for major depressive disorder, largely due to the demoralization, grief, and physical pain that medical disease brings (Cassem, 1995). In left-hemisphere strokes, multiple sclerosis, or Cushing's disease, however, either brain damage to emotion-regulating neurophysiological systems or hormonal effects on these systems produces depression regardless whether the patient's life world is a harsh one. In end-stage renal disease, the kidney disease itself can mimic depression. Within this single psychosocial phenomenon, depression, a half dozen or more relationships may hold between bodily disease and the psychosocial world, depending upon which medical illness is involved.

It is imperative for both medical physicians and psychosocial clinicians to be able to discern specific patterns of relationship between body and psychosocial world and to have competent skills in using these patterns to treat illness. Yet, the complexity of this task is daunting. Medical physicians and psychosocial clinicians study different domains of knowledge in their training, with medical training largely ignoring the psychosocial realm and psychosocial training largely ignoring the pathophysiology of disease. More importantly, medical physicians and psychosocial clinicians are each molded professionally by very different cultures, each with its own customs and habits for perceiving, thinking about, and treating ill patients.

A good biomedical clinician is driven by a scientist's passion for isolating single causes; a good psychosocial clinician relies on an aesthetic bent for seeing patterns as they emerge across different classes of details. When an ill patient presents a symptom for treatment, for example, the usual response of a biomedical clinician is to search for a single pathophysiological process that would link the symptom with a disease. This can work for diseases far toward the biomedical end of the biobehavioral continuum. However, it works poorly when psychosocial problems hold strong influence, since psychosocial problems typically consist of multiple small causes that, by interacting in complex patterns, undermine health. A psychosocial clinician routinely surveys the landscape for patterns of interaction between psyche, family, and culture that influence illness, but is typically ill-equipped to discern when abnormal anatomy or physiology generates symptoms by placing a ceiling on what is behaviorally possible for a patient in his or her psychosocial world. As neurologist Norman Geschwind once pointed out, "The strategy of 'looking at the whole patient,' which is often so useful to the [mental health clinician] in other circumstances, may be actively misleading when certain discharging or destructive lesions of the brain are present" (1975, p. 3).

Medical physicians and psychosocial clinicians tend to become wedded to divergent belief systems and ideologies. Biomedicine adheres to the values of empirical science, with diagnostic categories as its units of understanding. Empirical science has little use for the personal meanings with which a patient interprets an experience of illness. A psychosocial therapy, however, values most the unique meanings of illness for a particular patient and family, and its units of understanding are largely the stories that patients and family members tell. Clinicians from both camps become frustrated when these categorical and narrative understandings of illness proved to be nontranslatable one into the other.

Biomedical and psychosocial therapies each tend to bring forth a different quality of clinician-patient relationship. Biomedical understanding is best gained from a position of emotional distance from the patient. Narrative understanding is best gained from a close, empathic position. It can be difficult for biomedical and psychosocial clinicians to respect the kind of relatedness the other has with patients.

Finally, the routine clinical practices of biomedical and psychosocial clinicians are each so different that it is a challenge for one to understand the daily habits of the other. In a primary care setting, for example, a biomedical clinician spends an average of 8 to 12 minutes per visit. In order to preserve efficiency, a biomedical clinician is often preoccupied with how to contain or bring closure to talking with patients. Mental health clinicians spend 30 to 90 minutes with patients and families. They focus on opening a dialogue that will enable patients and family members to tell fully their accounts of illness, even if this takes much time.

While the task may be daunting, the time has come to search for a rapprochement between the worlds of biomedicine and the psychosocial therapies. As the chapters of this text illustrate, such a solution must incorporate ways to sustain cross-discipline dialogue, to value the contributions of each, and to share knowledge collaboratively. Toward this end we have much yet to learn.

REFERENCES

Andersen, B. L., Kiecolt-Glaser, J. K., & Glaser, R. (1994). A biobehavioral model of cancer, stress, and disease course. *American Psychologist, 49*, 389–404.

Andrews, H., Barczak, P., & Allan, R. N. (1987). Psychiatric illness in patients with inflammatory bowel disease. *Gut, 28*, 1600–1604.

Booth-Kewley, S., & Friedman, H. S. (1987). Psychological predictors of heart disease: A quantitative review. *Psychological Bulletin, 101*, 343–362.

Burton, H. J., Kline, S. A., Lindsay, R. M., & Heidenheim, A. P. (1986). The relationship of depression to survival in chronic renal failure. *Psychosomatic Medicine, 48*, 261–269.

Carney, R. M., Rich, M. W., Freedland, K. E., Saini, J., teVelde, A., Simeone, C., & Clark, K. (1988). Major depressive disorder predicts cardiac events in patients with coronary artery disease. *Psychosomatic Medicine, 50*, 627–633.

Cassem, E. H. (1995). Depressive disorders in the medically ill: An overview. *Psychosomatics, 36*(suppl), S2–S10.

Crouch, M. A. (1988). Irritable bowel syndrome: Toward a biopsychosocial systems understanding. *Primary Care, 15*, 99–110.

Dembroski, T. M., MacDougall, J. M., Costa, P. T., & Grandits, G. A. (1989). Components of hostility as predictors of sudden death and myocardial infarction in the Multiple Risk Factor Intervention Trial. *Psychosomatic Medicine, 51*, 514–522.

Esler, M., Turbott, J., Schwartz, R., Leonard, P. L., Bobik, A., Skews, H., & Jackman, G. (1982). The peripheral kinetics of norepinephrine in depressive illness. *Archives of General Psychiatry, 39*, 285–300.

Esterling, B. A., Kiecolt-Glaser, J. K., Bodnar, J. C., & Glaser, R. (1994). Chronic stress, social support, and persistent alterations in the natural killer cell response to cytokines in older adults. *Health Psychology, 13*, 291–298.

Fawzy, F. I., Fawzy, N. W., Hyun, C. S., Elasoff, R. Guthrie, D., Fahey, J. L., & Morton, D. L. (1993). Malignant melanoma: Effects of an early structured psychiatric intervention, coping, and affective state on recurrence and survival 6 years later. *Archives of General Psychiatry, 50*, 681–689.

Folks, D. G., & Kinney, F. C. (1995). Gastrointestinal conditions. In A. Stoudemire (Ed.), *Psychological factors affecting medical conditions* (pp. 99–122). Washington, DC: American Psychiatric Press.

Friedman, M. (1969). *Pathogenesis of coronary artery disease*. New York: McGraw-Hill.

Geschwind, N. (1975). The borderland of neurology and psychiatry: Some common misconceptions. In D. F. Benson, & D. Blumer (Eds.), *Psychiatric aspects of neurologic disease* (p. 3). New York: Grune & Stratton.

Goldstein, M. G., & Niaura, R. (1995). Cardiovascular disease, Part I: Coronary artery disease and sudden death. In A. Stoudemire (Ed.), *Psychological factors affecting medical conditions* (pp. 19–37). Washington, DC: American Psychiatric Press.

Greenberg, D. (1996). Systemic lupus erythematosus. In J. R. Rundell, & M. G. Wise (Eds.), *Textbook of consultation-liaison psychiatry* (p. 585). Washington, DC: American Psychiatric Press.

Greer, S., Morris, T., & Pettingale, K. W. (1979). Psychological response to breast cancer: Effect on outcome. *Lancet, 2*, 785–787.

Griffith, J. L. (1995). Physical symptoms result from unspeakable dilemmas. *The Menninger Newsletter, 3*, 4–5.

Griffith, J. L., & Griffith, M. E. (1994). *The body speaks: Therapeutic dialogues for mind-body problems.* New York: Basic.

Griffith, J. L., & Griffith, M. E. (1997, February 3–6). *Narrative therapy, unspeakable dilemmas, and the psychosocial treatment of cancer.* Symposium presentation at the Seventh International Congress on Anti-Cancer Treatments, Palais des Congres, Paris, France.

Helzer, J. E., Stillings, W. A., Chammas, S., Norland, C. C., & Alpers, D. H. (1982). A controlled study of the association between ulcerative colitis and psychiatric diagnosis. *Digestive Diseases and Sciences, 27*, 513–518.

Joffe, R. T., Lippert, G. P., Gray, T. A., Sawa G., & Horvath Z. (1987). Mood disorder and multiple sclerosis. *Archives of Neurology, 44*, 376–378.

Kathol, R. (1996). Endocrine disorders. In J. R. Rundell, & M. G. Wise (Eds.), *Textbook of consultation-liaison psychiatry* (pp. 579–584). Washington, DC: American Psychiatric Press.

Katon, W. (1996). Panic disorder: Relationship to high medical utilization, unexplained physical symptoms, and medical costs. *Journal of Clinical Psychiatry, 57*(suppl 10), 11–18.

Kirmayer, L. J. (1989). Cultural variations in the response to psychiatric disorders and emotional distress. *Social Science and Medicine, 29*, 327–339.

Kleinman, A., & Kleinman, J. (1985). Somatization: The interconnections in Chinese society among culture, depressive experiences, and the meanings of pain. In A. Kleinman, & B. Good (Eds.), *Culture and depression* (pp. 429–490). Berkeley: University of California.

Krantz, D. S., & Durel, L. A. (1983). Psychobiological substrates of the type A behavior pattern. *Health Psychology, 2*, 393–411.

Manuck, S. B., & Krantz, D. W. (1986). Psychophysiologic reactivity in coronary heart disease and essential hypertension. In K. A. Mathews, S. M. Weiss, T. Detre, T. M. Dembroski, B. Falkner, S. B. Manuck, & R. B. Williams (Eds.), *Handbook of stress, reactivity, and cardiovascular disease* (pp. 11–34). New York: Wiley.

Maricle, R. A. (1993). Psychiatric disorders in Huntington's disease. In A. Stoudemire (Ed.), *Medical psychiatric practice: Vol. 2* (pp. 88–99). Washington, DC: American Psychiatric Press.

Mathews, W. S., & Barbas, G. (1981). Suicide and epilepsy: A review of the literature. *Psychosomatics, 22*, 515–524.

McNamara, M. E. (1995). Neurological conditions: Depression and stroke, multiple sclerosis, Parkinson's disease, and epilepsy. In A. Stoudemire (Ed.), *Psychological factors affecting medical conditions* (pp. 57–79). Washington, DC: American Psychiatric Press.

Moran, M. (1995). Pulmonary and rheumatologic diseases. In A. Stoudemire (Ed.), *Psychological factors affecting medical conditions* (pp. 141–158). Washington, DC: American Psychiatric Press.

Niaura, R., & Goldstein, M. (1995). Cardiovascular disease, Part II: Coronary artery disease and sudden death and hypertension. In A. Stoudemire (Ed.), *Psychological factors affecting medical conditions* (pp. 39–56). Washington, DC: American Psychiatric Press.

Nunes, E. V., Frank, K. A., & Kornfeld, D. S. (1987). Psychologic treatment for the type

A behavior pattern and for coronary heart disease: A meta analysis of the literature. *Psychosomatic Medicine, 48,* 159–173.

Reich, P., DeSilva, R. A., Lown, B., & Murawski, B. J. (1981). Acute psychological disturbance preceding life-threatening ventricular arrhythmias. *JAMA, 246,* 233–235.

Richmond, J. M., Lindsay, R. M., Burton, H. J., Conley, J., & Wai, L. (1982). Psychological and physiological factors predicting the outcome on home hemodialysis. *Clinical Nephrology, 17,* 109–113.

Robinson, R. G., Bolla-Wilson, K., Kaplan, E., Lipsey, J. R., & Price, T. R. (1986). Depression influences intellectual impairment in stroke patients. *British Journal of Psychiatry, 148,* 541–547.

Robinson, R. G., Star, L. B., & Price, T. R. (1984). A two-year longitudinal study of mood disorders following stroke, prevalence and duration at 6 months follow-up. *British Journal of Psychiatry, 144,* 256–262.

Schiffer, R. B., Caine, E. D., Bamford, K. A., & Levy S. (1983). Depressive episodes in patients with multiple sclerosis. *American Journal of Psychiatry, 140,* 1498–1500.

Schulman, R., Price, J. D., & Spinelli, J. (1989). Biopsychosocial aspects of long-term survival on end-stage renal failure therapy. *Psychological Medicine, 19,* 945–954.

Siegman, A. W., Dembroski, T. M., & Ringel, N. (1987). Components of hostility and the severity of coronary artery disease. *Psychosomatic Medicine 49,* 127–135.

Smith, G. R., Rost, K., & Kashner, T. M. (1995). A trial of the effect of a standardized psychiatric consultation on health outcomes and costs in somatizing patients. *Archives of General Psychiatry, 52,* 238–243.

Spiegel D., & Kato, P. M. (1996). Psychosocial influences on cancer incidence and progression. *Harvard Reviews in Psychiatry, 4,* 10–26.

Spiegel, D., Kraemer, H. C., Bloom, J. R., & Gottheil, E. (1989). Effect of a psychosocial treatment on survival of patients with metastatic breast cancer. *Lancet, 2,* 888–891.

Wai, L., Richmond, J., Burton, H. J., & Lindsey, R. M. (1981). Influence of psychosocial factors on survival of home-dialysis patients. *Lancet, 2,* 1155–1156.

Weihs, K. (1996). *Survival in recurrent breast cancer patients predicted by patient coping style.* Research presentation at the Conference on the (Non)Expression of Emotions in Health and Disease, Tilburg, The Netherlands.

Weihs, K., Enright, T., Simmens, S., & Reiss, D. (1997). *Psychological distress and restriction of emotions as risks for recurrent breast cancer.* Manuscript submitted for publication.

Wise, T. N., Cooper, J. N., & Ahmed, S. (1982). The efficacy of group therapy for patients with irritable bowel syndrome. *Psychosomatics, 23,* 465–469.

Wood, B. L. (1993). Beyond the "psychosomatic family": A biobehavioral model of pediatric illness. *Family Process, 32,* 261–278.

Wood, B. L. (1994). One articulation of the structural family therapy model: A biobehavioral model of chronic illness in children. *Journal of Family Therapy, 16,* 53–72.

Zisook, C., & DeVaul, R. A. (1977). Emotional factors in inflammatory bowel disease. *Southern Medical Journal, 70,* 716–719.

3

The Community-Based Neighborhood Health Center HMO: An Available Alternative for Health Care Reform

E. H. Auerswald

The Gouverneur Health Services Program is an example of an attempt at integrated care within a much larger experiment in health care delivery. Auerswald's account can serve to keep the innovators of today from thinking that they are the first with the idea. It is also a cautionary tale about what happens to even very well-designed and very successful programs when they are far enough out of step with (some would say ahead of) the mainstream of health care delivery.

At the time of the Gouverneur program, the United States was undergoing a period of rapid and uncomfortable social upheaval. Revolutions and counterrevolutions in a number of areas of life were underway. Health care delivery, however, was not one of the systems undergoing rapid change. Although the new approach to delivering medical services that Auerswald describes was fully in step with the spirit of change, it was a poor fit with some of the day-to-day expectations of patients, providers, and larger institutions. Now the United States is in a period of relative stability and prosperity, and health care is undergoing a thorough, if unplanned, reorganization. It may be that now there is flexibility in a stable environment that makes change possible and less threatening.

Dick Auerswald died as this volume was in the final stages of preparation. It is my hope that its publication will introduce a new generation to his kindness, his humility, his humor, his power and clarity of thought, and his passion for social justice.

HEALTH CARE REFORM, as everyone knows who stops to think about it, is not new. Almost all of the industrialized nations of the world have gone through such a process and come out with a public single payer system that also leaves room for private care for those who want it and can afford it. The United States is a latecomer in this endeavor. Health care reform in the U.S. has not come up with a stable, comprehensive system that provides care for all citizens.

A laudable effort was made by the Johnson administration in the 1960s to develop such a system, but it resulted in piecemeal legislation designed to provide coverage only for the poorest of the indigent (Medicaid) and for the aged (Medicare). Care for the large number of nonaged people of limited income who lacked health insurance and who could not afford it was not provided. Also, these programs were constructed in such a way as to have little effect on the *structure* of health care delivery, where the primary problem is to be found.

However, one initiative that came out of the Office of Economic Opportunity, the administrative base of Johnson's "war on poverty," *did* allow for attention to structure. Fueled by the recognition that the standard model of health care delivery was not only inadequate but also *inappropriate* in the manner in which it dealt with the chronically poor, especially those of non-Eurocentric cultures, a grant program was established to assist innovative front-line health care facilities to develop new structures and methods of delivery. One of the recipients of such a "Neighborhood Health Center" grant was the program described in this chapter, the Gouverneur Health Services Program, that took shape on the Lower East Side of New York City.

THE SETTING

The quality of care delivered at the old city-operated Gouverneur Hospital, which served lower Manhattan and which was located on the East River just south of the Brooklyn Bridge, had gradually deteriorated over the years, and in 1958 a decision was made to close it. The city asked Beth Israel Hospital, which was further uptown and outside of the district that the old hospital had covered, to assume the provision of both inpatient and outpatient care for the population of that district, these services to be supported by money that had already been budgeted for the defunct hospital.

The district served, as most Americans know, had a very unique history. It had been the first stop upon arrival of millions of European immigrants. Remnants of this old immigrant population remained there, but there had also been an influx of Latin-Americans, mostly, but not all, from Puerto Rico, and of African-Americans, many from the South. There was also in this population a large percentage of single elderly people and fatherless households with several children. Not only that, but New York's Chinatown and a permanent Italian community known as "Little Italy" had become established in this area. The boundary between these two areas was The Bowery, notorious as New York's "skid row."

At the time that the decision was made to close the hospital, the Lower East Side Neighborhoods Association, a coalition of religious, business, cultural, and political leaders that had been established for many years and was supported by many of the old social agencies that had served the immigrants, was struggling to hold all this together in some more or less harmonious community form. This politically powerful group, representing the community-at-large, objected vigorously to the arrangement that would move the site of health care out of their community. Beth Israel Hospital, they argued, was too far away and could not, because of the range and size of its services, pay attention to the specific needs of their community. The Association mounted a campaign, replete with petitions and torchlight parades, to force the city to build a new hospital and to keep the "ambulatory care" portion of the Gouverneur Hospital open until the new hospital could be built. Faced with this politically potent challenge, the city's Department of Hospitals agreed to this course. Plans for the new hospital were formulated and the city contracted with Beth Israel Hospital to establish a community health center. The hospital was closed, the building was hastily refurbished, and the new center was formed from scratch. Thus, as the result of the actions of a group of people representing and deeply imbedded in their community, was born the Gouverneur Ambulatory Care Center, later to acquire the more appropriate name of the Gouverneur Health Services Program.

Community involvement preceded the program and was thus built in from the start. Although, strictly speaking, the organization of the program's base was not that of a community cooperative, it might as well have been, and the experience that ensued can be taken as an example of what could happen in a program organized as a community cooperative.

Given the vibrant heterogeneity of the area and beginning as it did at a time of increasing social awareness and unrest with a pot of money that had comprised the budget of the closed hospital pretty much available from the start, the program planning provided a fertile field for innovation — and innovative it was. So much so that in 1965, after the program was well underway, the Office of Economic Opportunity (OEO) took note of what was happening there and the Gouverneur program became one of the models for its federal Neighborhood Health Center program, and in 1965 the program was awarded a $661,000 annual grant, further enhancing the potential for innovation.

The degree of operational freedom afforded the program was remarkable. That the board of directors and the executive director of Beth Israel Hospital, Mark Freedman, working closely with the neighborhood association and the New York City Commissioner of Hospitals, Ray Trussel, accepted the task of sponsoring a "far out" innovative center was a tribute to them in itself, but they also granted nearly total autonomy to the medical director of the Gouverneur Program and his staff right from its inception. Furthermore, when the OEO grant was awarded later, it was delivered with only a couple of strings attached. One string, rightly, was that the way the money was spent must be recorded in detail, and the other, amazingly, was that the money must be used for a program that was "different" from standard practice.

Dr. Howard J. Brown, an internist by original training, who had been concerned with health care delivery for the poor for many years and who had been working for the Health Insurance Plan of Greater New York, was recruited to head up the program as medical director. Harold Light, a social worker by training, after a stint as the program's first director of social services, became the associate director. That a social worker assumed this position was at the time an innovation in itself, and it signaled the recognition of those involved in forming the program that social issues were as relevant to health as biological issues.

I became interested in the program when I heard that Dr. Brown was considering the idea of instituting a policy in which the family, not the individual, would be considered the "primary unit" to which health care would be delivered. I was, at the time in 1965, deeply involved in the growing family therapy movement and had developed the notion that human distress could be defined as ecological phenomena. Within this ecological framework, it had become clear to me that the family was the unit that assumed the primary responsibility for the maintenance of stability in the human ecological field. So I went to see Dr. Brown who, after a discussion, hired me as a planning consultant, and then, within a few weeks, hired me into a job he and I envisioned: director of applied behavioral sciences.

Following is a retrospective first person description of what happened after I accepted that job. It was first published in *Family Systems Medicine* (1983, 1[3], 5–24) under the title "The Gouverneur Health Services Program: An Experiment in Ecosystemic Community Health Care Delivery."

My involvement with the Gouverneur Program began about four years after its initiation, just prior to the granting of OEO funds. I assisted in the design of the program that was written into the grant proposal, and spent four-and-a-half years working in the program as director of applied behavioral sciences. Much happened in those years that defies description. Also, much went on outside my purview. For these reasons, I chose to write this article as a first-person narrative. Thus, I am writing as a participant/observer, and much of what I write is highly subjective, despite my effort to maintain objectivity. Also, my narrative is totally out of balance, since I thought it important to emphasize ideas basic to the program's design, its growth, and its ultimate decline. To do this, I have left out almost all of the exciting and highly rewarding relationships with people, both inside and outside the program, with whom I worked and thought together on a day-to-day basis during those years. The program belonged to all of us, certainly not to me, and not even to Howard Brown. That story is yet to be written.

ACT ONE: THE PROGRAM IS DESIGNED

I first heard about the Gouverneur Program in late August of 1964. I was in Washington talking with a friend who worked at the National Institute of Mental Health. I had been telling him about my conviction that illnesses should be conceptualized as ecological phenomena, especially in work with the economically poor and how, when one thought this way, socioenvironmental and family dynamics became visible as major etiological vectors in many of the presenting problems which were brought to health care facilities. He brought up the name of Howard Brown, who he said was interested in such ideas. Dr. Brown had been organizing the staff of his program at Gouverneur into teams, each of which would serve families in a census tract. He was calling these teams "family health units." Intrigued, I made an appointment to talk with Dr. Brown when I returned to New York.

Howard Brown turned out to be a round-faced bespectacled man with thinning hair, a ruddy complexion, and a gentle handshake. He listened politely as I presented my epistemological ideas. I don't think he was much interested. But when I began to share why I thought these ideas had pragmatic implications in the design of health and human services delivery systems, his polite detachment vanished entirely. His behavior — indeed, his whole appearance — changed. He became intensely involved in our conversation. When we discussed how the structure of the traditional health care delivery system mitigated against good health care for the economically poor, he made his points with restrained anger, and when we moved on to a discussion of alternative structures, he spoke with eager intensity. His extraordinary dedication to his work became very clear.

We found we were in agreement on three issues. One was that the health and human services system was in fragments as the result of specialization. Individual people and families with complex socioenvironmental, family, and individual problems had to shop for pieces of help. At the front door of each helping agency, in order to gain entry and get help, they had to define their problem according to the rule book of the helping system they approached. There was a great need for a system with a single point of entry which could respond in an integrated way to all the interrelated issues that created distress in each case. (At that time a popular phrase was "comprehensive." Many medical programs defined comprehensiveness by the number of fragments they had in operation: namely, how many specialty clinics. Many still use this definition.)

Second, we agreed that the idealized version of the old country doc who knew and understood the biological problems of his patients in the context of their families and social and physical environment was a valuable model which modern, technology-based, hierarchically-structured medicine could not obtain. However, an integrated front-line system made up of medical and behavioral science specialists who worked together as a team could be designed which could take the old doc's place, and could probably do his work even better. And the third issue was that the distress of an individual human being could never be fully understood outside the socioenvironmental context of his or her life, and that the most important system making up that context was the family.

In retrospect, I realize that, just as Howard failed to respond to the epistemological issues I brought to him during this first meeting, I, too, failed to respond to an idea he brought up repeatedly as we talked. He kept saying that we had to abandon the practice of referral. This seemed to me to be a semantic trick. It was much, much more than that, as I shall explain later.

At the end of that conversation, Howard asked if I would be willing to join the Gouverneur staff as a part-time planning consultant, which I readily agreed to do. The title of planning consultant, however, turned out to be something of a misnomer. What I subsequently did had less to do with planning in the traditional sense than it did with new program design and, as it turned out, implementation.

When we met the next day, Howard and I narrowed our discussion to the design of the proposed Gouverneur Program. Howard explained his concept of the family health unit. It was based, he said, on the ideas of abolishing the practice of referral and making the family the primary unit of health care. I, in turn, presented to him program ideas I had crystallized overnight which were also based on making the family the unit of health care and, in addition, on my conviction that it was useful to think of illnesses as ecological phenomena.

By the time we ended this second meeting, the rough outline of an alternative system of front-line health care had emerged. It looked like this:

The superstructure of the program would consist of a medical care program administration and an applied behavioral sciences program administration which would have equal status under the director and his assistant. Both program administrations would participate in formulation of overall policy and procedure.

The major tasks of the medical care program administration would be to obtain and maintain a high quality of biological medical care and to conduct a program of continuing medical education. The major tasks of applied behavioral sciences administration would be to train and provide ongoing consultation for an applied behavioral sciences staff.

The medical staff would consist of, as it already did, internists, pediatricians, nurses, and trained aides (family medicine was not yet a specialty). The applied behavioral sciences staff would consist of social workers, public health nurses, and trained aides with psychiatrists and psychologists available. These workers would be organized into family health units, each of which would serve a census tract. The medical staff of the team would be responsible for the biological issues, and the applied behavioral sciences staff would address the psychosocial-family-environmental issues in each case.

The teams would be organized horizontally and be responsible to a single leader. Each team would need a clerical staff. There would be no vertical specialty departments, but a corps of specialists would be available. People served by the family health units would not be referred to an array of specialty clinics. Although those specialties requiring space-containing special equipment would, of course, work in such space, procedures involving them in a given case would reflect the concept that they were being "pulled in" to the overall process of providing comprehensive care. (This was, of course, akin to what is now, 18 years later, the widespread concept of the primary care physician.)

In both components represented in the family health teams (medical and applied behavioral sciences), "indigenous" staff would be hired who came from the broad range of ethnocultural groups present in the census tract served. Also, since there were many people in the overall district served who were not proficient in English, multilingual capabilities would have to be built in, mainly Puerto-Rican Spanish, Chinese (of four different dialects), Yiddish, and Italian, in addition to English. In fact, all signs and materials providing instruction to users of services would have to be printed at least in English, Spanish, and Chinese. (This was already being done at the time of our discussion.)

Clients would be considered user-members of the family health units and, as much as possible, would be enlisted as families. Individual records would be combined in a family folder, which would contain a family life narrative. Individual records of those without family in the area would, nevertheless, be kept in a folder containing a narrative of the family story of that individual. Family life narratives would be written so as to include other sociocultural-environmental information. Specialty examinations, including psychological profiles done on individuals, and a record of specialty treatment rendered would be filed in the individual record within the family folder.

There would also be a system designed for making house calls to deal with medical, family, and socioenvironmental crises, and a home care program. And, finally, the evolution of the program would have to involve a representative group of citizens and other health and human service providers from the area served (again, Howard had already been heavily involved in developing such a group).

After this discussion, I left the building riding a high that was not to subside for three years.

Before going on to describe what happened, I would like to present some of the ideas which were immanent in the program design described in skeletal form above and the subsequent evolution of the program.

I mentioned above that in our discussion there were a couple of exchanges during which Howard and I did not connect. Howard was not much interested in my epistemological observations and I was unimpressed by his insistence that the most important pragmatic action to be taken was to abolish the traditional system of referral. At one point, I had made an effort to resolve what seemed to me to be a difference in our thinking. I remarked that in order to abolish the system of referral, the proposed family health units would have to use a patient care sequence rooted in a paradigm other than that used throughout the discipline of medicine. This medical paradigm is designed in a linear sequence to zero in on the site and nature of pathology inside the body. We would have to retrain the physicians in the program to think in a larger field, which to me meant, like epidemiologists in public health, they would have to look for ecological patterns, not for linear cause-effect relationships. Howard objected, saying that physicians should not and could not be expected to abandon a way of thinking which had produced such remarkable results over the years and in which they had been trained from the start. I had to agree with him, of course, thinking as I did, self-referentially, that this training had begun long before medical school, in infancy, when all of us in the Western world began to learn the rules used to define the occidental version of reality. We did not pursue this issue further but it posed a problem for me in my effort to design the applied behavioral sciences portion of the program, since the basic idea was to design an integrated delivery system.

To explain the problem, I must use an analogy.

Imagine four people, each of whom knows how to play only one card game. Let's say, for example, that two of them know how to play poker and two know how to play contract bridge. Imagine them alone in a room that contains a card table, four chairs, and a deck of cards. They decide to play a game of cards, and they cut for the deal. One of them begins to deal. Immediately, of course, two of them object to the way the cards are being dealt. If none of them is aware that there are other games than the one they know, they are at an impasse.

There are a number of sequences that can then follow: (1) They can argue until they are tired of the argument and give up, so that the game of cards will never come off; (2) they can discover each other's game and decide to discard one game and just play the other, or; (3) they can explore one another's game and decide to play both games. Choice 3 is by far the most interesting because, in order to arrive at it, they must in essence invent a new game by inventing a new rule. The rule which creates the new game is: "First, poker must be played by its rules, and then bridge must be played by its rules" (or vice versa). The new game might be called pokerbridge.

What is important to recognize is that pokerbridge is not poker, nor is it bridge; it is a new game, a new system, with poker and bridge as subsystems.

In the language of this analogy, the design problem I faced was as follows: If I designed an applied behavioral sciences program that hired people who thought ecologically (or trained them to do so), who would work side by side with others who thought in traditional medical ways, "poker" players would be working in he same room with "bridge" players. The two sections of the family health units would then inevitably engage in arguments about the "right way to deal the cards." To insure functional integration, I would have to find or invent rules that would create a pokerbridge game in which the ecological game and the medical game would become subgames, which could be played by the family health units, as called for in each case situation, without conflict.

It was not difficult to find the rule to create a pokerbridge game. It had already been invented in science during the emergence of quantum/relativity physics beginning with the work of Max Planck and Albert Einstein at the turn of the century. Out of their work had emerged a set of thought rules with which to define reality that were discontinuous with the thought rules of Newtonian physics. Over the intervening years, the thought rules of quantum/relativity physics had allowed for application of thought to a much expanded field without destroying the usefulness of the Newtonian thought rules. What happened, in fact, was that the thought system of quantum/relativity physics became the context within which the Newtonian thought system is used, in a selective way.

As ecological thought had later emerged from the thought system of quantum/relativity physics as part of "new science," while medical thought had, for the most part, remained rooted in the thought system that had produced Newtonian science, the rule I was looking for had already been invented. The rule is: "The ecological game played by the applied behavioral sciences program will furnish the context within which the medical game will be played."

I realized then, for the first time, how radical was the design we had proposed. The context used by health care delivery systems had always been medical with socioenvironmental issues seen as "ancillary." We were proposing a total reversal. I also realized why health care programs seemed so frequently incongruent to patients who brought their lives to doctors who had been trained to zero in on their livers. For affluent people whose lives as social beings were in reasonably good shape, this inconsistency would go unnoticed. But for people who lived under the social conditions of grinding poverty, the incongruity was clearly apparent.

Concurrently, my respect for Howard Brown grew. I now understood his emphasis on abolishing the system of referral. The idea was both strategic and tactical. Instead of identifying a problem and referring a whole person to a specialist who would ultimately only deal with a part of him, the physician first consulted would retain responsibility. He would have to consider a specialist's contribution as only one task in a case plan that might include many such tasks. The physician who was first contacted (at Gouverneur, an internist) would then have to become a generalist who would define what tasks were best carried out by what specialist. He would also become responsible for seeing to it that the various tasks were carried out. Howard's strategic goal was to plug the cracks in the system, thus preventing health care recipients from getting lost in the spaces between doctors' offices. Abolishing the referral system was a tactic within this strategy.

More important, however, from my point of view, was that under these conditions the internist would correlate all information concerning the biological state of the recipient in a manner that would expose patterned interrelationships. It would require a way of thinking congruent with that of the behavioral sciences program staff who could then expand the field of biological information to include that from family, culture, and socioeconomic environments, without getting trapped in poker/bridge games.

The next step, then, in the design of the applied behavioral sciences program was to make the family and socioenvironmental information in each case as visible as possible to the medical staff so that they could begin to see the connections between that information and the biological information they routinely collected. Strategically, we would follow Planck and Einstein, who never confronted the Newtonian physicists with the message that their thought system was no longer transcendent. They simply developed a new thought system, a new basis for rational definition of reality. They never responded to poker/bridge-type conflict. They simply demonstrated that the new thought system worked and that it shed light on phenomena that had baffled Newtonian physicists. A burst of creativity ensued, which Newtonian physicists scurried to join. With luck, we could create an analogous phenomenon in our funky old building on the Lower East Side. As I thought about this prospect, it became more and more exciting. It also frightened me some. Maybe this line of thought was simply inappropriate, even crazy. And even if it was on target, the unanswered question loomed large: Could we pull it off?

Six additional design ideas occurred to me at that time. One was already in place: a policy to train workers for each family health unit who would be specialists in exposing and dealing with the socioenvironmental problems of the people served. The ideas I added, each of which was designed to create an information feedback loop into the operational arena of the family health units, were as follows:

1. We would hire a writer who could think ecologically to document what happened when care was delivered in an ecological context.

2. We would place a one-way mirror observation room equipped for videotaping in the space occupied by each family health unit. Family therapy sessions and socioenvironmental planning sessions would be held

in this room, and all family health unit staff would be encouraged to spend some time observing the process. Videotapes would be used for family health unit training and in the training done by the applied behavioral sciences program.

3. Each day, family health units would have an early morning meeting at which biological, psychological, family, and socioenvironmental case data would be presented and plans constructed and reviewed.

4. Each family health unit would have a mobile team that could make house calls. The mobile team would be staffed by a medically trained psychiatrist (who was also a family therapist), a social worker, a public health nurse, and one or more indigenous workers. Medical staff could accompany mobile team members when needed. Situations requiring only home medical care would be channeled to the home care program, leaving the mobile team free to work with family and socioenvironmental problems. The work carried out by the mobile teams would be brought to the entire family health unit staff in case review and planning sessions.

5. We would develop a corps of volunteers, one from each block in the area we served, who would serve as "listening posts." We would train them briefly on how to spot individuals and/or families in distress in their block and how to approach them sensitively and diplomatically with the suggestion that there was a place where help was available and that they should give us a call or a visit.

From my perspective, the final scene of Act One began when Howard connected me with three very bright and accomplished social workers who were already on the Gouverneur staff: Harold Light, Jerry Adelson, and Margaret Dennis. Harold, who I had met briefly during my first visit with Howard, was Howard's assistant director; Jerry was director of social services, and; Margaret, who was an Englishwoman with experience in the integrated British health care system and in a special medical program for welfare recipients in New York City, was charged with developing liaison with social service organizations in the Gouverneur district, especially the New York Department of Social Services.

I first met several times with Jerry and Margaret to mesh my design ideas with theirs. To my delight I found we were substantially in agreement. Both turned out (as did Harold Light) to be ecological thinkers.

We then brought our proposed design to Harold Light, who was writing the OEO grant, for inclusion therein.

The grant was written, and subsequently funded. Before the money was in hand, I had joined the Gouverneur staff full-time as director of applied behavioral sciences, charged with the task of implementing the program as designed.

ACT TWO: THE PROGRAM TAKES OFF

It will come as no surprise to the reader that the implementation of our plan did not proceed as smoothly as we had hoped. When the OEO grant was funded, it became immediately apparent that our design had been too ambitious. There was not nearly enough money to carry out all the plans we had made.

Furthermore, the need surfaced for a number of fairly expensive and necessary services which had not been fully planned for. It had been planned, for example, to run a 24-hour seven-day/week emergency room. Utilization of that service turned out to be much greater than had been anticipated, and thus more expensive.

There was not enough space to set up all the specialty services, which needed separate space; so to begin with, specialty clinics at Beth Israel Hospital had to be used. Transportation for users of the program to these specialty services was needed. Also, when a decision was made that people needed hospital care, again transportation was needed. An expensive 24-hour jitney service had to be established.

There was not enough space to house the medical components of the four family health units, much less a one-way mirror family therapy complex and an applied behavioral sciences staff for each. One family health unit became a satellite, moving into a building that had housed the Judson Health Center, an old established visiting nurse program in "Little Italy" on the Lower West Side portion of the district. There were still not enough partitioned spaces. Considerably more money had to be spent for renovation than had been planned.

The upshot of all of this was that in the beginning we were able to fully staff and equip only one family health unit, which we decided to make into a demonstration unit to test our original family health unit design. Hopefully, we could also show what could be done with a fully staffed unit in a manner that would attract additional funds. We wound up with a single one-way mirror room, one mobile team, and one behavioral sciences team of our original design attached to one family health unit. The dream, it seemed, would be considerably attenuated. But serendipity, it seemed, came to our rescue. A behavioral sciences program staff appeared from other directions to revive the dream.

Henry Street Settlement, a dynamic community service program only a few blocks from Gouverneur, had received a large grant from the Office of Economic Opportunity to establish a program known as Mobilization for Youth (MFY), Inc., which had become a sponsor of the grant received by Gouverneur. A proposal was submitted and funded by

OEO in which MFY, Inc. and Gouverneur would collaborate in the training of "indigenous" applicants for a category of job to be called "social health technician." Training costs and salaries for this group would be picked up by a category of OEO funding known as a "new health occupations grant."

Social workers for the family health units also appeared when an unusual field placement arrangement was worked out with the School of Social Work at Adelphi University. Social work students in training as "generic" social workers would be placed at Gouverneur during the entire two years of their matriculation for an MSW.

Public health nursing students from New York University also appeared to do their field placement at Gouverneur, although the length of their placement and their weekly time commitment were not sufficient to fully integrate them into the family health units.

Of course, I don't really believe these developments were at all serendipitous. They were, I think, the result of three conditions. One, of course, was the attitude then prevalent in the OEO, which awarded the grant with the expectation that something new would be tried. Strings on use of the grant money were minimal. Akin to this was the support of Dr. Cecil Sheps, then director of Beth Israel Hospital, who had been instrumental in development of the original Gouverneur program.

Another condition was the careful and thorough groundwork of community involvement that had been laid by Howard Brown, with the help of others, such as Harold Light and Jerry Adelson, in the early days of the program, which was expanded as a result of the OEO grant and other OEO-funded activities in the district. Relationships with a large variety of organizations and citizens' groups had been established, including Henry Street Settlement and Mobilization for Youth, Inc.

The third condition was the use of the ecological systems thought rules. I must explain what I mean at some length. Western (Cartesian-Newtonian) thinking contains a rule of dualism. Ultimately, all situations are thought of as either this or that. People are either sick or well, rich or poor. Governments must be either communist or capitalist, dictatorial or democratic. We are either at peace or at war. These dualisms are built into our language. We all know that they are simplistic and don't really conform to experience. We usually talk about "shades of grey" and "exceptions to the rule." But when push comes to shove, the either/or dualism emerges. When this happens we are forced to choose sides and engage in conflict. If the conflict is of the poker/bridge type and a lot is at stake, cold wars, and even hot wars, can ensue. Each side defends its own territory, at least, and if the fight heats, tries to eradicate or disempower the other. This rule creates societies that arc held together more by blame systems than by unifying human values.

Another rule of Western thinking is that space is a vacuum filled with things. It is no accident that Newtonian science spawned a technological explosion. Very complex things can be designed. Instruments and machines, in fact, have been designed which have greatly extended the senses, the mobility, the speed of thought, and the productivity of humankind. In this respect, the outcome of this rule of thought has been truly amazing. But it is a mechanistic rule and, as a result, has limited use in understanding life. We do ourselves a disservice when we think of living systems as things. A person is not a thing. When we try using Newtonian thought to design a person, we come up with a robot.

We know better than to treat people like robots. Doctors may discuss patients among themselves as if they were robots that need to be fixed, but when confronting the patient they usually don't behave this way. Usually, not always, they will transcend the mechanistic nature of the thought system.

A concomitant outcome of this rule also is that Western thinkers tend to see understanding of a phenomenon in the same way they seek understanding of a machine — by breaking it down into parts. When we do that, what we get is a list of parts, not understanding. We understand each part better because we know where it fits in the whole. We have contextualized the part. But we do not gain much useful understanding of the whole phenomenon we set out to understand until we put it in context and can see, from outside the phenomenon, how the parts articulate with each other and how the whole articulates with its environment.

Yet another rule of Western thinking is that things are naturally arranged in vertical hierarchies with each level of the hierarchy controlling the levels below. Once a hierarchy is formed, we tend to think of it as permanent. Although this view is changing, we still almost always set up organizations this way. The larger and more complex the organization, the more levels it contains and the more it demonstrates the outcomes of the Western thought system. The organization will not only engage in dualistic either/or poker/bridge games with other organizations, but such games will also show up internally. In order to gain more control (and the rewards of a "higher" hierarchical position), people within the organization will play "king on the hill." The people who get high on the hill are considered "successful." In an effort to keep these phenomena from getting out of hand, those at the top invent management rules designed to force the organizational machine to run smoothly. These rules robotize people, etc., etc., etc. That this happens is no longer news.

The ecological thought system of "new science" is profoundly different. There is no dualistic rule — no either/ors. Instead, based on a view that the universe is monistic, the rule is: Think both/and. This does not mean "everything goes." Elements that enter an ecosystem must join in supporting the viability of the system. If the new system element does not achieve a sufficient degree of supportive integration and synchrony with the ecosystem it has entered, it loses its own viability. It will change, leave, or die. Occasionally, a new element will result in profound change in the ecosystem. Viability of the ecosystem is maintained by this process of selection, not by protective wars at system boundaries. Everything is allowed in, but only those elements that "fit" and contribute stay.

There is also no rule that space is a vacuum filled with things. In fact, space is not thought of as separate from time. Instead, the rule is that spacetime contextualizes patterns of interaction. This does not mean that we cannot describe things, but that things are defined as clusters of events which take on substance and boundary as a result of density and patterned structure (event shapes).

Also, there is no rule that states that understanding is achieved by breaking a thing or phenomenon into its parts. Instead, the rule is that understanding is achieved by locating the thing or phenomenon in context. In other words, in order to understand a phenomenon, one must station oneself both inside and outside the phenomenon. An accompanying rule is that to contextualize the phenomenon in question, it must be viewed from at least two vantage points, preferably more.

What I am saying, in summary, is that built into the predominant thought system used in the Western world are rules of thought that preclude unification, and promote fragmentation, territorial chauvinism, duplication of effort, and confrontational conflict. When that conflict is of the poker/bridge type, there is no solution other than that in which one set of game players eradicates or disempowers the other. The ecological new science thought system, on the other hand, promotes growth and synthesis, which together create synergy. The rule that creates the new game of pokerbridge is built in.

What happened in the Gouverneur program, where the ecological thought system was used, I believe, illustrates my point. An amazing network of cooperating people formed in what seemed like an instant. Information began to flow within the network, which allowed for quick, often unusual, solutions to many problems. Poker/bridge conflicts, when they began to form, were abandoned. The network quickly included ecological thinkers from well outside the boundaries of the program, even lower Manhattan. I cannot begin to describe the burst of synergy that occurred, centered in our decrepit old building on the Lower East Side of New York, in the two and a half years following the receipt of the OEO grant. Creative people, it seemed, came out of the woodwork to join the effort.

Among these events were those mentioned above: the appearance of applied behavioral sciences staff, indigenous social health technicians via Mobilization for Youth, Inc. and the New Health Occupations Grant, social work students from Adelphi University, and public health nursing students from New York University. What seemed like serendipity was actually, I believe, the outcome of the thought system we were using, together with the atmosphere created by the general expectation of the enabling organizations that something different be tried. An open system was created that attracted creative people with creative ideas. Most of the usual organizational and hierarchial restrictions were, for a while, suspended. Instead of a mechanistic program tied to those restrictions, a growing aesthetic endeavor, tied to the varied pragmatic requirements of the multicultural population served, ensued. The program never became static. It evolved.

Some of this evolution just seemed to happen. For example, when Howard hired a podiatrist, the waiting room in the podiatry clinic became a hangout for elderly people who lived nearby. We moved in a coffee pot and a volunteer who was a retired group worker, and we had a group counseling program for the aged.

When one family health unit began providing medical care for residents of a nearby nursing home, attention was automatically paid to the socioenvironmental conditions within the home. The isolation and loneliness of the residents were exposed and a whole new program of social activities and family participation sprang up, which transformed the nursing home.

A program dealing with the total lives of handicapped persons grew out of a program that began simply to provide various appliances to them.

When the interrelationship of socioenvironmental and health components in the lives of welfare recipients was exposed in Margaret Dennis's liaison project, it became expedient for the welfare unit serving this group to move into the Gouverneur building. Space was found for this purpose. The welfare workers began to attend the family case review meetings, which resulted in case plans that integrated health and welfare issues.

Other programs evolved out of the emergence of problems for which there were no established answers. We had to seek out answers. For example, we quickly discovered that the family and sociocultural information we needed to identify ecological patterns was, in some cases, scattered in bits and pieces over a large network of people. To collect it we had to expend considerable time contacting all these sources, one at a time. So we developed a technique in which the entire network was convened at one place and time to share information and to construct a shared plan of action. In addition to the families and Gouverneur staff, an astounding variety of people came to these meetings — extended family, clergymen, welfare workers, teachers, employers, policemen, neighbors, friends, even neighborhood grocers and bartenders. I haven't named them all. Most of those who attended took on some task in the case plan. A case "chairman" was elected at these meetings, whose task was to see to it that the plan was carried out. We began to call such a meeting a "chairman of the case conference."

We also discovered that the data of the ecosystems perspective were found in the case story. As the program evolved, we began to see clusters of similar stories that exposed the need for policy and operational changes both in our own organization and in other organizations dealing with our clientele. For example, one cluster of stories concerned women who had come from Puerto Rico and had become isolated in tenement apartments as a result of their inability to cope with the complex New York City environment. Personality disorganization occurred in many of these women, and others developed physical symptoms. These phenomena could be frequently prevented by getting them a telephone; they would use the telephone to consult with other Puerto Rican women they had known back home who had also migrated to the city. Unfortunately, recipients of public assistance were not allowed the luxury of a private telephone. However, our data convinced the Department of Social Services to allow telephones for such women.

Using another example, we brought a cluster of stories to the New York City Housing Authority that demonstrated how relocation efforts carried out without attention to the social networks that existed in a relocation area created serious problems for those being relocated and the relocation workers assigned to the area. The Housing Authority began to relocate in a manner that would keep such networks intact.

In a third example, another cluster of stories showed us that a large number of children from chronically poor families who did not engage in planning got into serious trouble in school when they reached third grade. The stories were remarkably similar, as were the third-graders sent to us. They came bearing an amazing variety of diagnostic labels. When we explored this observation, we discovered that the diagnostic label each child had acquired depended on the discipline of the professional who had made the diagnosis. Psychiatrists diagnosed them as "behavior disorders"; psychologists who did IQ tests applied the diagnosis of "borderline retardation"; and pediatricians applied the diagnoses of "hyperactive," "dyslexia," or "minimal brain dysfunction."

We hypothesized that there was a mismatch between the cognitive skills of these children and the requirements of the third-grade curriculum. We hired a psychologist who was trained in the theories of cognitive development of Jean Piaget, and who proceeded to test all children who came to our program between the ages of 6 and 12. We discovered that the children in question developed the cognitive tools they needed to deal with the third-grade curriculum at about the age of 10, at least two years after they needed them. We brought these findings to the principal and teachers of one of the elementary schools who struggled with these children, and established a cooperative project using specially designed exercises and teaching machines to speed up cognitive development. Instead of procedures that saddled these children with labels that affected their lives in negative ways, a process ensued that recognized the mismatch. The project worked well.

For me, perhaps the most important observation as the program evolved was that, as I had hoped, the ecological view of reality we had adopted quickly pointed out how frequently symptoms that were reported in the physician's office were actually a facet of a larger set of life conditions that remained invisible to the physician. There were two cogent reasons for this. One was that the busy physician simply could not afford the time to seek out these sometimes complex stories, even when he had been taught how to do so. Even more important, however, was that the people themselves did not see the connections between the events that made up the story of which the symptom was a part. Lynn Hoffman, who was hired as the writer to chronicle the program, and who turned out to be a major contributor to other facets of the program as well, put it this way: "The doctor was often in the position of a man trying to get the lights back on by replacing a fuse, when it was the whole power grid which had broken down."

Hundreds of stories illustrating this point unfolded when applied behavioral sciences staff, working with the medical staff, sought them out. Space allows me to present only two.

One story concerned a 32-year-old Puerto Rican woman with three very young children, abandoned by her husband, and on welfare. The woman (Juanita, I shall call her) was being treated unsuccessfully by an internist in her family health unit for hypertension. Her blood pressure readings were averaging about 185/100. Diuretics had no effect, and the drug of choice at that time, reserpine, produced a slight drop that proved temporary. Kidney function tests were normal, and there was no evidence of pheochromocytoma.

Juanita's story unfolded when she appeared one day in the internist's office and presented him with a dirty paper bag containing a dead rat, chattering as she did so in Spanish, which he could not understand. The internist, recoiling, told her with some force to get the dead rat out of his office. She then marched down the hall to the office of the pediatrician who took care of her children, where the scene was repeated. The pediatrician, however, called in the family health unit's social worker who, in turn, enlisted the help of a Spanish-speaking aide.

It turned out that Juanita had brought in the rat to illustrate her contention that she was living in a tenement apartment that had been invaded by rats. Sometimes, she said, there were as many as 20 rats there. She had not slept much for weeks, she said, because she was afraid the rats would attack her children. Instead, she dozed sitting in a chair with a broom in her hands. Before coming to the doctor, she had taken her dead rat to the guidance counselor at her children's school. The guidance counselor spoke Spanish and understood Juanita's story, but told her that there was nothing she could do. She had suggested that Juanita take her story to the New York City Housing Authority. For reasons later understood, she had chosen to go to her doctor instead.

The family health unit social worker then enlisted the mobile team that made house-calls. One of the team accompanied Juanita to her home after she had collected her children from the health center's baby-sitting nursery. The woman's story checked out. The worker helped her chase several rats back into their holes. The rest of the story then became apparent.

Juanita was living in the last occupied apartment in a block that was being torn down to make way for a crosstown expressway (which, incidentally, was never built). In their effort to relocate her, the NYC Housing Authority had offered her an apartment in Brooklyn. The woman, however, did not want to move to Brooklyn for two reasons. One was that she wanted to keep her child in the school he was attending, where he had a Spanish-speaking teacher. The other was that her only close friend, a woman with whom she had grown up in her village in Puerto Rico, lived nearby with her four children. The two women provided support for each other, an arrangement which would be lost if she moved to Brooklyn. In fact, she would not even be able to call to her friend since the Department of Social Services (DSS) did not allow recipients of public assistance the luxury of a telephone. (The policy change described above had not yet taken place.) She could not move in with her friend, who had a tiny apartment, so she had been looking for a nearby apartment on her own without success. She had refused the Brooklyn apartment much to the annoyance of the relocation worker.

The mobile team worker called the relocation worker from a street telephone. The relocation worker was indeed annoyed. She felt she had done Juanita a great favor by finding her a much nicer apartment in a safer neighborhood. Such an apartment, she said, was a rarity within the

DSS rental allowance. She also said Juanita had gotten her in trouble with her supervisor. Juanita's continued presence in the rat-infested apartment was holding up demolition.

The mobile team worker arranged a temporary shelter for Juanita in the parish house of a local church, and consulted the cop on the beat that included the building in which Juanita's friend lived. The police officer showed her two apartments where no one was living. Both, on further exploration, turned out to be for rent. Two days later, Juanita moved into one of them. When she next visited her doctor, her blood pressure was 128/82. It remained within normal limits, at least for the next two years.

Some family stories were signaled by distress in several family members.

At a morning case review conference, it was noted that three members of a family were in trouble. The family was a three-generation Italian family who lived together over the Italian bakery that supported them.

Giovanni, 58, and Donna, 57, had emigrated from Italy to New York in 1936, with their two-year-old son, Mario, now 31. Six years later, their daughter Anna, now 25, was born. Both children had grown up and married children of other Italian immigrants. Mario had been married for two years to Marisa, now 26. They had a five-month-old daughter. Anna had been married for less than a year to Joseph, age 24. They had no children.

The bakery Giovanni had started had supported the family reasonably well over the years. But three people had been added to the menage, and Giovanni found his savings dwindling. He voiced his resulting anxiety daily to his family, and family concern over money had been rising.

The three members of the family who were having trouble visible to the medical staff were Giovanni, Mario, and Marisa. The first problem appeared when Marisa consulted her obstetrician to get his opinion about whether another immediate pregnancy would harm her. She said she was under much pressure from her family to have another child straightaway. The obstetrician told her it was too soon after her recent pregnancy for her to get pregnant again. She had begun to cry and left his office.

Next, Mario had consulted his physician with a complaint of impotence of recent onset. Routine physical exam and blood chemistry turned up no abnormalities. The internist had made an appointment for Mario to see the unit's psychiatrist. This meeting had not yet taken place at the time of the case review.

The day after Mario's visit, Giovanni appeared in the same doctor's office with complaints of frequent heartburn and late afternoon and early morning epigastric pain. Fluoroscopy had revealed a duodenal ulcer and treatment had been prescribed. The internist also recorded that Giovanni seemed very depressed.

It was the juxtaposition of the visits of Mario and Giovanni to his office that had led their physician to place the family on the list for family case review. At the family case review meeting it was decided that applied behavioral sciences workers should convene the family in their home and attempt to get the rest of the story.

At the subsequent family session, the story unfolded quickly. Shortly after the birth of his grandchild, Giovanni had offered Mario and Marisa $5000 if they would have another child immediately. This strange offer, plus Giovanni's refusal to share the reason for it, had thrown the family into turmoil. Anna and Joseph were furious, considering the offer a clear sign of favoritism. Donna was also furious and seriously worried about her husband's sanity. Mario and Marisa were at first bemused, but they, too, became angry. Marisa did not want to have another child right away. Neither did Mario, but he also had never before acted against his father's wishes. In short order, the whole family was angrily wanting Giovanni to divulge what his offer was all about. When he would not, the whole family had fallen into a state of depressed silence.

As this story unfolded in the family meeting, the visiting therapists zeroed in on Giovanni's secret. They, too, pressed him to reveal it. Giovanni, looking on the verge of tears, got up and left the room. One of the therapists followed. When he promised not to share the secret unless Giovanni agreed, Giovanni unloaded. Crying, he confessed that he considered himself a fool. An old obsession, he said, had led him to make the disrupting offer. He wished he had never made it, but now it was too late. He could never tell his family about his obsession, and they would never respect and love him again until he did. The therapist said he did not see how any obsession could be that bad, and pressed Giovanni to reveal it. Giovanni sobbed out the following story: Back in Italy, a few months after he and Donna were married, he had one day seen Donna talking to an old suitor on the street. He had felt a strong surge of jealousy and later had angrily told Donna that she must never talk to his former rival again. They had quarreled. Donna took the position that she would not be married to a man whose unfounded jealousy restricted her freedom. The argument simmered for several days and then flared up again. In anger, Donna packed her clothes and left. Giovanni was astonished. Such an action was nearly unheard of in Italy in their time.

They remained stubbornly apart for a week. It was Giovanni who gave in. He went to Donna and apologized. They had a tearful and passionate reunion.

Nine months to the day after their reunion, Mario was born. Mario, it turned out, had a light complexion, green eyes, and straight hair. He looked slightly like his mother, but he bore no resemblance to Giovanni, who had a dark complexion, brown eyes, and curly hair. For years, as Giovanni watched Mario grow, he had been obsessed by the thought that Mario might not be his child. Could it be that, during the week of their separation, Donna had seen her former suitor again and conceived the child? Gradually, however, over the years, he had put his obsession aside — until Mario had married, that is. As Mario and Marisa stood at the altar making their marriage vows, it occurred to Giovanni that they would have children. His obsession came rushing back. Perhaps they would have a son who would resemble him, and his doubts could be set aside forever. He had urged the newlywed couple to have children, assuring Mario that he would always have a place in the business.

Marisa, of course, had given birth to a daughter, not to a son. The child did not resemble Giovanni who was stuck, once again, with his obsession. One day, tortured by his thoughts, he had blurted out his offer, and the fat was in the fire.

Having finished his story, Giovanni fell silent, looking haggard and depressed. "There is nothing to be done," he said. The therapist later reported that, for a couple of minutes, he had shared Giovanni's despair. But then he had hit upon an idea, which he shared with Giovanni. What he said was this: "Why don't I share part of the truth with your family? What I could say to them is that they must understand that you are an Italian man from the old country who puts much emphasis on maintaining your family bloodline through sons. You wanted a son to be born to your son. I can say that you and I talked about that, and that you agreed that perhaps the younger members of the family did not feel he same as you, and that the way you had tried to make that happen was wrong. You could then agree with me, withdraw your offer, and apologize for letting your old country ideas cause so much upset.

Upon hearing this idea, Giovanni brightened, and agreed. The plan was carried out. After Giovanni and the therapist had each made their speech, there was silence. Then Donna broke into laughter. Mario began to grin and, mimicking a well-known spaghetti-sauce TV commercial, said to his mother, "Eh, Mama, that's Italian!" and the family began to chatter.

Before the session ended, the therapist led the members of the family into affirming their love for one another, making sure that Giovanni had ample opportunity to tell Donna what a good wife and mother she had been over the years.

During this session Giovanni's depression and his ulcer, Mario's impotence, and Marisa's conflict with her obstetrician were never explicitly mentioned. With relief from the contributing stress, Giovanni's depression and gastrointestinal symptoms disappeared immediately. Two weeks later, on fluoroscopy, no trace of his ulcer could be seen. Mario's potency returned on the night following the session. He canceled his appointment with the psychiatrist. Marisa, no longer under pressure to have another baby, decided to wait at least another year.

Review of the family record a year later revealed that there had been no recurrence of symptoms. The family narrative, however, was revealing. Mario had concluded, a few months following the above events, that the bakery simply could not support so many people. He had decided to strike out on his own. He, Marisa, and their daughter had moved to the Bronx, where with help from Giovanni he had opened another bakery. The family was doing well. This information created a minor crisis in the family health unit. Although Mario and his family were now living out of Gouverneur's district, they continued to come to the program for health care, thus breaking a rule. The staff of the family health unit decided to ignore the infraction.

ACT THREE: THE PREDOMINANT "REAL WORLD" MOVES IN

I wrote above that I walked away from my second meeting with Howard Brown in 1965 riding a high that was to last for three years. As I write, looking back, it becomes more and more clear that the events which ended my high were predictable. I am older and, I hope, wiser now, and I know that foreign body reactions are not restricted to physiology. They also occur in social, cultural, and even abstract ideational portions of the human ecosystem.

Remember, ecosystems are not concerned with dualisms such as who are the "good guys" or the "bad guys." They react to how a newcomer subsystem "fits," to how well it can establish congruence and synchrony with the larger environment that surrounds it.

A system that does not fit will experience much pressure to make changes so that it will fit. As in the poker/bridge analogy, the fit can be made by the invention of a new rule which licenses the newcomer system to remain as is. Unless it is extremely powerful, in the absence of such a rule, in order to survive, the newcomer system will have to change, and fit or move to a more cordial environment.

In the context of our society, which constructs reality using Newtonian thought rules, the Gouverneur program was clearly a "misfit." However, it gained support and was able to survive and grow because a new rule had surfaced in Washington in a climate of change. The new rule was, in 1965, part of Lyndon Johnson's "war on poverty," and stated, "Money will be provided for programs which find new ways to benefit poor people." It called for innovation. What was extraordinary at OEO was that, for awhile, the definition of innovation included real structural, or even epistemological, change. It was a both/and rule. It did, however, create a disturbance in the power hierarchies of our society in which either/or thinking predominates. It enhanced the power of the people at the bottom of the socioeconomic ladder. In either/or thinking, this upset the whole ladder. If it should happen that the bottom rungs disappear, there is, of course, no ladder. But as long as the new both/and rule was backed by the power of money and political and moral support, programs like ours at Gouverneur could flourish.

There was even a growing climate of acceptance for the form of our program. A glimmer of ecological consciousness was abroad in the country, created by the expansion of the field of human activity into space outside our planet.

By 1968, however, all this had changed. Catalyzed by the conflict over the war in Southeast Asia, the nation had polarized. Richard Nixon was on his way into the White House. The both/and rule had been withdrawn. Innovation meant, once again, old wine in new bottles. The polarized factions became involved in a massive, occasionally violent, argument over how to play the game of life in our country, a massive either/or poker/bridge type of confrontation. Ecological both/and thinkers often found themselves attacked from both sides. This is what happened at Gouverneur.

Prior to the receipt of the OEO Grant and in the years following, demands on the Gouverneur program had come from the organized health care advocacy groups in the community served. The policy was always to respond to the best of our ability, even when those demands were sometimes unreasonable. For example, at one point a strong demand was made that we get the junkies off the streets of the Lower East Side. We responded by saying that we didn't see any way to do that by ourselves, but that we would pull together a task force of people from agencies and the community who could address the problem. As the task force was formed, it became clear to those who had made the demand that the roots of the problem extended far beyond our health care arena. The demand, accordingly, changed. It became reasonable. We were no longer asked to "fix" the problem, only expected to participate with others in a search for a way to fix it.

The demands from the community, as we responded to each of them, became more and more reasonable and fewer and fewer. By the end of 1967, most of the messages coming to us from the community were laudatory. Complaints concerned minor issues such as the abrupt behavior of a staff member on a day in which he/she was in a bad mood. Our program now fit the needs of our community and, under the both/and rule, it was also accepted in general by our sponsoring agencies, if not entirely without protest.

In 1968 when the both/and rule changed back to either/or and the definition of innovation changed, it felt to us like an invasion — sudden, not gradual. Instead of spending our time directing and fine-tuning our program, we found ourselves attending meetings in a profusion that rapidly made it difficult to schedule them all. In virtually all of these meetings, some facet of our program was being questioned. Immanent in the questioning was a demand that we abandon whatever the facet was and go back to a standard practice that fit the traditional health care delivery structure.

Prior to this invasion we had always been able to handle the occasional question of this type. The question was always an either/or question, and we would give a both/and answer. When the invasion came, this no longer worked. An example that comes to mind is as follows:

The administration of our sponsoring hospital, in response to pressure from the hospital's department of orthopedics, raised the question, "Why do you need a podiatry clinic, when you also have an available orthopedic clinic?" As always, the question was an either/or question and, as such, quite legitimate. As usual, instead of responding with an either/or answer that would have required us to defend podiatry as opposed to orthopedics, we gave a both/and answer. We said: "The podiatry clinic serves a function for elderly people, most of whom have rather vaguely defined trouble with their aging feet that the orthopedic clinic does not have time to attend to. By attending to their feet, we have been able to collect elderly people in one site and to involve them in group discussions. In these discussions, they have formed mutual support networks, which overcame the conditions of social isolation under which many of them lived. This, in turn, cut down on the number of visits they made to physicians, many of which were made more to make human contact than to seek medical help. This answer satisfied the hospital administrators the first time around. In 1967, the issue would have been dropped. In 1968, it was not. Continued pressure from the hospital's department of orthopedics, where the doctors considered podiatrists to be less than professional, led to a series of meetings. These meetings culminated in an order to us from the hospital administration to close the podiatry clinic, because having both podiatry and orthopedic clinics was not "cost-effective"—this, despite the fact that it was OEO grant money that supported the podiatry clinic and that money was lost with this action.

And so it went. Little by little, we found ourselves forced to "fit" into the predominant thought system and its traditional structures. Here is another example, this one occurring at the interface of our program and the OEO. Late in 1968, one of the OEO consultants suggested to me over lunch, in a kind of conspirational way, that what we ought to do to preserve our "innovative" image, was to abandon our current program and set up our internists in storefronts around the district. I agreed with the idea, which we had long since discussed at planning meetings. However, I had missed his point. When I began to talk about how such a move would facilitate the work of the family health units, he broke in. In an almost condescending way, he made it clear that he had not meant that we would move family health units into storefronts; when he had said internists, that's what he had meant. He told me I was a naive idealist to think that there would be any way to continue to fund family health units, as the major source for ongoing fiscal support of the program would have to be medicaid. Medicaid would only pay doctors to treat diagnosed illnesses and no more. Moving the internists into a storefront, he said, would keep the program's image as "innovative." But anything more was too "radical" to be acceptable. When I countered by saying that I was talking about health care, not radical politics, he responded that the two arenas could not be separated.

Unfortunately, of course, he was right. Any idea or social structure which implied a change in rules of thought had been relegated to the realm of radical politics. The new rule was: Innovation will be acceptable as long as nothing significant is changed. Real change was now defined as political radicalism.

I have written above that the Gouverneur program, in its halcyon years, fit the world of its impoverished clientele. When, in order to survive, the structure and function of the program had to revert to a more traditional model, the fit was lost. Predictably, an answering crescendo of complaints and demands came at us from the community groups we had organized. It is slightly gratifying to report that we did not for long remain the target of these attacks. The leaders from the community had become sophisticated observers. They moved past us to attack our sponsoring agency. They realized that we were being forced to play our health delivery game by an old set of rules. They sought to wrest control of our program from the hospital, and the politics of confrontation took over. The final poker/bridge game had become a battle, and the battleground was our program. Like many of the confrontations of that time, the battle reached ugly proportions. At its peak, police were guarding the hospital administrative offices. It was clear from the start which combatant had most power.

In the vanguard of the community's "troops" were the indigenous workers we had trained as social health technicians. They had, after all, the most to lose. If their role in the Gouverneur program was lost, they had no place to go. In the traditional health care system, they were misfits.

ACT FOUR: AFTERTHOUGHTS

I believe the major lesson to be learned from these events is that there is a gap in the socioeconomic ladder in our country. There are rungs missing between the poor at the bottom and those in the middle and at the top. And, there is a qualitative difference between the segments below and above that gap.

This means that whenever people from the top segment design programs that are the same for both segments, such programs will not fit the bottom segment. The Gouverneur program was designed with only the bottom segment in mind, in cooperation with people from that segment. It did fit. And it can be replicated. Furthermore, though I cannot prove this contention, I am convinced that the widespread use of this model, which would provide free front-line health care for poor people via lump-sum grants to communities, would certainly require no greater expenditure of funds than is now being spent on the health of the economically poor. I strongly suspect it would result in considerable savings. It would also eliminate many of the problems that now beset the nation's Medicaid and Medicare programs. Here is why I believe this to be so:

1. The considerable cost of administering Medicaid and Medicare programs would disappear.
2. Separate funding for community mental health centers would be unnecessary in areas served by Gouverneur-type programs.
3. A large volume of unnecessary and expensive doctor visits would be prevented.
4. A large volume of expensive psychiatric admissions to hospitals would be prevented.
5. Medical personnel costs could be controlled since workers in Gouverneur-type programs are salaried employees.

6. There is, in this arrangement, no opportunity for misuse of funds, such as that which exists in Medicare and Medicaid systems.
7. Data can be collected on interrelationships between social conditions, psychological states, and biological symptoms that could suggest ways to use so-called "social services" funds in more appropriate and more cost-effective ways.

Of course, there are those who will object violently to this proposal. They will say it is fully socialized health care. It is, of course, though only for the economically poor. And my suggestions will never find acceptance in our society as long as dualistic either/or thinking predominates.

The either/or rule creates considerable irony in the predominant thinking of our land today. For the most part, we rail a way at doctors and rising health care costs, while at the same time resisting change and supporting the very system that creates the conditions we are railing away at. My hope is, of course, that this paper will demonstrate to some the pragmatic value of both/and thinking, and that a few more ecological both/and thinkers will be born.

The Gouverneur story ended for me in late 1969. Having myself become a "misfit" there, I left to seek out a more cordial environment in which to work. So, the party ended.

I believe, however, that the dream lives on. From time to time, I run into people with whom I shared the Gouverneur experience. Most of them are busy bringing the ideas we developed there to some other health or human services system, despite their perception that the climate for such a transformation is not now abroad. Even now, after more than a decade, there is a tie that binds us — a kind of network of nostalgia in which we wait. The trends in health care today seem to me to presage a day when a front-line system like that which flowered and died on the Lower East Side of New York can once again find support.

HMOs have sprung up across our country. Family medicine is growing and, more and more, family therapists are bringing ecosystemic ideas to the training of family practitioners. The idea of the primary health care practitioner is fully accepted; holistic medicine, despite its sometimes foolish assertions, nevertheless signals a broadening of the field of thought, which can move on to an ecological perspective. The winds of change are rising in health care. And, in the larger arena of our world, ecological consciousness is growing and accelerating. I think it is just possible that those of us who share nostalgia for the Gouverneur days will, before too many years, find a place where our work will make us high again.

AFTERTHOUGHTS, 1997

As I have already stated, I wrote the above retroview in 1982 and it was published the next year, 12 years after the Gouverneur program died. Fifteen more years have passed, and another retroview is now possible. Sadly, I must say that the hopes I expressed in that last paragraph of the above article have not really materialized. There is, however, good news and bad news.

The good news is that many of the ideas realized in the Gouverneur program have now become institutionalized. The notion of the HMO made up of teams is solidly in place. The primary care physician has become the central figure in the delivery of health care. A training sequence in family medicine is now an established element in medical training. And, with the recent growth of the collaborative care movement in the field of health care, there is some movement toward the dissolution of traditional hierarchies, and increased focus on family, psychosocial, and environmental factors in routine health care delivery in some programs.

The bad news is that health care has been taken over by profit-oriented corporations in the private sector who ultimately base decisions on the bottom line of the financial balance sheet. There has been almost no acceptance of ecological thinking. Managed care is the buzz-phrase of the day, and this means that the structure of health care programs has come to revolve around standard business methods. In this regard, the current thrust of health care reform is 180 degrees away from the thrust of the Gouverneur program. Whereas in the Gouverneur program the ecological paradigm provided the contextual thinking in planning, development, and practice, in the current managed care facilities the mechanistic reductionist paradigm determines what goes on. Ecological thinking is inclusionary and allows for reductionistic thinking when called for, making creative evolution possible. Mechanistic/reductionistic thinking, on the other hand, is exclusionary, ultimately labeling creative ecologically conceived ideas as irrational. I find this developmental direction unfortunate to say the least.

It is not the purpose of this chapter to do a critique that exposes the difference between the Gouverneur model of the HMO and the current managed care model. Such a critique is the topic of another chapter, at least. However, I cannot end without presenting the contrast between the two in some fashion. Thus, I have chosen to end this chapter with a table that outlines some of the differences. In the service of brevity, the table will have to speak for itself.

TABLE 3.1
Comparison of the Community-Based HMO
and the Corporate HMO

POLICY/FUNCTION	Community-based HMO, ecologically conceived	Corporate HMO, mechanistically, redutionistically conceived
PRIMARY FOCUS	Effective health care for all	Profit
ULTIMATE CONTROL OF DECISIONS	Community board	Corporate representative
DEFINITION OF HEALTH CARE	Human right	Product
RANGE OF CARE	Integrated biopsychoso-cial/environmental	Biological care plus limited ancillary care
PRIMARY DISCIPLINE	None/multidisciplinary team	Medicine
BIOLOGICAL HEALTH/ MENTAL HEALTH	Integrated	Separated
PRIMARY PATIENT	Family/individual in context	Individual
RANGE OF ACCESS	All community members	Insured only
MOBILITY/HOME VISITS	24-hour mobile team	Certified home care only
SOURCE OF REVENUE	Sliding scale and government supplement	Insurance premiums and government (Medicare, Medicaid, etc.)
FOCUS OF PRE-VENTION	Biopsychosocial/ environmental	Biological health only
RELATION TO OTHER HELPERS	Integration of help is goal	Separated — little contact
IATROGENESIS	Low incidence	Restrictions create high incidence

BIBLIOGRAPHY

The article that forms the core of this chapter was written without recourse to references. However, the following articles were also written during or about the Gouverneur experience. Some have been published; some have not.

Auerswald, E. (1996). Interdisciplinary versus ecological approach. *Family Process, 7*(2), 202-215.

Auerswald, E. (1969). Cognitive development and psychopathology in the urban environment. In P. S. Graubard (Ed.), *Children against school: Education of the delinquent, disturbed, disrupted* (pp. 181-201). Chicago: Follet.

Auerswald, E. (1971). Families, change, and the ecological perspective. *Family Process, 10*(3), 263-282.

Auerswald E. (1971). The non-care of the underprivileged: Some ecological observations. *International Psychiatric Clinics, 8*(2), 42-63.

Auerswald, E. (1974). Thinking about thinking about health and mental health. In S. Arieti (Ed.), *American handbook of psychiatry: Vol. 2* (pp. 316-338). New York: Basic.

Auerswald, E. (1968). *The Gouverneur applied behavioral sciences program.* Unpublished manuscript.

Auerswald, E., & Notkin, H. (1969, November). *Psychosocial services in a comprehensive health program — An ecological view.* Paper presented at the meeting of the American Public Health Association, Philadelphia.

DeMeuron, M., & Auerswald, E. (1969). Cognition and social adaptation. *American Journal of Orthopsychiatry, 39*(1), 56-67.

Dennis, M. (1966, May 28). *Family-centered medical care.* Paper presented at the annual meeting of Medical Social Consultants in Public Health Programs, Chicago.

Hoffman, L., & Long, L. (1969). A systems dilemma. *Family Process, 8*(2), 211-234.

Long, L. (1969). *The Gouverneur history.* Unpublished manuscript.

4

Integrated Primary Care in Rural Areas

Tillman Farley

Most of the chapters in this book describe the improvement that comes by having the mental health or behavioral health professional in the primary care site as opposed to located in another building or in an office across town. Tillman Farley reminds us that for 25% of the population in the United States, the mental health provider could be not just across town but across the county or across the state. In most primary care practices, mental health services are not possible for 30–50% of the patients with diagnosable mental disorders because of the stigma they perceive to be associated with a referral. They will not accept a referral for counseling or therapy. In rural communities, the stigma of referral is higher while access to mental health providers is lower.

In areas in which there has not been a sufficient concentration of patients to induce private mental health practitioners to locate there, it has been state-funded mental health and health bureaucracies which have had to see that some minimal level of service was provided. As Farley describes, because health services and mental health services are usually provided by entirely different state bureaucratic structures and funding streams, coordinating services between mental health and medical practitioners in rural areas has been particularly difficult.

It is in rural care that patients are most likely to bring every problem to one door. Therefore, it is in rural areas that integrated primary care is most necessary to meet the needs that patients present. It is necessary to concentrate services at the door that people in the area are most likely to use to find help with their problems and pain. Locating a mental health provider in a primary care office makes utilization much more likely and helps to ensure a patient flow that can make services in a rural area viable. Only when the mental health professional is located in the physician's office, can patients who are seeing mental health professionals have some level of confidentiality about what sort of service they are receiving.

In rural areas, providers are less protected by anonymity when they are off duty. Farley describes the way in which small communities require a physician to be all things to all people. In this situation, a mental health person who works as a team member in the same office can provide a much needed second point of view and a confidante for the physician, which can greatly enhance the work life and private life of both providers.

Dr. Farley gives a powerful and personal description of the way he went about setting up an integrated practice in a rural Texas town we call "Tount." He makes the case for the importance of integrated care in rural settings at the same time that he gives an honest account of the difficulties and challenges involved in setting up such a practice. Since one-fourth of the population in the United States lives in rural areas, it is an account that could prove important to the health care of a significant portion of the population.

THE UNITED STATES is becoming more and more urbanized, yet 25% of our population is still classified as rural (U.S. Department of Commerce, 1990). Access to health care, particularly mental health care, in rural areas is a major problem (Philbrick, Connelly, & Wofford, 1996; Shelton & Frank, 1995; Yuen, Gerdes, & Gonzales, 1996). Geographical isolation, lack of transportation, lack of local mental health providers, inadequate insurance coverage, poverty and increased stigmatization combine to present significant obstacles to proper mental health care in rural areas (Hargrove, Fox, Blank, & Eisenberg, 1995; Philbrick et al., 1996; Shelton & Frank; Yuen et al., 1996). Specialized mental health services in rural areas are more likely to be provided solely by county or state health departments and to be intermittent and episodic, without full-time staff onsite (Hargrove et al.; Shelton & Frank).

Unfortunately, the barriers to mental health care in rural areas have not come about because of a low prevalence of mental health problems. Although data on mental health problems in rural areas is sparse, several studies support the idea that urban and rural areas do not differ significantly with regard to incidence and prevalence of mental health problems (Kessler et al., 1994; Philbrick et al., 1996; Robins & Regier, 1991). Just as in urban areas, a high percentage of visits to rural health care providers have a significant psychosocial component (Human & Wasem, 1991; Philbrick et al.). Epidemiological Catchment Area (ECA) data indicates that as many as 22% of users of general medical services have a diagnosable mental disorder (Robins & Regier). An even higher percentage will have subthreshold conditions over the course of their lifetime, which are associated with impaired function and overutilization of the health care system (DeGruy, 1996; DeGruy, Dickinson, Dickinson, & Hobson, 1994). There are data to suggest that these numbers are generalizable to rural areas (Philbrick et al.). Because of the lack of mental health resources in rural areas, mental health care is either left to the primary care physician, or even more likely, not provided at all. Patients with mental health problems visit their doctor about twice as often as do those patients without mental health problems, placing further strain on rural health care systems which are already stressed to the breaking point (DeGruy, 1996; DeGruy et al., 1994; Fox, Merwin, & Blank, 1995). Integrated care — the close collaboration between colocated mental health providers and medical care providers — can eliminate most of the obstacles to proper mental health care in rural areas, relieve pressure on rural physicians, and provide for better outcomes in those patients with mental disorders and subthreshold conditions (Boydston, 1983).

DIFFERENCES BETWEEN RURAL AND URBAN COMMUNITIES

In order to understand the importance of integrated primary care in rural communities, one must first understand the unique aspects of rural communities. Rural and urban communities differ in terms of structure of the community, the doctor's relationship to the community, the doctor's relationship with his or her patients, resources available for patient care, and confidentiality (Coward, DeWeaver, Schmidt, & Jackson, 1983).

Community Structure

Many urban dwellers have an idealized and inaccurate picture of life in a rural community. Although rural communities differ in significant ways from urban ones, some commonly perceived differences are not supported by objective data. For example, the ideas that rural communities are more closely knit or provide more support and assistance to their inhabitants have generally been shown to be false (Blank, Fox, Hargrove, & Turner, 1995; Coward & Jackson, 1983). In fact, much more significant than whether a community is rural or urban, is the "psychological sense of community" (Blank et al.). Many rural communities tend to have a diluted psychological sense of community. The economic decline that has affected most rural communities over the past 20 years has led to a serious decline in the quality of rural life and a sense of loss of control of their lives among rural residents (Hill & Fraser, 1995). Because of high unemployment and lack of opportunity, there is an outmigration of young, educated people, leading to a decreasing population and tax base (Hill, 1988). Many rural communities are rapidly becoming bedroom communities of urban areas. This detracts from the sense of community, since these commuters generally define themselves as residents of the urban area rather than the rural area (Fox, Blank, Kane, & Hargrove, 1994). Finally, rural areas tend to have a high "dependency ratio," defined as the proportion of residents either under the age of 18 or over the age of 65 (Coward & Jackson). All these factors contribute to an increase in general community stress and its attendant psychological and behavioral difficulties among the residents of rural communities (Hill & Fraser).

The Doctor's Relationship to the Community

Because of the difficulty rural areas have recruiting doctors, and because of the sense of "esteem" that a rural community gets from having a doctor in residence, individual doctors are valued much more highly in rural areas than in urban areas. The more rural the town, the more its growth and prosperity are tied to having a doctor live and work there. Rural doctors are much more likely to live in the community in which they work, although they may be less likely to be a native of that community. They are much more likely to be known by many, perhaps most, of the people in their community. A rural doctor is more likely than his urban counterpart to involve himself in other aspects of community service, such as school board, county board, etc. Since the community plays a large role in determining the nature of the health care system, having a doctor integrated into the community influences community and individual health.

Although the rural doctor is a highly valued person in the community, the value is primarily in terms of what he or she can do for the community. Patient needs, no matter how trivial, always outweigh the doctor's needs, no matter how great. This is a lonely position and it can be very isolating. Small-town doctors, therefore, tend to be in the seemingly contradictory position of having tremendous power and influence over all parts of the community, but not over their own lives.

The Doctor's Relationship to Patients

Perhaps the greatest difference between urban and rural doctors is the prominence of boundary issues in relationship to patients. A rural doctor is more likely to know his or her patients outside of practice. Compared to urban doctors, rural doctors are much more likely to care for their family and close friends, and therefore more likely to know things about the patient that go beyond what is learned in the typical biomedical interview. This forces an integrative approach to medicine, even if one were not already disposed to it. Knowledge of complex psychosocial issues in individual patients and families is automatically incorporated into any diagnostic or treatment plan. The option of ignoring psychosocial issues, consciously or unconsciously, is not available. Unfortunately, rural doctors in general have inadequate options to deal with psychosocial issues, given the fact that in 1994 most rural counties had no qualified mental health professionals of any kind (Blank et al., 1995). Rural physicians must therefore incorporate a great deal of mental health care into their practices. However, because rural doctors tend to be busier than their urban counterparts, doing more housecalls, seeing more patients, and being on call more often, the responsibility for care of mental health problems adds markedly to the already difficult job. Many studies demonstrate that because of inadequate training and insufficient time, primary care physicians in general underdiagnose and undertreat mental health problems (Higgins, 1994; Main, Lutz, Barrett, Matthew, & Miller, 1993; Simon & von Korff, 1995).

Sara, a close friend of ours in the small town in west Texas in which we practiced, suffers from depression. In a larger town, we would have suggested another doctor for Sara, but here my wife, also a family physician, assumed her care herself. She began seeing Sara in counseling, and eventually started her on Prozac. Sara remained close friends with our family, and would often come over to visit. Clearly the formal counseling sessions were somehow different from the casual visits. Yet information gained in casual conversation is useful in therapy, and information gained in therapy promotes a bond that makes casual conversation easier, at least in this case. Several months after starting therapy, Sara

developed an acute life-threatening GI bleed of unknown etiology. Nota-
bly, Sara's mother had died during routine surgery at the age of 35,
Sara's age at the time of the bleed. My wife was acutely aware of this as
she struggled desperately to get Sara stable enough to airlift to the big
city hospital 120 miles away. Because of her intimate knowledge of Sara's
life, she was able to anticipate particular areas of concern as she guided
the family through the frightening experience. On the other hand, because of her close friendship with Sara, my wife did not have the benefit
of detached professional objectivity. She was exceedingly anxious during
this entire emergency. Had there been a bad outcome, her guilt would
have been far out of proportion to her culpability. This phenomenon has
been well described by David Hilfiker (1985) in his years as a rural family
doctor in northern Minnesota.

Available Resources

Doctors in rural areas are less likely to have easy access to the latest
technological advances, and so are more likely to rely on total information about a patient's life in arriving at diagnoses and treatment plans.
Rural patients are less likely to sue their doctors, so there is less defensive
medicine. When I was in practice in upstate New York, with MR scan-
ners ubiquitous, I sent lots of patients for MR scans. In rural Texas,
where patients were less likely to have the money for the test or the
inclination to drive 240 miles to have it done, I found that I ordered very
few of these expensive scans.

Since there are fewer doctors in rural areas, patients are less likely to
"doctor shop." The doctor, therefore, is more likely to be stuck with
"difficult" patients for a longer period of time and with less chance to
continually pass the patient on to specialist consultants. Difficult patients have a much higher incidence of mental distress as a component of
their visits (DeGruy, 1996; DeGruy et al., 1994). If the doctor is able to
employ an integrated approach, working in concert with a mental health
professional onsite, he or she has the chance to develop a truly therapeutic relationship with the most difficult patients.

Confidentiality

An interesting and important fact of life in rural communities is the
relative lack of confidentiality. Residents of rural areas are likely to be
secretive regarding sensitive personal issues, knowing that if they talk to
someone about a problem today, the whole town is likely to be talking
about it tomorrow. Jim Burden, narrator of Willa Cather's *My Antonia*,

describes rural living as a "guarded form of existence" and likens it to "living under a tyranny." "People's speech, their voices, their very glances [become] furtive and repressed. Every individual taste, every natural appetite [is] bridled by caution" (Cather, 1918, p. 219). Because everyone knows everyone else, the secretiveness is usually only partially successful, which leads to an extensive, powerful, but largely inaccurate rumor mill. Concern about this rumor mill can lead to a style of indirect communication with which the doctor may not be familiar. In the words of Cather's Jim Burden, rural life is "made up of evasions and negations . . . devices to propitiate the tongue of gossip." It is particularly important to pay attention to subtle comments and references, which may in fact be highly significant.

A locally prominent businessman presented to my office with new onset atrial fibrillation, which shortly thereafter spontaneously converted to normal sinus rhythm. Within 90 minutes of presenting to my office, a good portion of the town had heard that something was wrong with his heart. Much like the childhood game "Telephone," the story of his predicament changed a bit with every retelling, until the version his wife finally heard was that he was on life support in the hospital and she needed to go over to decide whether to turn off the machines.

Efforts to set up practice in a rural area must take the above factors into account. Rural residents are likely to seek out their local physician for any required health service, be it for mental health problems or physical health problems. In rural areas, there is a greater likelihood that any problem not dealt with in the primary care provider's office will not be dealt with at all. Given the high stress of rural communities, the work load of rural physicians, the fact that patients don't have the option of choosing another doctor, and the tendency for patients with psychosocial problems to overutilize the health care system, an integrated care practice seems critically important.

SETTING UP INTEGRATED CARE IN RURAL AREAS

Community Preparation

The organization of health care in a community often reflects the perceived compartmentalization of problems by community health planners. Interestingly, most rural residents intuitively integrate mental health, social health, and physical health (Hill & Fraser, 1995). Unfortunately, health policy planners at various levels have forced an artificial separation of services onto most populations, both urban and rural. This artificial separation does not fit with either the experience or the intuition of rural residents, who tend to get all their care from a single primary care provider. The resulting conflict leads to underutilization, inappropriate utilization, and noncompliance (Hill & Fraser).

This conflict can be resolved by changing the way the larger system is organized. In rural communities it is especially important that change come from within the community rather than from an outsider. Outsiders can nudge the process along, but cannot be seen as taking control or making all the decisions unilaterally. Techniques of community-oriented primary care (COPC) are quite helpful in changing community health systems. As one tries to change a rural system, consensus building is critical. Hierarchical decision-making processes are destructive. Doctors that fight against community systems without support from the community itself are unlikely to last long in that community.

The formation of a patient advisory council may also be helpful in the struggle to reorganize a community health care system into a more integrated system. A community-based board that advises operations of the clinic helps people take charge of their own health care and of the total health care system of the community. A patient advisory council with a good understanding of integrated primary care would also be quite helpful in promoting the idea to the community at large.

Office Preparation

Integrated health care demands a systems-oriented, biopsychosocial approach (Engel, 1977). Office staff must be prepared for such an approach, sufficiently knowledgeable about mental health care and mental health providers to be able to answer questions and schedule clients appropriately. In rural areas, staff are unlikely to have had prior experience with specialized mental health care and mental health providers, and will need to be educated. When not at work, the staff will be interacting with the community. If the staff doesn't buy into the concept of integrated care, then neither will the community. Conversely, if the staff has a good understanding of integrated care, and talks about it, the marketing battle is mostly won.

There are several concrete tools that facilitate an integrated approach to patient care. These include family charting, the use of genograms, and waiting room and exam room setups that encourage patients to bring family members to visits. These tools develop the kind of information needed to identify potential psychosocial or mental health problems, help create systemic associations for the patient, and keep the discussion with the mental health provider from being a dysjunction for the patient.

Family charting encourages family visits by allowing easy access to family member charts when more than one family member is in the room. Each family member should have an individual file within a larger cover file. Family charting should in no way compromise the confidentiality of each individual file. Many physicians prefer "household" charting, whereby each cover file contains the individual chart of every person living in the household. These may or may not be family members.

Genograms are a visual picture of a person's history. They can be as simple as a two-generational nuclear family tree showing a medical history, or complex enough to show multiple relationships among many generations and branches of the family. Genograms provide an easy mechanism by which to move from "safe" medical history to more difficult and "dangerous" relationship information. Genograms often reflect the patient-physician relationship, since they grow and change over time as the patient gains trust in the doctor. One may choose not to use genograms, but if there is not some mechanism by which to easily capture and record the relationship information that a genogram contains, then one is not practicing in a sufficiently biopsychosocial, systemic way.

Waiting rooms and exam rooms need to be big enough and with sufficient seating that patients feel comfortable bringing a family member or other support person to the office with them. Many visits to the doctor are prompted by relational problems at home; often the identified patient and the true patient are two different people. Furthermore, having support people in the room helps correct the tremendous imbalance of power that is always present between the doctor and the patient. The physician and staff should not only tolerate, but actually encourage, family visits. This may entail enlarging the waiting area.

Patient Preparation

As noted earlier, rural patient populations are unlikely to have had much experience with mental health care and mental health providers. For the most part, rural patients with mental health problems seek help from friends, family, pastors, etc. (Fox et al., 1995). However, rural patients intuitively understand the link between mental health and physical health (Hill & Fraser, 1995). It will take little effort on the part of the primary care provider to educate patients as to the purpose of an integrated practice. A biopsychosocially oriented physician will already have gone a long way toward remerging the mind-body split through the use of genograms, family visits, brief counseling, etc. Adding a therapist to the office staff is then seen as a natural progression. The more difficult job is to convince rural residents with mental health problems that formal therapy can be helpful, and that the therapist, who is probably an outsider, can be trusted.

Phraseology is important when talking about mental health services to anyone, but perhaps particularly to rural patients, who are more likely to see mental health care as necessary only for "crazy" people. Use of nonjudgmental language is critical. When bringing up the idea of seeing a therapist, I generally use nonthreatening, affirming statements such as, "Some people find it useful to talk to someone when faced with problems as difficult as yours." If they are receptive, I then follow with a statement like, "We actually have a person in this office that I work with very closely who is quite skilled at helping people with problems similar to yours." I try to bring the idea of counseling up casually, and let the patient "discover" the idea as if it were his or hers rather than mine. I let the patient know that the therapist is someone I trust and whose services I think are quite valuable. I find it helpful to introduce the therapist to the patient at the visit in which I first discuss the possibility of therapy. When the therapist and I meet with people for the first time together, I introduce him as someone particularly skilled in listening and helping people with the stress caused by whatever problem they have. I find that people are much less distrustful of psychologists than they are of psychiatrists. I tend to use an inclusive comment like "Not many people need to see a psychiatrist, but we could all benefit from seeing a psychologist sometimes." I also try to informally "advertise" the presence of the therapist as much as possible, in order to demystify him or her. It is helpful to have the therapist participate in community functions, self-help groups, and school activities, as a means of getting him or her accepted by the community. Using these techniques, I find that people are quite accepting and that there is a very low no-show rate for therapy appointments.

Mrs. Jones, a 33-year-old woman who had recently moved to town from east Texas, brought her 8-year-old daughter to see me, who was complaining of cold symptoms. Mrs. Jones was very distraught by what seemed a minor illness. During construction of a basic genogram, the following story came out.

Mrs. Jones was a successful big-city realtor. She moved here with her fiancee to live and work on a remote ranch 14 miles out of town, which her fiancee, a successful Houston attorney, had just bought. Neither of them had any ranching experience. Her plan was to marry her fiancee if she liked the rural ranch life and to leave him and go back to Houston if she didn't. To complicate the situation, Mrs. Jones had been married until less than a year earlier when her husband, the father of her child, committed suicide.

She was quite guilt-ridden over her husband's death. She also felt badly that she had abandoned her career to move to a remote area in a different part of the state, where she would have no opportunities to work in her profession. She was concerned about her child's well-being, having lost her father and then moving into a strange new environment. Mrs. Jones and I talked about these issues briefly, before I mentioned that we had a therapist in the office who was quite skilled in helping adults and children deal with such difficult events. She agreed that this might be helpful, so I immediately brought the therapist in to meet her. The three of us met for another 10 minutes or so, and then Mrs. Jones made an appointment to follow up with the therapist. He met with her and her child three or four more times. Ultimately, she made the decision to move back to Houston and continue with her career.

TOUNT, TEXAS

Tount* is a small town in Texas that prior to 1993 illustrated quite well a medical service system with an institutionalization of the mind-body split. The town consists of 3,000 people, mostly quite poor, with a per capita income about half that of the rest of the state. There is no town of comparable or larger size for over 100 miles in any direction. In 1993, the various health care services in town, all under completely separate auspices, included:

- an elderly GP in private practice
- a small 25-bed district hospital
- a public health clinic, run by the Texas Department of Health (TDH)
- TDH Mental Health and Mental Retardation offices (MHMR), in a completely different building than the TDH Public Health Clinic, offering psychiatric services by a visiting doctor every three months
- a home health agency owned by Columbia/HCA

Splitting of services had always been the defining concept of health care here. Children were delivered by the GP, and received their acute care from him, but received their well child exams and immunizations

---

*Due to confidentiality concerns, the name of the town and all inhabitants referred to in this chapter have been changed.

from the TDH Public Health Clinic. Low income women got their acute care from the GP, but their health maintenance care from the TDH Public Health Clinic. The TDH medication payment program for low income patients did not pay for psychiatric medications. To get psychiatric medications, a patient would be referred to TDH Mental Health and Mental Retardation (MHMR). All MHMR clients, whether self-referred or referred by a doctor, whether experiencing acute psychosis or mild adjustment disorder, were required to see the psychiatrist who came from a city 120 miles away every few months, undergo a complete physical exam by that doctor, and have a full set of blood tests. None of this information, or any subsequent information about diagnosis or treatment, was generally relayed to the primary doctor.

This system did a better job of keeping people away from mental health care than it did getting them into it. The mind-body split was entrenched, with separate buildings, separate budgets, and separate doctors for those complaining of mental health problems. Even the psychiatrists "medicalized" mental health concerns by requiring physical exams and blood work when a client entered the system. The system worked fairly well for patients with major psychoses and chronic schizophrenia, but it did not work at all for the far more numerous people with lesser mental health problems. Few people with marital problems, adjustment disorder, or subthreshold conditions were willing to go through the machinations and humiliations required to navigate this system.

In the summer of 1993, the local hospital district opened a federally qualified rural health clinic. From its inception, the Tount Rural Health Clinic worked to put together an integrated system of health care. Much of the initial work was directed toward consolidating the health care in the community and introducing a clinic based on the biopsychosocial model. Indigent care, family planning, and well child care, all previously done by the state health department in a separate facility, were taken over by the Tount Rural Health Clinic. Household charting, family visits, and genograms were all used extensively from the first day the clinic opened. The two doctors running the clinic examined the psychosocial aspects of each visit, and even did some formal counseling. Neither of us was a trained family therapist, but we had gained enough exposure to this field that we felt somewhat competent to conduct therapy with selected patients. The patient-centered approach to medical care used by the Tount Rural Health Clinic was new to the community, which was used to a very old-style paternalistic model.

From the start, our efforts at the Tount Rural Health Clinic were hampered by the lack of qualified mental health care providers in the community. Like many rural communities, the county in which Tount resides is quite poor, with a high percentage of uninsured people. A self-employed therapist would have difficulty generating a sufficient income. Nor did the hospital district have sufficient funds to cover the therapist's salary. It seemed equally clear, however, that the entire community could benefit from the presence of a qualified therapist in the community.

Before we could recruit a therapist, we first had to obtain funding to pay his or her salary. We needed to identify a problem that would generate grant funding and the solution of which would benefit the community as a whole. We decided to concentrate on family violence, a widespread problem that affects every community. In conjunction with the school principals, the Tount Rural Health Clinic conducted a survey of all students in the junior and senior high schools, looking at the problem of family violence as reported by those students. The results were striking and supported our supposition that family violence was prevalent and underrecognized.

The next step was to get community support for a family violence intervention program. We took our findings to the county long-range planning committee meeting. Based on the findings of the school survey, the committee identified family violence as the number one health problem facing the community over the next five years. We then put together a task force to begin to examine the problem and come up with an intervention plan. There was tremendous support for this project among all sectors of the community, including the schools, law enforcement, city and county government, and the local judges. A community-wide plan was formulated, a major part of which was the recruitment and hiring of a family therapist. The community supported the project to the extent that each of the four taxing entities in this very poor community agreed to put up money to hire a therapist until other funding could be secured.

The search for funding then began in earnest. We decided to concentrate on federal grants, although other options would have included private donations from local businesses, state mental health money, and private foundation grants. We managed to secure a federal grant from the Office of Rural Health to fund the project for three years. Based on the money offered up front by the local taxing entities, therapist recruiting efforts had already begun. One month after the grant was secured, we had hired a community family therapist to work out of the Tount Rural Health Clinic.

Recruiting mental health providers into rural areas is difficult. There is generally not a pool of qualified applicants living within the community, so candidates must come from the outside. There are real and valid reasons that most health care providers do not want to live in rural areas. Rural areas have less "culture," fewer educated people, fewer activities and resources, fewer job opportunities, and higher poverty rates than do urban areas (Fox et al., 1994). Rural mental health providers often face professional isolation and limitations on reimbursement (Shelton & Frank, 1995). Clearly, a doctor in search of a mental health provider for his or her office is not going to change these problems. However, one can look for and emphasize the advantages of living in a rural area. For us, the most important selling point was the integrated, collaborative nature of the practice. Most mental health providers are not in an integrated environment, but many may find such a philosophy of care quite attractive.

In our advertising, we emphasized the remote, frontier nature of the community, and advertised for highly motivated, self-directed people interested in cutting edge work providing integrated care to a poor, cross-cultural clientele. We decided to expand our search to include family therapy and psychology interns for several reasons. We thought we would have a larger pool of applicants if the term of the job was for a defined, relatively short period. We also reasoned that an intern might be less encumbered by dogma about "the way it is supposed to be done," and more able to adapt to a relatively new paradigm. We interviewed several excellent candidates, and hired a mature, self-motivated psychology intern from out of state. We arranged for a psychologist from the nearest city to supervise this intern once a week and be available by phone the rest of the time.

Day-to-Day Operations of an Integrated Practice

Once a mental health provider is established in a physician's office, there are several important and ongoing steps to ensure success of the integrated system. The most important component to a successful integrated practice is adequate communication between mental health providers and physicians. To this end, the psychology intern that we hired was put into an office directly across the hall from our office. This allowed and encouraged constant communication among all of us. Formal meetings were planned weekly, during which time discussion of ongoing and upcoming cases took place. We also had far more numerous informal discussions, which were facilitated by the close physical colocation.

In order to work together, it is important that physicians and mental health providers each learn how the other functions. In particular, the mental health provider will have to adapt to a more chaotic office environment. Mental health providers work in a different world than do physicians. Mental health professionals have a limited number of clients who schedule in advance for 50-minute visits, during which interruptions are not tolerated. The typical primary care physician's world is one of barely organized chaos, as he or she tries to orchestrate the health care of 3,000+ patients in 15-minute visits, constantly interrupted by phone calls, nurse questions, acute unscheduled visits, hospital crises, etc. We found it useful for the psychologist to spend some time actually seeing patients with a physician. This served several purposes. Besides allowing the psychologist a glimpse into the work world of the physician, it was helpful to have an independent and objective observer watch the interaction between patient and physician. Particularly with difficult encounters, the psychologist was able to offer observations that helped get relationships "unstuck." The interview process was more informative in general when conducted by both a physician and a psychologist. Finally, seeing the physician and therapist working together demonstrated to the patient the high value the physician placed on the therapist.

Others have experimented with a model in which all patients are seen initially by a therapist/physician team (Dym & Berman, 1986). Although this model has significant merit, we found it difficult to accomplish in our rural setting, given the demands on both the physician's and the therapist's time. We used a modified version of this model, in which some patients were seen by the therapist first, some by the physician first, and some by the physician and therapist together. The decision as to which provider the patient saw first could be made by the patient, the receptionist (based on reason for visit), the therapist, or the physicians. The end result of the scheduling process was that some patients were seen primarily by the therapist, some by the physicians, and some by both. There were frequent formal and informal consultations back and forth between physician and therapist as each recognized the need for the other's services with particular patients.

Mrs. Lyons was a 62-year-old woman who had been seen by our clinic on numerous occasions for several medical problems, including ataxia of uncertain etiology. Her husband, a savage wife beater, died in 1982. Her son had been convicted of burglary and was serving time in jail in another town. Prior to the arrival of our therapist, and concomitant with the sentencing of her son, Mrs. Lyons developed acute psychotic depression, but adamantly refused hospitalization. Because she was so well-known to our practice, we decided to follow her ourselves, rather than transport her against her will to the nearest psychiatric facility—120 miles away. The physicians saw her seven days a week for two months, during which time she slowly improved. We relied heavily on a neighbor to help Mrs. Lyons around the house and to keep an eye on her.

After two months, Mrs. Lyons was well enough that we could space her visits out to once weekly. When our therapist arrived, we immediately involved him in Mrs. Lyons's care. Mrs. Lyons was seen by the physician/therapist team several times, after which the therapist began seeing her alone. Her medical issues were ongoing. However, instead of scheduling separate visits for her biomedical care, the therapist and physician continued to work in concert at each visit, although the physician did not stay in the room for the entire counseling session. At some point during the therapy sessions, sometimes at the beginning, sometimes in the middle, and sometimes at the end, the physician would come into the room. Because the physician was well-versed in Mrs. Lyons's mental health problems, he could keep track of the progress in that arena at each visit. Similarly, because the therapist was aware of the medical problems Mrs. Lyons faced, he was able to keep track of those and advise the doctor of new developments and concerns. Mrs. Lyons did very well under this arrangement. Her psychotic depression resolved with help from the antidepressants prescribed by the physician and the excellent counseling she received from the therapist. She regained her baseline level of functioning and avoided what would certainly have been a long and difficult psychiatric hospitalization.

In a rural practice, the issue of confidentiality must be continually stressed. I recommend an entirely different charting system for therapy notes, kept under lock and key by the therapist. These notes should be available to the physician and the therapist, but absolutely to no one else. In rural areas it is quite likely that the patients and staff know each other outside of work. Staff should not be filing the notes from therapy sessions, since the temptation to read them is too great. Moreover, if records are requested to be sent elsewhere, the therapy notes should not be sent unless specifically requested by the patient. These confidentiality safeguards should be described to patients who are considering entering into counseling. One must be continually aware of the small-town rumor mill and its effect on patients' willingness to divulge sensitive information.

One obstacle to a true collaborative relationship between a mental health provider and a physician is the initial inherent imbalance of power. The mental health provider has moved into the physician's office and has to adapt to that environment. Patients are initially much more distrustful of a mental health provider than they are of a doctor. A physician's work is seen as more important and more difficult than the work of a mental health provider. Many times, patients are referred to a mental health provider only after a doctor has determined that "nothing is wrong with you." The system values physicians more, as evidenced by the salary differentials between physicians and mental health providers. The success of an integrated practice depends to a large degree on one's success in correcting this imbalance of power. The physician must believe in the integral importance of the work of the mental health provider. The mental health provider must not be treated as ancillary staff. The value of the mental health provider must be accurately and successfully conveyed to the staff and to the community.

The most difficult logistical problem for mental health providers in rural areas is the issue of billing. Unless one has outside funding, the therapist will have to support him- or herself through billing. Rural areas have a high percentage of uninsured patients, without the funds to pay for mental health care. Many of those who do have insurance will not have mental health coverage. Any capitated or managed care plans in the area will likely have a mental health carve out, or not cover mental health at all. It may be difficult for a therapist to generate a living wage working in a rural area. This problem needs to be approached creatively. There may be grant money available for provision of mental health services in areas where none exist. Other organizations, such as the school or the hospital, may be willing to fund part of the therapist's salary. In the absence of grant money or other outside funding, the physician may decide that a colocated therapist is valuable enough that it is worth subsidizing the therapist's salary alone. Therapy interns are generally quite inexpensive, while experienced therapists are relatively expensive. In our case, the federal grant covered the entire salary for three years, during which time we would gather data on how much money the therapist could actually generate as well as data on cost-effectiveness which we could show to the community at large. I would propose that since the community at large benefits from the presence of a therapist, each taxing entity in the community should share in the expense of subsidizing the therapist. This may be a difficult proposal to sell to the community, however.

Miss Rooney heard about our therapist from other people in the town. She had recently been promoted to a new job, which required her to travel away from Tount quite frequently. Prior to the job change she had been quite active and influential in town and had been selected as Citizen of the Year one year earlier. Now she was quite distant from the town and her friends, and was feeling depressed. To complicate things, her best friend and roommate had started an affair with Miss Rooney's ex-boyfriend. Miss Rooney scheduled an appointment to see our therapist. He saw her for several visits, during which time it became clear that she might benefit from antidepressants. He discussed the case with me and then had me see her with him during the next session. I agreed with his assessment, and started Miss Rooney on Prozac. Our therapist continued to see her in counseling, and over the next few weeks she improved dramatically. The therapist ended up seeing Miss Rooney, her roommate, the ex-boyfriend, and the ex-boyfriend's daughter together in counseling to try to work out the family issues. All parties did well over the next six months. Miss Rooney's job continued to take her away from town more than she wanted, but she figured out ways to stay involved from a distance while she worked with her company to decrease the amount of time she was required to travel. She took the Prozac for six months and then stopped, with no further problems from depression.

Caveats and Cautions

It is worth paying attention to several potential trouble spots when setting up an integrated rural practice.

First, although expanding the recruitment search to include interns will allow for a greater number of applicants, and therefore a greater choice in selection, there will also be an increased supervision burden. I would suggest that the primary care physician choosing to work with an intern should have a great deal of comfort in working with mental health issues him- or herself. Supervision from a qualified mental health professional will need to be arranged, and time away from the practice for this supervision will need to be part of the intern's weekly schedule. Interns will tend to be younger than experienced therapists, and may need more prodding to start community work. It makes sense to have a specific plan in place detailing the intern's duties with the schools, courts, etc. The Tount Rural Health Clinic was fortunate to be able to hire an extremely self-motivated, mature, and enthusiastic intern who was specifically looking for such a collaborative practice. This may not be the general case.

Second, therapists and physicians have a different definition of confidentiality, which should be addressed immediately. Physicians tend to work in groups, where case consultation is the norm. Since doctors don't discuss cases with non-doctors, all information shared with other doctors is still confidential. Therapists, on the other hand, tend to work alone, and do not consult as often. From a therapist's point of view, release of any information, even to another doctor, is a breach of confidentiality. This conflict needs to be worked out in order for a true collaborative practice to unfold, with each member of the collaborative team having full access to all information.

Third, doctors document all patient encounters on paper, in the chart. Notes are written with the idea that another doctor (or a lawyer) might read them. Therapists do not expect another doctor to read their notes, and have much wider variability in quality of notes. Again, for ideal flow of information to all members of the collaborative team, agreements will need to be reached regarding written notes. I would suggest that the therapist notes be written with the idea that the collaborating doctor will indeed read them.

Fourth, the issue of billing needs to be looked at carefully, particularly if one hires an intern. Certain third party payors will not allow mental health visits. Medicare will only reimburse if the therapist has a Medicare number. When the doctor and the therapist see patients together, the visit can be billed by the doctor as an extended visit. For patients seen by the therapist alone, the billing strategy will need to be decided on a case-by-case basis.

Finally, data collection should be an integral part of the program. Sustaining a therapist in the community will probably not be budget neutral, for the reasons discussed above. In order to generate the degree of community support needed for the community to agree to subsidize the therapist's salary, data will need to be collected on a whole range of parameters, depending on which issues the community considers most important, and in which settings the therapist is working. For example, if the community feels that teenage vandalism is a major problem in the community, part of the therapist's time should be spent on this problem. If prospective data shows that collaborative interventions are successful in reducing the burden of teenage vandalism, the community may see this as a reason to keep the therapist in the community.

Expanding the System

In rural areas, an integrated health care system has the potential to affect the larger community system. This requires expanding the scope of integrated collaboration outside of the office and into the community. Getting the therapist out into the community is helpful for several reasons. Working with the school system or the legal system or providing community-wide classes on various psychosocial topics not only renders a needed service, but also helps get people into contact with the therapist who might not otherwise be so inclined. This is particularly helpful in rural areas where people are more likely to use the informal mental health system, consisting of friends, pastors, family, etc., than they are to seek out professional help (Fox et al., 1995). Because our therapist was part of a family violence intervention project, it was understood from the beginning that he would be involved with the school system and the legal system. He worked extensively with troubled kids from the school. Both the physician and the therapist met frequently with the high school principal and the life skills teacher to discuss health-related curricular issues (including such things as societal violence, teenage pregnancy, etc.) as well as specific children that might benefit from contact with the therapist/physician team. The project also called for the therapist to work with the legal system to set up a mandated counseling program for batterers. By expanding the role of the physician/therapist team to include working directly with the school and the legal system, the Tount Rural Health Clinic was able to have a much greater impact on the community as a whole.

Oscar was a 16-year-old high school freshman when he was arrested for vandalism. This was not his first problem with the law. Oscar was also chronically in trouble at school. He had numerous absences and had been held back several grade levels. Oscar was not considered an instigator of trouble, but he was always quick to go along with whatever mischief his friends had planned. Per school regulation, because of his arrest, Oscar was expelled from school. His mother appealed his expulsion to the school board. As part of the resolution, the school board mandated that Oscar start seeing the Tount Rural Health Clinic therapist. Over the course of the next several months, Oscar and the therapist met weekly. Oscar began attending class every day and worked hard on football training during the offseason so that he could rejoin the team the following year. Toward the end of the school year, a group of Oscar's friends vandalized the high school, causing $20,000 damage. Uncharacteristically, and as evidence of the success of the therapy sessions, Oscar had declined to join in this crime when entreated to by his friends.

SUMMARY

There are many models for integrated care (Blount & Bayona, 1994; Dym & Berman, 1986; Glenn, Atkins, & Singer, 1984; Seaburn, Lorenz, Gunn, Gawinski, & Mauksch, 1996; Mueller & Williams, 1985; Zimmerman & Wienckowski, 1991). The Tount Rural Health Clinic is one such model. Rural areas require a slightly different approach than do urban areas when putting together an integrated practice. Whatever the final shape of the rural integrated practice, however, certain elements seem necessary (Goldman, 1982). Colocation is important. The community as well as the office staff need to understand and accept the process. The physician/therapist team should not be confined to the office practice, but should expand their activities out into the community. Both the physician and the therapist need to understand and respect rural life and culture. Boundary issues and confidentiality concerns, more problematic in rural areas than urban ones, need to be addressed.

Integrated primary care should be the norm in rural areas. Rural residents have an intuitive understanding that mental health and physical health are inseparable (Hill & Fraser, 1995). The local doctor's office is the place where rural residents go for whatever ails them, be it a physical problem or a mental problem. Yet rural physicians tend not to have the training or the time to adequately deal with the volume of psychosocial problems that present to any general practice. Rural areas generally have a dearth of mental health providers (Blank et al., 1995) and rural residents are not likely to drive to a city to see a mental health provider. For this reason, mental health carve outs make particularly little sense in rural areas (DeGruy, 1996). Access to mental health care is a huge problem in rural America. Any attempted solution to this problem short of integrated practice will likely cause more barriers to mental health care for rural residents. As Frank DeGruy (1996) states so well in his recent treatise on mental health in the primary care setting, "Mental health care cannot be divorced from primary medical care, and all attempts to do so are doomed to failure" (p. 311).

REFERENCES

Blank, M. B., Fox, J. C., Hargrove, D. S., & Turner, J. T. (1995). Critical issues in reforming rural mental health service delivery. *Community Mental Health Journal, 31*(6), 511–524.

Blount, A., & Bayona, J. (1994). Toward a system of integrated primary care. *Family Systems Medicine, 12*(2), 171–182.

Boydston, J. C. (1983). Rural mental health: A partnership with physicians. *Practice Digest, 6*, 23–25.

Cather, W. (1918). *My Antonia*. Boston: Houghton-Mifflin.

Coward, R. T., DeWeaver, K. L., Schmidt, F. E., & Jackson, R. W. (1983). Distinctive features of rural environments: A frame of reference for mental health practice. *International Journal of Mental Health, 12*(1–2), 3–24.

Coward, R. T., & Jackson, R. W. (1983). Environmental stress: The rural family. In L. McCubbins, & C. R. Figley (Eds.), *Stress and the family, Vol. I: Coping with normative transitions* (pp. 188–200). New York: Brunner/Mazel.

DeGruy, F. (1996). Mental health care in the primary care setting. In M. Donaldson, K. Yordy, K. Lohr, & N. Vanselow (Eds.), *Primary care: America's health in a new era* (pp. 285–311). Washington, DC: National Academy.

DeGruy, F., Dickinson, L., Dickinson, P., & Hobson, F. (1994). *NOS: Subthreshold conditions in primary care*. Presented at the Eighth Annual NIMH International Research Conference on Mental Health Problems in the General Health Care Sector, McLean, VA.

Dym, B., & Berman, D. (1986). The primary health care team: Family physician and family therapist in joint practice. *Family Systems Medicine, 4*(1), 9–21.

Engel, G. (1977). The need for a new medical model: A challenge for biomedicine. *Science, 196*, 129–136.

Fox, J. C., Blank, M. B., Kane, C. F., & Hargrove, D. S. (1994). Balance theory as a model for coordinating delivery of rural mental health services. *Applied and Preventive Psychology, 3*(2), 121–129.

Fox, J. C., Merwin, E., & Blank, M. B. (1995). De facto mental health services in the rural south. *Journal of Health Care for the Poor and Underserved, 6*(4), 434–468.

Glenn, M. L., Atkins, L., & Singer, R. (1984) Integrating a family therapist into a family medical practice. *Family Systems Medicine, 2*, 137–145.

Goldman, H. H. (1982). Integrating health and mental health services: Historical obstacles and opportunities. *American Journal of Psychiatry, 139*, 616–620.

Hargrove, D. S., Fox, J. C., Blank, M. B., & Eisenberg, M. M. (1995). Introduction to special issue: Rural mental health theory and practice. *Community Mental Health Journal, 31*, 507–510.

Higgins, E. S. (1994). A review of unrecognized mental illness in primary care: Prevalence, natural history and efforts to change the course. *Archives of Family Medicine, 3*, 908–917.

Hilfiker, D. (1985). *Healing the wounds: A physician looks at his work.* New York: Pantheon.

Hill, C. E. (1988). *Community health systems in the rural American South: Linking people and policy.* Boulder, CO: Westview.

Hill, C. E., & Fraser, G. J. (1995). Local knowledge and rural mental health reform. *Community Mental Health Journal, 31*(6), 553–568.

Human, J., & Wasem, C. (1991). Rural mental health in America. *American Psychologist, 46*(3), 232–239.

Kessler, R. C., McGonagle, K. A., Zhao S., Nelson, C. B., Hughes, M., Eshleman, S., Wittchen, H. U., & Kendler, K. S. (1994). Lifetime and 12-month prevalence of DSM-IIIR psychiatric disorders in the United States: Results from the National Comorbidity Survey. *Archives of General Psychiatry, 51*(1), 8–19.

Main, D., Lutz, L., Barrett, J., Matthew, J., & Miller, R. (1993). The role of primary care clinician attitudes, beliefs, and training in the diagnosis and treatment of depression. *Archives of Family Medicine, 2*, 1061–1066.

Mueller, T. V., & Williams, D. M. (1985). The social worker in the family physician's office. In L. R. Jones, & R. R. Parlour (Eds.), *Psychiatric services for underserved rural population* (pp. 103–117). New York: Brunner/Mazel.

Philbrick, J. T., Connelly, J. E., & Wofford, A. B. (1996). The prevalence of mental disorders in rural office practice. *Journal of General Internal Medicine, 11*, 9–15.

Robins, L. N., & Regier, D. A. (1991). *Psychiatric disorders in America: The Epidemiologic Catchment Area study.* New York: Free.

Seaburn, D., Lorenz, A., Gunn, W., Gawinski, B., & Mauksch, L. (Eds.). (1996). *Models of collaboration: A practical guide for mental health professionals working with health care providers.* New York: Basic.

Shelton, D. A., & Frank, R. (1995). Rural mental health coverage under health care reform. *Community Mental Health Journal, 31*(6), 539–52.

Simon, G., & von Korff, M. (1995). Recognition, management, and outcomes of depression in primary care. *Archives of Family Medicine, 4*, 99–105.

U.S. Department of Commerce, Economics and Statistics Administration. (1990). *Census of Population.* Washington, DC: Government Printing Office.

Yuen, E. J., Gerdes, J. L., & Gonzales, J. J. (1996). Patterns of rural mental health care: An exploratory study. *General Hospital Psychiatry, 18*, 14–21.

Zimmerman, M. A., & Wienckowski, L. A. (1991, Winter). Revisiting health and mental health linkages: A policy whose time has come again. *Journal of Public Health Policy,* 510–523.

5

Developing a Behavioral Health System of Care Within an Integrated Delivery System: The Primary/Behavioral Health Care Connection

Robert E. Simpson, Jr.

Robert Simpson has been at the business of integrated primary care as a provider, trainer, and manager for over 15 years. In talking with him about his chapter as it was being written, I found that he took for granted patterns of interaction between providers that others of us thought we were articulating for the first time. His world presently is the world of corporate policy and health system organizational decisions that support integrated primary care and a behavioral health service system as a whole.

His perspective is unique in this volume both for his particular position within a large health system and for the type of health system that he represents. Unlike HealthPartners in Minneapolis and Group Health Cooperative in Seattle, Baystate Health Systems, of which Simpson is Vice President for Behavioral Health, is not an HMO. It is a regional, comprehensive health system serving patients with various public and private health plans. The behavioral health services system has matured in an environment in which there were multiple payors with no coordination of regulations and payment structures. It is significant that the incubator of integrated primary care in the early days in this system was a capitated contract for the largest payor in a small, well-defined geographic area.

In addition to his experience with integrated care, Simpson provides us with an important look at the development of a behavioral health system outside of primary care. He describes the acute inpatient services, "step down" or intensive outpatient services, and specialty outpatient mental health services which are still needed in a large health system, even when integrated primary care has been implemented.

The development of behavioral health services in this system parallels the development of medical services more generally in respect to the relationship of generalist and specialist services. The generalist in primary care handles a broad array of problems and presentations that formerly would have gone to the "general specialist" (e.g., dermatologist, urologist, obstetrician, cardiologist, or mental health practitioner). Specialist services are provided by increasingly subspecialized providers focusing on smaller populations of more complex problems. Each subspecialist serves a much larger number of potential patients or "covered lives" than did the general specialist because a smaller percentage of patients are referred for specialist care. Simpson's reorganization of the outpatient mental health clinic from a group of generalist specialists into more specialized teams to serve the cases that could not be treated in primary care is the behavioral health version of this ubiquitous pattern.

THIS CHAPTER DESCRIBES the history, key strategic initiatives, and decisions that lead to the development of an integrated continuum of behavioral health services within Baystate Health Systems, Inc. (BHS). The role of integrating behavioral health services within primary care practice sites is particiularly emphasized.

Baystate Health Systems is a large multihospital system managing a coordinated continuum of health care services, physicians, facilities, and education and research programs producing over $500 million in annual revenues. BHS includes Baystate Medical Center, a 700-bed tertiary care level I trauma center and major teaching hospital; Franklin Medical Center, a 164-bed rural community hospital with extensive community-based ambulatory programs; Mary Lane Hospital, an 80-bed rural hospital with strong community ties and programs (Table 5.1); the Pioneer Valley and Franklin County Visiting Nurse Associations; Baystate Affiliative Practice Organization; Health New England, a 70,000-member HMO, and a large number of other health-related organizations and services.

The vision of BHS is to become a regional, not-for-profit, integrated

TABLE 5.1
Hospitals within Baystate Health Systems, Inc.

	Baystate Medical Center	Franklin Medical Center	Mary Lane Hospital
SERVICES			
Central intake	Y	Y	Y
Emergency services	Y	Y	Y
MENTAL HEALTH			
Respite services	Community contract	Community contract	Community contract
Inpatient, adult	32 Beds	26 Beds	N
Inpatient, child	12 Beds	5 Adolescent beds	N
Partial hospital, adult	Y	Y	N
Partial hospital, child	Y	N	N
Neuropsych testing	Y	Y	Y
Medical behavioral input	N	Y	N
Outpatient, child/adult	Y	Y	Y
Behavioral medicine	Y	Y	Y
SUBSTANCE ABUSE			
Inpatient detoxification	Y	Y	N
Acute residential	Y	Y	N
Residential	Y	Y	N
Outpatient	Y	Y	Y

delivery system that is the acknowledged provider of the region's highest quality health care. To accomplish this vision, senior management at BHS has been reorganizing and investing in the development of major clinical service lines. In 1995 BHS's senior management consolidated the behavioral health programs within the system under the leadership of the vice president for behavioral health services and the chairman of the department of psychiatry. What follows is an account of the background and implementation strategies that have led to the successful development of the BHS behavioral health product line.

FIRST STEPS: THE INITIAL PRIMARY CARE INTERFACE

In 1979 I became one of the original owners of Comprehensive Health Systems, Inc. (CompHealth) in Salt Lake City, Utah, a practice management and physician placement company that owned medical clinics throughout the western United States and placed locum tenems physicians throughout the country. I knew from that experience that a significant portion of a physician's day was spent seeing patients who present with medical complaints that stem from psychological factors.

When I moved back to Massachusetts in 1987, I joined Deerfield Valley Internists, a physician private practice group consisting of specialists and primary care physicians, as the mental health clinician in the group practice. In my role as vice president of medical services for Comp-Health, I had previously hired and worked with one of the Deerfield Valley Internists physicians. He and I shared a belief in the positive benefits of mental health and primary care providers working closely together. With my CompHealth experience in mind, I provided consultation services for the physicians and brief psychotherapy treatment services for their patients. I grew increasingly convinced that this integration was good for physicians and patients alike. It reduced physician anxiety about the most appropriate course of treatment for their patients while also reducing patient anxiety about receiving mental health treatment, because patients could enter treatment in their doctor's office without having to accept a referral to the psychiatric clinic. Many patients agreed that they had stress in their lives or that they felt anxious or depressed, but they didn't think they were "crazy," something a referral to the psychiatric clinic connoted to them.

In 1988, I accepted an offer from the president of Franklin Medical Center in Greenfield, Massachusetts, to direct their behavioral health services and had the opportunity to begin the process of integrating behavioral and primary health care within a rural health care setting. At that time, Franklin Medical Center was already part of Baystate Health Systems, but its behavioral health services were run completely separately from those at the much larger Baystate Medical Center, located in Springfield, 35 miles to the south. A year earlier, Franklin Medical Center had entered into a capitated arrangement with Community Health Plan, a Northeast regional HMO with a local membership of 17,000 members, to deliver behavioral health ambulatory services. As the newly hired division executive of behavioral health services, I made the decision to integrate behavioral health clinicians into Community Health Plan medical practices as well as other community medical practices as a key strategy to deliver services within the capitated budget. Community

Health Plan is an independent practice model HMO that owns and operates its own staff model health centers while also contracting with independent private physicians. On behalf of Franklin Medical Center, I approached private physician groups and Community Health Plan administrators, explained our concept, and negotiated to lease available discrete space in primary care settings or to use physician office space that became available for reasons such as hospital rounds, days off, meeting time, etc. In all cases the lease costs were extremely reasonable, as the physician groups and Community Health Plan administrators recognized the mutual benefit to all concerned, that is, patients, administrators, behavioral health clinicians, and physicians.

We believed that controlling access and referral rates to behavioral health services is key to maintaining fiscal control over capitated budgets. Utilization must be well matched to appropriate and effective services. On the other hand, we knew that access to behavioral health treatment has been historically difficult, even in cases in which these services are clearly warranted. There are several reasons for this, including the lack of training for primary care providers (PCPs) to recognize mental health and substance abuse disorders, the stigma associated with these disorders, and the fact that the relationship between PCPs and behavioral health clinicians in general has not historically been strong, often due to the geographical distance often separating PCPs and behavioral health clinicians. Our review of the relevant literature at the time confirmed my previous experience and demonstrated that 15–45% of the visits to a PCP are for medical complaints that stem from psychological factors (Barrett, Barrett, Oxman, & Gerber, 1988). In fact, recent work by Kroenke and Manglestorf (1989) suggest that these percentages may be conservative.

We felt strongly that early identification of mental health and substance abuse disorders was key to controlling the higher downstream costs of untreated mental health and physical illness. Research has demonstrated that untreated mental health and substance abuse illnesses are up to four times more costly than treating the disease at an early stage (Borus & Olendzki, 1985). We also reasoned that if stigma played a role in keeping patients away from the mental health or substance abuse clinic, then providing access to behavioral health care at their doctor's office would reduce stigma and increase early access to care. This would decrease the potential for more lengthy treatments and more costly higher intensity levels of care. While we were not yet in a fully capitated all-inclusive budget for both medical and behavioral health illnesses, we also believed that resolving behavioral health disorders in the general medical setting would drive down the demand for medical care and promote a more efficient use of medical resources by both patients and family members.

We also believed that this integration would provide opportunities for cross training between PCPs and behavioral health clinicians and that practicing together would insure opportunities for providers to recognize what patients were already experiencing clinically: the joining of the mind and body in the course of their presenting complaints. Practicing together would also improve overall patient care. The patient who returned to their PCP for somatic complaints with no known underlying physical disease would be provided a bridge to appropriate care through the presence of the behavioral health clinician in the physician's office. We would provide the opportunity for the patient to improve his or her life while also making the PCP's professional life easier in the process.

In fact, referral rates from physicians increased dramatically. Previously, patients with behavioral health disorders complained that their PCP did not take enough time with them. Often, the nature of the behavioral health disorder was either undisclosed by the patient to the PCP, the patient was unsure of the relationship of his or her presenting medical symptoms to a potential underlying depressive or anxiety disorder, or the PCP was not sufficiently skilled in the diagnosis of behavioral health disorders. PCPs also felt that they did not have time to sufficiently open up the behavioral health issue in a brief medical visit. We made it easy for them to identify the issue and then walk the patient down the hall for a behavioral health consult with a "fellow clinician." Anecdotal reviews from patients and physicians revealed high satisfaction with this model of integrated care. Community Health Plan administrators were also pleased with the model. As customer satisfaction has been shown to be the primary determinant of future enrollment or disenrollment in a health plan, we believed that our model contributed to the strong Community Health Plan gain in local market share—triple its nearest competitor.

TRAINING FOR CLINICIANS

In 1988, behavioral health managed care was in its infancy in western Massachusetts, but the directions that the future would take were clear. We knew that we needed to provide training for all behavioral health clinicians in brief models of care. In addition, the move of some clinicians into primary medical practices created additional training needs for them and for their colleagues who continued to practice in the general outpatient mental health unit at the Franklin Medical Center. Both of these groups of clinicians consisted of psychologists and clinical social workers with similar training. "Medical practice behavioral health clinicians" were selected solely on the basis of their interest in working in a medical setting.

We needed to provide training for our medical practice behavioral health clinicians in brief consultation models of care in order to preserve their availability for the PCP referrals. If they filled their time with the same sort of therapy cases they were used to in the mental health clinic, they would be unavailable to the physicians and patients they were relocated to serve. If they kept a great deal of time open so that they would be available, their work would not be viable financially. They needed to learn to do extra brief interventions with patients on a consultative basis to physicians.

Recognizing that some patients require more than a brief consultation session followed by a brief treatment intervention, we created specialty teams back at the hospital behavioral health clinic to develop brief treatment modalities in various specialty areas, including eating disorders, substance abuse, children's therapy, psychopharmacology, geropsychiatry, group therapy, family therapy, and behavioral medicine. The teams also provided opportunities for team members to develop "best practices" approaches to specific problems and to teach these practices to members of other teams and to the medical practice behavioral health clinicians. The team structure proved to be a powerful way to develop new and stronger services while upgrading the generalist skills of a whole staff. Teams also became a strong support system for the members and had a significant positive impact on morale.

As part of the team structure, our medical practice clinicians created the "brief therapy team." These clinicians tended to be more cognitive-behaviorally trained, though that was not required for their selection to be medical practice clinicians. The team structure was particularly important to the medical practice behavioral health clinicians because it gave them a group of colleagues to meet with regularly for case discussions and to share ideas about working in primary care. The rigorous demands for brief responses in their settings helped to create ways of working that they could teach to the clinicians of the mental health clinic. These practices were very helpful as everyone learned to cope with the demands of managed care.

Additionally, we developed an extensive training program for all behavioral health clinicians on the treatment of patients with dual diagnoses (concomitant mental health and substance abuse problems). We incorporated into the training the exploration of mythologies carried by our mental health and substance abuse program staffs. These two worlds had been somewhat separate, with both staffs believing that the other was not adequately doing the job. Mental health staff tended to think that substance abuse staff focused too narrowly on substance issues and the substance abuse staff thought that the mental health staff overlooked or downplayed substance abuse problems. The training greatly increased the standing of substance abuse staff members in the eyes of behavioral health staff and vice versa. Mental health staff became much more attuned to uncovering and treating substance abuse problems. This training was particularly important for the medical practice behavioral health clinicians because substance abuse is so common and so undertreated in primary care.

Since 1988 in the Franklin Medical Center behavioral health system, a consistent statistic has been that the average number of visits per episode of behavioral health treatment in physician's offices has been 3.2 while in the clinic it has been 6.2. These numbers underscore the consultative focus of the physician office behavioral health practice.

In order to help staff stay motivated to go through all of the changes they were enduring, we provided financial and strategic information to them on a regular basis, stressing the importance of developing a continuum of most to least restrictive programs for patient care. We stressed our fundamental belief that the future of our services in a highly competitive and capitated health care environment lay in having a continuum of behavioral health services in place that could demonstrate the impact of medical cost offsets associated with the integration of behavioral health and medical care. We also took every advantage to formally educate senior BHS management of this opportunity.

DEVELOPMENT OF A MEDICAL-COST-OFFSET MINDSET

Our initial decision to place behavioral health clinicians in primary care practice sites was driven by a decision to provide better services to our local physicians and to provide easier access points for patients with behavioral health disorders. As we gained experience both with capitation and in working within primary care office settings, we began to focus our thoughts on the role of behavioral health services in reducing the total costs of medical care. Over several years we followed the literature and began to present the argument to senior management at BHS that simply reducing the costs in the delivery of behavioral health services would not be sufficient as BHS moved to total risk contracting. We argued that the costs related to untreated mental health and substance abuse disorders were significantly higher than direct treatment costs and that the effective treatment of behavioral health disorders would influence savings in the treatment of other medical disorders.

Additionally, we knew that employers were becoming increasingly sophisticated purchasers of behavioral health services and recognized that untreated mental health and substance abuse disorders adversely affected their work environments. Studies demonstrated that job productivity is 33% lower, workers' compensation costs are 3 times higher, off-job accidents are 4–6 times higher, and absenteeism is 2–3 times higher for employees who suffer from mental health and substance abuse disorders (American Hospital Association, 1993).

We argued that resolving addictive and mental disorders in the general medical setting would not only drive down the demand for medical care but also promote a more efficient use of medical resources by both patients and family members (Langenbucher, 1994a, 1994b). We also presented information to senior management regarding substance abuse and its relationship to medical illness, noting that more illnesses, deaths, and disabilities result from substance abuse (including tobacco) than other preventable disorders (American Hospital Association, 1993). Nationwide, one in four deaths is related to substance abuse (American Hospital Association). We emphasized that early case identification and aggressive intervention should exponentially improve clinical outcomes. To bring the point closer to home, a review of BHS hospital admissions revealed that up to 25% of all patients admitted had substance use and abuse as the underlying cause of their admission, mirroring national statistics (Fox, Merrill, & Chang, 1995). This same study revealed that there was no substance abuse documentation in 60% of the charts reviewed for medical conditions with a high correlation to substance abuse and that 95% of these patients were not referred for follow-up. These facts reinforced the need not only to bring more education to the medical staff regarding the identification of substance abuse, but also to develop greater substance abuse treatment resources than existed within BHS at the time.

In addition, we offered studies that suggested that mental and addictive disorders were underrecognized by primary care physicians (Jencks, 1985) in order to demonstrate that our integrated model of primary care made both clinical and economic sense. Fifer and colleagues (1994), for example, reported that up to a third of patients present in primary care with anxiety disorders that are often unrecognized and untreated. These same patients reported reduced levels of functioning within ranges that would be expected for patients with chronic physical diseases such as diabetes and congestive heart failure.

As Baystate Health Systems' senior management began large-scale development of BHS physician-owned practices, I felt that it was important to continually remind managers at all levels that research findings repeatedly show that patients with untreated anxiety and depression are more likely to present to their primary care provider with somatic complaints for which there is little or no underlying medical illness (Katon et al., 1990). In fact, individuals with panic disorder have the highest risk of presenting with multiple medically unexplained symptoms and of being high utilizers of medical ambulatory services, emergency, and inpatient services (Katon et al.). These patients present to their primary care physician with somatic complaints, including cardiac (tachycardia, chest pain), GI (epigastric pain, irritable bowel syndrome), or neurologic (headache, dizziness, or syncope) symptoms (Simon, Ormel, von Korff, & Barlow, 1995).

We also reviewed studies that looked at the health care costs associated with depressive and anxiety disorders in primary care. Simon et al. (1995) found that primary care patients with depressive or anxiety disorders at baseline had markedly higher baseline health care costs ($2,390) than patients with subthreshold disorders ($1,098) and those with no anxiety or depressive disorder ($1,397). Additionally, large cost differences persisted after adjustment for medical morbidity. These cost differences reflected higher utilization of general medical services rather that higher mental health treatment costs. Overall, we believed strongly that the literature supported our primary care/behavioral health partnership.

We trained our clinicians working in our primary care practices in the identification and treatment of substance abuse. We had developed strong competence in substance abuse treatment. We believed that we should give special attention to a review of the literature with regard to substance abuse in the primary care setting. Our review demonstrated that the following five major assumptions should guide the design of a cost-effective care program for the treatment of alcohol and drug abuse and dependence.

1. *Early case identification and aggressive intervention exponentially improves prognosis and outcome.* Individuals in early stages of abuse and dependence rarely present with stated alcohol and drug problems. Rather, they often present to their physician with symptoms of insomnia, anxiety, and depression in addition to evidence of impulsiveness, job problems, school problems, etc. It is an accepted fact that alcohol abuse leads to frequent use of medical services. And yet primary care providers become frustrated by patient noncompliance and are unprepared to facilitate steps to insure recovery from addictions. They typically are not trained to recognize mild to moderate alcohol-related problems in patients being treated for other primary diagnoses. PCPs need training in early identification of substance use and abuse.

Our medical director of substance abuse services at Franklin Medical Center is certified in internal medicine and is also board certified by the American Society for Addiction Medicine. He began our "A-Team Consultative Service," which offers attending physicians an alcohol and drug consultation initiated by a specially trained nurse for patients presenting on the medical floors with diagnoses closely associated with an underlying substance abuse problem. The A-Team has helped our PCPs recognize substance abuse problems in their office-based practices. The PCPs can follow up their suspicions with a referral to a behavioral health clinician assigned to their practice.

2. *Treatment works.* The guiding principle of any successful substance abuse treatment program is that even though alcohol and drug abuse and dependence is a progressive disorder marked by the deterioration of psychological, social, financial, occupational, and medical status, we also know that treatment works and that recovery is marked by substantial periods of improved functioning, occasional relapses, and remission. The reality of successful treatment is often at odds with biases concerning treatment outcome. We have consistently attempted to correct these biases in the hospital setting and it has been enormously beneficial for educating practitioners in the primary care practices so that we can test the reality of provider biases and demonstrate treatment successes.

3. *Reduced total health care costs can be achieved through the delivery of treatment services to alcohol and drug abusing and dependent patients and to their families.* Studies support the finding that substance abuse treatment reduces medical utilization, decreases patient morbidity, and significantly reduces the total dollars spent on medical costs (Hayami & Freeborn, 1981; Holder, 1987; Holder & Blose, 1987, 1992; Holder & Shachtman, 1987). High-quality treatment services for substance abuse stand up to cost-benefit analysis better than many other areas of medical care.

4. *Employers and employees want treatment services for alcohol and drug abuse covered in health care plans.* Workplace substance abuse treatment programs significantly lower medical expenses for employees who complete them (Worner, Chen, Ma, Xu, & McCarthy, 1993). Studies support the finding that treatment reduces workplace costs of doing business by reducing absenteeism and sick time and by increasing productivity.

5. *The literature on addictions treatment medical cost offsets suggests that resolving addictive disorders in the general medical setting will drive down the demand for health care, promote more efficient use of care by both patients and their families, and preserve scarce resources that can be deployed more wisely elsewhere.* The demand to reduce waste and trim health care expenditures challenges the historic gulf between general

medical practice and the management of addictive behavior. Addictions treatment is often viewed by policy makers as a costly and inefficient add-on to an already overburdened system. This view contradicts a large body of literature on addictions treatment cost-offsets, which shows that treatment for addictive disorders drives down the demand for health care and promotes more efficient use by both patients and their families (Longenbucher, 1994a, 1994b). A 14-year longitudinal study of the medical and treatment costs of alcoholics enrolled under an HMO health plan (3,068 alcoholics received treatment, 661 did not) revealed that the total medical costs of treated alcoholics were 24% lower than comparable costs for untreated alcoholics (Holder & Blose, 1992).

Our ongoing review of the literature on the relationship of mental and addictive disorders to the costs of overall medical treatment in a given population continued to suggest two key strategies. First, the integration of primary care and behavioral health care make financial and clinical sense and we should, therefore, continue the expansion of these services. Second, the impact of managed care in behavioral health services demands that we also expand our continuum of available treatment options in behavioral health services.

FURTHER DEVELOPMENT OF BHS BEHAVIORAL HEALTH SERVICES 1990–1996

Following up on the early movement of behavioral health into primary practice sites and recognizing that managed care was making significant inroads in the behavioral health care market, senior management at BHS engaged a consultant in 1990 who made the following recommendations:

1. BHS must develop a plan to become the provider of choice for mental health and substance abuse services by broadening its services through direct contracting with community behavioral health providers along with internal development of its own services.
2. BHS must move toward centralizing the management of its behavioral health services and develop a culture where pleasing the customer is as important as providing high-quality care. To accomplish this task, a continuum of outpatient-based treatment modalities must be developed.
3. BHS must also focus on providing cost-effective services with a vision toward entering and managing at-risk contracts.

In 1991, BHS's senior management commissioned the behavioral health committee to respond to the 1990 consultant's report and to recommend strategies to implement a BHS coordinated continuum of behavioral health services.

Findings of the Behavioral Health Committee

The committee recognized that purchasers of behavioral health services were extremely concerned about the rising costs of health care services in general. Total health care costs as a percent of the gross national product were 6% in 1965, 11% in 1990, and 12% in 1992. For employers the mental health and substance abuse portion of total plan costs grew from 8.2% in 1988 to 9.6% in 1989 and 11.4% in 1990, an overall percentage growth increase of 47% (American Hospital Association, 1993). In response to these unabated health care cost increases over the past decade, both the private and public sector were looking to managed care to provide solutions for cost containment and quality control. In addition to rapidly rising costs, purchasers identified several quality-related problems as they were considering available behavioral health services.

For example, the committee noted that purchasers believed that behavioral health services were purchased without indication of clinical effectiveness, making it difficult to identify good care and good providers. While the scientific literature has demonstrated that a variety of biopsychosocial interventions are effective, there have been few accepted guidelines to direct purchasers to appropriate treatments. It has also been true that indemnity plans have been designed with the assumption that individuals are knowledgeable about their choices of appropriate providers for care. Purchasers were reporting that this naiveté and lack of clarity has resulted in inefficient and inappropriate choice of services.

The committee also noted that purchasers believed that inpatient hospitalization, the most costly and restrictive treatment setting, has been overused. Traditional benefit plans have contained a financial incentive to use hospitalization rather than diversionary and ambulatory services. These plans were designed to protect those most in need of services and often discourages early intervention and effective case management. Traditional indemnity plans approach cost containment by limiting coverage in inpatient and outpatient care while excluding such intermediary services as respite, partial hospitalization, residential care, intensive day or evening treatment programs, and in-home family counseling.

The committee additionally reported that purchasers believed that the service delivery system has been extremely fragmented in behavioral health services. Not only has there been a lack of coordination between the hospital and ambulatory follow-up care, there has also been a general lack of coordination between medical and support services and between mental health and substance abuse services, decreasing the effectiveness of the treatments provided. It has also been true that case management, an approach that works to ensure the kind of effective coordination that matches the costs of care with the appropriate level and intensity of care, has been unavailable in traditional indemnity plans.

Public and Private Managed Care Initiatives in the Marketplace

The committee reported that the response of both public and private purchasers has been to restructure the manner in which they purchase services. The committee underscored that the present behavioral health care market is a payor-driven, outcome-oriented market that is designed to aggressively contain costs through the purchase of services that provide a step-down continuum of care approach that places the patient in the least restrictive clinically appropriate treatment setting. Both public and private purchasers are interested in pursuing risk-sharing contracts with providers who demonstrate the ability to focus on a long-term approach to cost management that emphasizes total cost rather than single components (e.g., inpatient hospital costs). The overall treatment approach is one that ensures a focus on brief, intermittent, solution-focused, targeted interventions. This payor-driven managed care market is highly focused on utilization review that ties clinical outcomes to the least-cost approach to care.

It is important to note that the application of managed care principles to mental health and substance abuse services paid for with public funds is a relatively new concept. The committee reported that they believed that this public trend toward managing behavioral health services would augment and accelerate the managed care trend in the private pay market. Individual private payers do not manage enough volume of patients to guarantee a diversionary program's success, but the sheer force of the volumes that the public sector (Medicaid, the Department of Mental Health, and the Department of Public Health) controls would allow managed care vendors in the public sector to encourage providers to set up diversionary programs that would also attract private pay business. The committee reported that local public and private purchasers expressed strong interest in contracting for diversionary programs that would be coordinated by a single provider.

In summarizing the behavioral health market forces, the committee noted that while contracting for public services can provide some volume guarantees, the level of reimbursements has traditionally been lower than those provided in the more dispersed private sector, which has historically paid at higher rates in the absence of significant volume guarantees. However, recent reimbursement trends demonstrate that managed care has pulled private reimbursement rates down. The committee felt strongly that BHS must be able to position itself to obtain both public and private volumes at reasonable rates.

This competitive trend in the managed care arena suggests that the small community providers would be moving quickly to create stronger affiliation networks. The larger hospital systems would be either downsizing or exploring opportunities for building diversionary programs of their own or through affiliation agreements in order to remain competitive.

Specific Recommendations of the Behavioral Health Committee in 1992

In 1992, the Behavioral Health Committee made several recommendations to senior management to ensure success in the payor-driven managed care market (Table 5.2).

1. Build linkages between hospital clinical programs and purchasers, including insurance companies, managed care entities, and the business community, by offering a behavioral health plan that would link primary care to the BHS employee assistance program and BHS behavioral health services.
2. Create diversionary programming emphasizing a step-down continuum of care within the BHS system to include respite care, partial hospitalization, intensive outpatient, detoxification and recovery programs, and case management services.
3. Focus on quality outcomes that would demonstrate both cost- and quality-effective care to purchasers of service.
4. Train staff in consumer-oriented strategies in the marketing and delivery of behavioral health services.
5. Develop a fully relational management information system that would coordinate financial and clinical outcome data to enable successful contracting, utilization management, and clinical programming.
6. Create training programs for staff in effective managed care treatment. These programs should educate staff in the values and policies of managed care which emphasize that there are finite, not infinite, resources, that treatment should be brief and solution-focused, and that aggressive utilization management will match patients to the least restrictive level of care.

TABLE 5.2
Recommendations of the Behavioral Health Committee

**BHS BEHAVIORAL HEALTH STRATEGIES FOR THE 1990S:
AN INTEGRATED SYSTEM OF CARE**

1. Create an integrated system to respond to payor-driven, outcome-oriented, consumer-oriented, consumer-sensitive, managed behavioral health care market.

2. Create a managed system designed to contain costs and assure standards for quality assurance that are outcome-based.

3. Accelerate the development of resource-sensitive, clinically-effective, step-down continuum-of-care models with a competitive pricing strategy.

4. Evaluate the role of horizontal and vertical business alignments, blurring distinctions between public, private, and nonprofit sectors.

5. Capture the market share and expand revenue by pursuing risk-sharing capitated contracts with insurers *and* employers.

6. Demonstrate the ability to focus on a long-term approach to cost management, emphasizing total costs rather than single components (e.g., inpatient hospital costs).

7. Demonstrate the ability to respond to demographically driven increases in high-risk, high-need populations — elderly, HIV, chemical addition.

8. Stress a consultative participatory leadership and management style with a multidisciplinary team approach to program management and development.

9. Stress leadership that expresses a consistent demonstration of commitment to a proactive change strategy necessary to survive in an increasingly competitive managed market.

10. Educate staff that survival is predicated on programs that are margin-driven where profits are achieved through capturing market share and control of costs.

**MANAGEMENT INFORMATION SYSTEMS
AND UTILIZATION REVIEW**

1. Develop a management information system that addresses efficiencies and effectiveness of services.

2. Insure an overall treatment focus on brief, intermittent, solution-focused targeted interventions.

TABLE 5.2
Continued

3. Redefine internal utilization review to focus on clinical outcomes and pro-
    ductivity management through improved assessments tied to efficient case
    management.

4. Refine utilization review system to assure that treatment criteria match pa-
    tients by medical necessity to treatment in the least restrictive setting.

CUSTOMER SATISFACTION FOCUS

1. Create regional and managed systems that are insurer, employer, and pa-
    tient-customer "user-friendly."

2. Demonstrate to consumer and payor the ability to focus on value, effec-
    tiveness, and efficiency.

3. Create integrated satellite and centralized intake system designed to assure
    both clinical access to appropriate program or service in the system *and*
    contract managment.

4. Develop consumer orientation among staff throughout system and assure
    a focus on consumer satisfaction.

The Results: BHS Behavioral Health Services, 1992–1996

The implementation of the behavioral health committee recommendations has been enormously successful. Ambulatory visits at BHS (including traditional outpatient mental health, substance abuse, behavioral
medicine, and partial hospitalization for adults and children, and intensive outpatient and emergency service intervention) grew from 36,000 in
1990 to 111,000 in 1996. Inpatient mental health and substance abuse
volumes remained stable at approximately 26,000 inpatient days, which
represented a significant increase in market share given that average
lengths of stay in that same period dropped by 40% and diversions to
step-down, less intensive levels of care also increased dramatically.

By developing a "one stop shopping" broad continuum of ambulatory
behavioral health services, BHS was able to capture additional market
share, increase physician satisfaction with our services, and thereby increase physician referrals. Our belief that many patients initially find
their way to mental health and substance services through contact with
their primary care physician was supported by our substantial market

share gain. Contracting opportunities with managed care organizations naturally increased as we were able to demonstrate a "one stop shopping" opportunity by offering a full continuum of services. Several key initiatives added to our success, including the creation of central intake (described below), the development of a fully relational data base, expansion of substance abuse recovery services, the building of alliances with community behavioral health organizations for the provision of emergency and respite services, and the development of a continuum of geropsychiatric services. In 1997 we significantly expanded our substance abuse services capability in our flagship hospital, Baystate Medical Center, by acquiring Alcohol and Drug Services of Western Massachusetts (ADS). ADS is the largest provider of substance abuse services in western Massachusetts, providing 60,000 units of inpatient, outpatient, and residential services.

Creation of Central Intake

A series of planning task forces led to the creation of central intake and the reorganization of secretarial support services at each hospital campus by organizing the work flow within behavioral health cost centers. The central intake system services approximately 1800 new referrals per month. Services include initial screening, insurance verification, prior authorization, triage, appointment scheduling, and preregistration. Physician office practices are high utilizers of central intake services.

Development of a Relational Data Base

We developed a fully relational data base that allows us to track behavioral health patient care across all of our facilities from intake to discharge, provide prior authorization and concurrent review (utilization management) functions, capture billing and cost per episode per case per insurer information, and provide management tools to account for clinician productivity and other management reports, including no-show rates by diagnoses and insurer, preregistration successes, etc. We could not function adequately nor compete effectively in a managed care market without this capability. The hospital management information system did not offer sufficient rigor to capture essential information to manage successfully in our highly competitive managed care environment. We built our data base using Microsoft Access software and integrated it into the hospital financial accounting software. Our data base also tracks physician referrals from PCPs and specialists allowing us to be aware of changes in physician referral rates.

Recently we entered into a full-risk behavioral health capitation for a local 25,000-member HMO. Our data base provides a significant piece of the necessary infrastructure to do effective utilization management and case management. We run daily reports targeting potential patient high utilization of multiple services and have developed a utilization and case management system to manage their care. An important component of this utilization and case management function is to ensure that the behavioral health and primary medical care are coordinated. Our data base and clinician placement in primary care offices provides a set of unique tools to ensure integrated care across both behavioral health and primary care medical services.

Integration of EAP and Behavioral Health Services

In 1992, we consolidated the employee assistance program (EAP) at the BHS corporate level and expanded our internal and external EAP services. When the BHS human relations department recognized in 1995 that the behavioral health component costs of its self-insured employee health insurance (administered by an outside contractor) was growing disproportionately to its other plan costs, they turned to behavioral health's senior management for a proposal to manage this care. In 1995, BHS spent approximately $1 million or $11 per member/per month for behavioral health treatment services to approximately 7,000 covered lives. We recommended consolidating the utilization management functions through EAP. We established a preferred network of facilities, diversionary programs, and providers, negotiated preferred rates, and included all BHS behavioral health program components. Instrumental to our program was the use of deductibles to encourage the network utilization of BHS behavioral health outpatient clinicians coupled with the placement of these clinicians in BHS primary care medical practices, allowing employees confidential access to behavioral health care in their physician's office.

In the first year of operation, we reduced the total BHS dollar spent on behavioral treatment costs by $442,000, spending $6 per member per month, a reduction of $5 per member per month. This program has been a major success from a clinical, financial, and operational perspective.

Integration with Community Behavioral Health Organizations

A key part of our development strategy was to look for opportunities to develop diversionary programs through collaboration with community behavioral health organizations. At Franklin Medical Center we entered into a partnership with Community and Support Options, Inc., the local county mental health center, to merge our emergency service clinical teams and to develop respite care beds in a joint venture. By agreeing to deliver these services jointly, we offered a more comprehensive service, provided more cost-effective care, and brought a valued community partner into the BHS System. Our PCPs at Franklin Medical Center were pleased with this collaboration, as it eased the burden on their patients by merging the hospital and community emergency services teams. At Baystate Medical Center we are presently in discussions with a community behavioral health organization to promote a similar joint venture.

Geropsychiatric Service Expansion

During this same period we significantly expanded our geropsychiatric services. We developed a geriatric nursing home team to provide consultation to nursing home personnel and our PCPs caring for their patients in the nursing homes. This program was extremely successful and we expanded these services throughout our primary BHS service area. This program led to the decision to open a medical-behavioral unit at Franklin Medical Center to provide specialized medical psychiatric care to patients with primary medical disorders complicated by behavioral disorders.

Team Building

Central to our growth and development has been our emphasis on building a strong management team. In 1995, senior management at BHS initiated behavioral health services as the first integrated product line across all BHS facilities and created a senior matrix management structure with the vice president of behavioral health and the chairman of the BMC department of psychiatry, sharing strategic and operational authority. Similarly, program managers and medical directors of major program areas are paired with program managers focusing on day-to-day administrative functions and medical directors focusing on direct clinical care. Administrative meetings stress team building and group problem solving.

The Formation of Baycare Behavioral Health

In 1995, BHS developed the Baycare Health Partners, Inc., a physician-hospital organization joining community physicians and BHS employed physicians and hospitals to market health care services to managed care organizations and general insurers of health care. In 1996 Baycare

Health Partners agreed to form Baycare Behavioral Health, a consolidation of private behavioral health providers, community behavioral health organizations, and Baystate Health Systems' behavioral health services. Baycare Behavioral Health fosters the cooperation of existing community behavioral health providers and BHS behavioral health services to provide a truly integrated continuum of behavioral health services that can be marketed to purchasers of behavioral health services who are interested not only in a continuum of behavioral health services but also behavioral health services that are linked to general medical services through Baycare Health Partners. We believe that our strategy to form linkages to primary medical care will foster the further development of highly integrated medical care necessary for success in a risk-sharing capitated environment.

As the integration of behavioral health and primary care is a major driving strategy, future tasks to strengthen our integration with primary care throughout Baycare Health Partners include refining our primary mental health delivery model. We have watched with interest the development of the primary mental health delivery model at Group Health HMO in Puget Sound, Washington. Our consultation-based model will need further refinement to more formally structure training modules and clinical roles for both primary and behavioral health care providers.

SUMMARY

In this chapter, I have tried to outline the progression of key strategic initiatives that led to the development of a comprehensive continuum of behavioral health services within an integrated delivery system, Baystate Health Systems. The comprehensiveness of our behavioral health services allows us to compete across the spectrum of behavioral health programs in our geographic area. Behavioral health is not a sideline. We focus a great deal of energy and resources of the Baystate health system in this area. Central to our conceptualization of the delivery of these services has been the integration of behavioral health clinicians within a primary care medical practice site because of our strong belief that this integration enhances quality and cost-effective care. We believe that we have developed a strong continuum of behavioral health services, managed to be responsive to the rapidly changing health care environment — one that will be increasingly dominated by the spread of full capitated contracts. Our commitment to the integration of behavioral and primary health care will enhance our ability to provide an integrated case management system necessary to prosper in a health care world increasingly dominated by shared-risk across providers and hospitals. It also greatly enhances our primary care medical services and improves our competitive position in this most central area of health care delivery.

REFERENCES

American Hospital Association. (1993). *Mental health and substance abuse report.* Washington, DC: Author.

Barrett, J. E., Barrett, J. A., Oxman, T. E., & Gerber, P. D. (1988). The prevalence of psychiatric disorders in a primary care practice. *Archives of General Psychiatry, 45,* 1100–1106.

Borus, J. F., & Olendzki, M. C. (1985). The offset effect of mental health treatment on ambulatory medical care utilization and charges. *Archives of General Psychiatry, 42,* 573–580.

Fifer, S. K., Mathias, S. D., Patrick, D. L., Mazonson, P. D., Lubeck, D. P., & Buesching, D. P. (1994). Untreated anxiety among adult primary care patients in a health maintenance organization. *Archives of General Psychiatry, 51,* 740–750.

Fox, K., Merrill, J. C., & Chang, H. H. (1995). Estimating the costs of substance abuse to the Medicaid hospital care program. *American Journal of Public Health, 85,* 48–54.

Hayami, D. E., & Freeborn, D. K. (1981). Effect of coverage on use of an HMO alcoholism treatment program, outcome and medical care utilization. *American Journal of Public Health, 71,* 1133–1143.

Holder, H. D. (1987). Alcoholism treatment and potential health care cost saving. *Medical Care, 25,* 52–71.

Holder, H. D., & Blose, J. O. (1987). Changes in health care costs and utilization associated with mental health treatment. *Hospital & Community Psychiatry, 38,* 1070–1075.

Holder, H. D., & Blose, J. O. (1992). The reduction of health care costs associated with alcoholism treatment: A 14-year longitudinal study. *Journal of Studies on Alcohol, 53,* 293–301.

Holder, H. D., & Shachtman, R. H. (1987). Estimating health care savings associated with alcoholism treatment. *Alcoholism, Clinical & Experimental Research, 11,* 66–73.

Jencks, S. (1985). Recognition of mental distress and diagnosis of mental disorder in primary care. *JAMA, 253,* 1903–1907.

Katon, W., von Korff, M., Lin, E., Lipscomb, P., Russo, J., Wagner, E., & Polk, E. (1990). Distressed high utilizers of medical care: DSM-III-R diagnosis and treatment needs. *General Hospital Psychiatry, 12,* 355–362.

Kroenke, K., & Mangelsdorff, A. D. (1989). Common symptoms in ambulatory care: Incidence, evaluation, therapy and outcome. *American Journal of Medicine, 86,* 262–266.

Langenbucher, J. (1994a). Rx for health care costs: Resolving addictions in the general medical setting. *Alcoholism, Clinical and Experimental Research, 18,* 1033–1036.

Langenbucher, J. (1994b). Offsets are not add-ons: The place of addictions treatment in American health care reform. *Journal of Substance Abuse, 6,* 117–122.

Simon, G., Ormel, J., von Korff, M., & Barlow, W. (1995). Health care costs associated with depressive and anxiety disorders in primary care. *American Journal of Psychiatry, 152,* 352–357.

Worner, T. M., Chen, P. J., Ma, H., Xu, S., & McCarthy, E. G. (1993). An analysis of substance abouse patterns, medical expenses and effectiveness of treatment in the workplace: Long-term follow-up. *Employee Benefits Journal, 18,* 15–19.

6

Integrating Behavioral Health and Primary Care Services: The Primary Mental Health Care Model

Kirk Strosahl

Kirk Strosahl's distinction between primary care behavioral health services and specialty mental health services is extremely important and may be one of the most fundamental contributions in this volume. He points out that the behavioral health services that some have wanted to bring into primary care, in which the patients are treated in psychotherapy or family therapy separately from their medical care, is inevitably a specialty service with the different language and routines that go with a specialty service. Primary care behavioral health services as he describes them are a different kind of service than most mental health providers have ever practiced.

His clarification of the role of the behavioral health provider as being a consultant to the physician's treatment of the patient is a fundamental shift from the early attempts at collaborative care. It helps resolve the problem that patients do not want to be referred to a "shrink" by eliminating the referral. His way does not require a change in the definition of the kind of treatment the patient is receiving. It faces squarely the reality that in the future there may be more times that a psychologist or other psychotherapist in primary care is functioning as a mid-level provider on a team lead by a physician than times when they are separate providers billing from separate benefit pools.

The distinction he proposes is one that fits my own experience and that of a number of other behavioral health providers who practice in primary care. Working in a primary care setting, the word "therapy" is rarely heard. Instead, medical and behavioral health providers talk to patients about visits to address a particular problem, deal with stress, or help them cope with the challenges of a particular medical condition. The self-identification as "psychotherapist" or "family therapist" begins to attenuate, and the identity of "health care provider" becomes more central to how we describe ourselves.

While Strosahl's delineation of the difference between specialty mental health and primary care behavioral health is telling and clearly put, I admit I had more trouble with his distinction between integrated care and collaborative family work in primary care. As I explained in Chapter I, I consider collaborative and integrated care to be parts of a continuum while Strosahl defines them as dichotomous. As a person who has identified himself as a family therapist all of his twenty plus years of professional experience, initially I was not comfortable with the side of the dichotomy to which I perceived myself to be assigned.

As I have considered the chapter further, I find myself agreeing with Strosahl's distinctions in this area as well, but wanting to clearly note that a number of practitioners who got into this work from positions as behavioral science faculty in family residency programs, who originally saw "collaborative family health care" as the goal toward which they were working, have become primary care behavioral health providers as Strosahl defines the role, after a period of time working in a primary health care setting. They may continue to use "collaborative health care" as the term for their work, as the specifics of their practice are in many instances similar to the practice that Strosahl advocates. Because Strosahl is so clear, his work pushes others to clarify their own thinking.

T HIS CHAPTER INTRODUCES the primary mental health care service delivery model, a population-based approach to integrating health and behavioral health care. To understand this new paradigm of behavioral health care, it is first necessary to appreciate the primacy of mental disorders and psychosocial stresses as determinants of medical utilization and health care outcomes. It will then be possible to look at potential impact areas for integrated behavioral health services in primary care. Finally, the defining features of primary mental health will be discussed, how it differs from specialty mental health care as a service delivery philosophy, and why it holds promise as a solution to the integration dilemma.

The setting in which the primary mental health care model was derived is Group Health Cooperative (GHC) of Puget Sound, a consumer-owned, staff and network model HMO with a membership of approximately 460,000 consumers in the Puget Sound region. For eight years, the GHC mental health department has been in the process of developing and implementing integrated behavioral health services within the GHC primary care system, using the primary mental health care approach as the overriding framework. At this point, nearly 15% of GHC behavioral health staff resources are devoted to providing integrated primary care services, with a goal of increasing this percentage to 20% by the end of 1998. In this sense, GHC may be more "evolved" in its integration efforts than may be true in other behavioral health settings. Direct experience with large-scale program planning, design, and evaluation, as well as eight years of direct clinical experience delivering services in this framework, set the context for many of the concepts expressed in this chapter.

THE PRESSURE TO INTEGRATE SERVICES

Fundamental socioeconomic forces are leading to the reform and re-engineering of both the health and mental health delivery systems in the United States. Generation one of managed health care, with its emphasis on cost containment strategies, is simply an omen of the more drastic changes to come. In generation two, not only will there be an intense focus on developing cost- and quality-oriented delivery systems, but also on *integrated services* (cf. Cummings, 1995; Strosahl, 1994a, 1995, 1996a). Formerly segregated delivery systems will be pressured to merge as a way of reducing redundant administrative and infrastructure costs as well as addressing consumer demands for simpler "one stop shopping" service delivery venues (Strosahl, 1996b). Most importantly, the emphasis on integrated delivery of services will emerge primarily because there is a "floor" beyond which using strictly cost containment strategies will begin to damage cost, quality, and satisfaction outcomes (Sobel, 1995). Health care purchasers and providers alike will gain firsthand appreciation of the fact that health care costs cannot be contained as long as health and mental health care are structured as a nonoverlapping enterprise. Such a great proportion of medical care is driven by psychological and psychosocial concerns that the ability of the two systems to contain utilization (and cost) ultimately hinges on their ability to integrate services (Friedman, Sobel, Myers, Caudill, & Benson, 1995). The pressure to integrate services will arise from the widespread implementation of at-risk financing models, such as capitation. Capitation and similar health care financing strategies will radically change the rules of the health care service delivery "game." Instead of being profitable by delivering more services (many of which have marginal utility), delivery systems will survive based upon their ability to provide only those services that are actually needed. Many of the external cost controls evident in generation one (i.e., third party utilization management, carve outs, benefit limits) will be phased out, as financial risk for managing care is shifted directly to providers (Strosahl, 1995). Currently, this part of the health care industry represents a significant source of "overhead," which reduces the total potential impact of the health care dollar. Significant cost savings are likely to be achieved simply by eliminating "third party" cost control systems and moving to direct, at-risk contracting with health care provider groups.

The main argument here is that meaningful health care cost containment cannot occur without the integration of behavioral health and primary care into a consolidated system. However, to achieve this objective, many obstacles will need to be overcome, including financing issues, "turf" struggles, culture clash, and decades of mutual negative stereotyping. The most formidable challenge is to develop an integrated service delivery model that is affordable, logistically practical, and consistent with the goals, strategies, and gestalt of primary care medicine.

PRIMARY CARE MEDICINE: THE REAL MENTAL HEALTH SYSTEM IN THE UNITED STATES

The *defacto* mental health system in the United States is primary medical care (Reiger et al., 1993). The term *primary care provider* refers to a number of medical disciplines (e.g., family practice, general internal medicine, obstetrics-gynecology, pediatrics) and allied health care specialists (physicians' assistants, clinical nurse specialists, registered and licensed nurses, women's health care specialist). Typically, primary care practice is organized around the health care team, which may include any number of primary care providers. Usually, at a minimum, the team is comprised of a single physician and one or more nurses, but team membership can expand to include other allied health providers in larger practice settings. Any member of the health care team provides routine medical care and is likely to encounter patients with mental disorders or significant psychosocial stresses. Research indicates that half of all the formal mental health care in the United States is delivered solely by these providers (Narrow, Reiger, Rae, Manderscheid, & Locke, 1993). Nearly half of all individuals with a diagnosable mental disorder seek no mental health care from any professional, but 80% will visit their primary care physician at least once yearly. For many patients with psychological or psychosocial concerns, medical visits are generated by the physical symptoms of distress (Smith, Rost, & Kashner, 1995). For example, a recent study of the ten most common physical complaints in primary care revealed that 85% end up with no diagnosable organic etiology during a three-year follow-up period (Kroenke & Mangelsdorff, 1989).

Primary health care providers have been criticized for being unable to recognize and effectively treat mental disorders or psychosocial complaints (Bolestrian, Williams, & Wilkinson, 1988). However, in the majority of cases, most provide both medical and psychosocial interventions to their patients. Nonpsychiatric physicians prescribe approximately 70% of all psychotropic agents in America (Beardsley, Gardocki, Larson, & Hidalgo, 1988). Research looking at physician-patient interactions in the treatment of depression indicate that many physicians use behavioral interventions with their patients and encourage their patients to use behavioral strategies outside the confines of the physician's office (Robinson et al., 1995; Robinson, Katon, et al., 1996). Taken as a whole, these findings remove any doubt that a major characteristic of primary care medicine is addressing the psychological needs of the medical patient, often without access to behavioral health support.

This alone would make a compelling case for integrating behavioral health interventions into the daily practices of primary care physicians. However, the "straw that stirs the drink" is the huge medical cost offset potential of integrated care. For example, research has consistently shown that untreated depressed primary care patients use two to three times the annual medical services as their nondepressed counterparts (Simon, VonKorff, & Barlow, 1995). Studies of physician decision making suggest that only 15–25% of medical decisions are based upon health morbidity; the remaining decisions revolve around psychosocial needs, patient preferences, and the doctor-patient relationship (Friedman et al., 1995; Sobel, 1995). There have been several meta-analyses of studies looking at medical cost offsets achieved through integrating health and behavioral health service. While the cost offset literature is still in its methodological infancy, various meta-analyses have indicated that provision of behavioral health services to medical patients may result in cost offsets in the range of 20–40% (Friedman et al.; Sobel; Strosahl & Sobel, 1996). Properly done, integrated primary care and behavioral health services can *achieve significant medical cost offsets and improve the quality of mental health care delivered by primary care providers* (Strosahl, 1996b; Strosahl & Sobel).

POPULATION-BASED CARE: THE FRAMEWORK FOR INTEGRATED SERVICES

Before examining the particulars of an integrated primary care behavioral health service delivery model, it is important to understand the philosophy of population-based care and its pivotal role in the primary health care system of today and the future. Population-based care is derived from an epidemiological, public health view of service delivery planning. Rather than focusing on the health of the individual, population-based care emphasizes the importance of processes that address the health and behavioral health care needs of the entire population. For example, the key population question always is, "What are the needs of the population to be served by this system of care?" A primary care provider's "mission" is not only to address the health needs of the patient in the office, but also to think about similar patients in the population who are under the "care umbrella" of that provider. Are there other patients like this who are not coming in for care? Are there variations in the way care is being provided for patients like this that result in differential health outcomes? How can we prevent conditions like this in patients who have similar risk factors? Can a consistent process of care be organized that addresses the needs of this patient class in the population we serve? From a public health perspective, a population-based service delivery model needs to have case-rate capacity (capable of seeing a large number of cases) and case-rate turnover (the ability to finish cases quickly). In primary care medicine, capacity is created by using 10- to 15-minute visit intervals, so that 30 to 40 patients can be seen each day. The primary care service delivery model involves treating common causes of medical problems first, then moving to more elaborate medical solutions only if the quicker fix fails. This approach addresses the requirement for rapid turnover, in that on the average a large percentage of medical concerns respond to general primary treatment strategies. Those who don't respond are quickly moved though an algorithm involving more specialized secondary treatments. If these treatments fail, the patient is no longer seen by the primary care provider, but is referred on for specialty medical consultations and treatment.

When developing a framework for integrating behavioral health services into primary care, the same public health perspective applies. For example, what types of behavioral health service needs exist in the population of patients served by this primary care team? What type of service delivery structure will allow maximum penetration into the whole population? What types of service interventions work with the "common causes" of psychological distress? What secondary, and more elaborate, interventions are appropriate for a primary care setting? At what level of complexity is a patient better treated in specialty mental health care? These are pivotal service delivery planning questions.

The percentage of a population accessing fee-for-service mental health services seldom exceeds 3–5% in any given year, but fully 80% of that population will make at least one visit to a primary care provider. While the 3% of the population who seek specialty mental health care tend to have elevated symptom levels and are more likely to have specific mental disorders, the behavioral health needs of the 80% who visit a primary care provider are tremendously diverse and are more likely to involve lower proportional rates of diagnosable mental disorders, while exhibiting higher rates of life stress, life transitions, and other forms of distress. The 80% is more likely to have some form of complicating medical condition. With 80% annual penetration, the case rate (i.e., patients who qualify for some form of behavioral health service) is going to be vastly greater in an integrated setting than in a specialty setting, simply because of the volume of patients in the system. Like primary care medicine, integrated behavioral health systems need to have both the case capacity and turnover rate to manage this significantly increased demand for services.

HORIZONTAL AND VERTICAL INTEGRATION: TWO TEMPLATES FOR INTEGRATIVE PRIMARY CARE

The population-based care framework also incorporates two different approaches to improving the health of the population being cared for. Planning services designed to impact the behavioral health needs of the entire primary care population is an example of *horizontal integration*. Horizontal integration is the platform upon which all other forms of integrated behavioral health care reside, because there are many members of the primary care population who can benefit from "generic" behavioral health services. A distinguishing feature of horizontal integration is that it casts a wide net in terms of how it defines health care needs and how it defines the population to be served. Traditional primary care medicine is largely based upon the horizontal integration approach. The provider delivers a wide array of services across his or her "panel," with the goal of improving the health and well-being of the entire cohort of patients under his or her care. In this approach, every member of the panel is encouraged to have a primary care visit. Services are provided to patients based upon unique needs but, in the aggregate, regular visits from most panel members allow the primary care provider to "tend the flock."

Vertical integration involves providing targeted behavioral health services to a well-defined, circumscribed group of primary care patients. This is a major contemporary development in primary care medicine, and behavioral health as well. Targets for vertical integration are usually high-frequency and/or high-cost patient populations, such as patients with depression, panic disorder, chemical dependency, and certain groups of high medical utilizers. A complaint that occurs frequently in the population, such as depression, is a good candidate for a special process of care. Some conditions, although rare in the general population, are so costly that they require a special system of care. A good example of this type of problem involves patients with acquired immune deficiency syndrome (AIDS). In the behavioral health arena, high utilizers of medical care, by definition, are a small but costly group that often are the targets of vertical integration programs (Strosahl & Sobel, 1996). "Critical pathways" are one way vertically integrated care processes are developed to optimize clinical outcomes for a particular target group. By systematizing assessment, treatment, and follow-up care, systems can deliver better care overall for a selected condition. Critical pathways may not guarantee more intensive care for each individual because a major goal is to match the level of care with an established level of clinical need. Patients with subthreshold depressive symptoms, for example, may receive a more abbreviated "care package," when compared to patients with chronic, treatment-resistant depression. Because the goals of population-based care are to provide services to and raise the health care outcomes of the entire population, some individuals may actually experience a reduction in level of care, or receive a substitute (and in theory equally effective) form of care. Other examples of vertical integration initiatives include classroom programs for high utilizers of care, wellness programs for patients who report problems with stress management, and lifestyle classes for postsurgery heart disease patients, to name a few.

TARGET AREAS FOR INTEGRATED SERVICES

Well-integrated primary care behavioral health services should be focused on controlling medical costs that arise directly from psychosocial or mental health factors while optimizing both health and behavioral health care outcomes. Maximizing the impact of integrative services involves capitalizing on both horizontal and vertical opportunities for service integration. There are three health/behavioral health outcome arenas where this impact can be achieved:

1. improving the immediate clinical outcomes of primary care health and/or behavioral health interventions for patients with mental health or medical concerns,
2. producing better outcomes over time in those patients with recurrent, chronic or progressive medical or mental health disorders, and
3. limiting unnecessary medical utilization and costs in patients who have dramatic social support needs and/or chronic and treatment-resistant health or mental health problems.

Improving Acute Care Outcomes

The acute episode of care provided by the general health care provider often involves attempts to stabilize a mental health or health care concern. An integrated service should assist primary care providers in the recognition and treatment of mental disorders and psychosocial stresses at the point of initial presentation. The key goal is to support the primary care provider in intervening early, appropriately, and aggressively to address the patient's concerns. Integrated behavioral health services have much to offer in this area, for success in the acute care phase requires some expertise in screening, differential diagnosis, clinical competence in delivering effective treatments for particular conditions, as well as the ability to tailor treatments to fit the fast pace of primary care visits. There is an unavoidable cost in failing to properly diagnose and treat acute mental health concerns. For example, in medical settings, the average patient with panic disorder is seen by nine specialists before a definitive mental health diagnosis occurs (Strosahl, 1994a). As noted previously, undiagnosed depression leads to elevated medical utilization for the duration of the depressive episode. More unsettling is research indicating that minor depression and dysthymia, conditions that are the most difficult to recognize, are associated with long-term patterns of elevated medical utilization (Robinson, Wischman, & Del Vento, 1996).

It is possible to influence the course of treatment provided by primary care providers when integrated behavioral health services are available. Recent research has suggested that an integrated approach leads to superior outcomes for depressed primary care patients in a wide range of areas; including use of coping strategies, compliance with medication, and use of relapse prevention strategies. This same research suggests integrated services lead to a greater likelihood of using an appropriate dose of antidepressant medication, discussing behavioral and relapse prevention strategies with clients and, most importantly, increased patient and provider satisfaction (Katon et al., 1996; Robinson, Katon, et al., 1996).

There are many acute concerns that patients present to their nurse, physician's assistant, or doctor, ranging from troublesome stress-related physical symptoms (i.e., headache, irritable bowel, dizziness) to problems with a spouse, children, or job supervisor. In each of these circumstances, the primary care provider usually feels obligated to do something to help. Integrated services can focus the primary care providers on strategies that will work within the confines of the "15-minute hour." Done properly, a secondary impact of integrated care with "garden variety" psychosocial stresses is to resolve them before they lead to more significant mental health problems. Preventing mental health morbidity is a very wise and humane "health care investment" and is rarely achievable in segregated delivery systems.

Improving the Long-Term Course of Problems

It is in the area of long-term health outcomes that the best research exists to support the clinical and cost efficacy of the integrated primary care behavioral health approach. For conditions such as heart disease, cancer, diabetes, and arthritis, management outside the acute specialty phase of treatment often falls to the general health care provider. Often, many of the most salient interactions about lifestyle and stress management issues occur after the acute medical crisis is over and the patient is no longer facing a life-threatening condition. Coronary artery disease is an excellent case in point. Several well-conducted studies have shown that depression, anger, and a socially isolated lifestyle are associated with decreased survival time following heart surgery (e.g., Frasure-Smith, 1991). An integrated service approach emphasizes working with both the patient and primary health care providers to effectively isolate and address factors that promote the likelihood of long-term lifestyle changes. Since decreased survival time is associated with repeated hospital admissions and expensive secondary surgeries, integrated care not only results in an enormous cost savings, but also in a huge increase in the patient's quality of life.

Some mental health conditions are likely to recur and worsen without appropriate relapse prevention efforts. The best example is major depression, in its untreated or improperly treated state, a recurrent condition that leads to progressive deterioration of social and role functioning.

Indeed, results of the Medical Outcomes Study (Wells et al., 1989) indicate that the social, physical, and occupation role loss in depression is greater than any other chronic disease, except end-state coronary artery disease. Research indicates that depressed patients who are treated solely with an antidepressant medication, and have no exposure to cognitive behavioral coping strategies, have a very high likelihood of relapse following discontinuation (cf. Shea et al., 1992). It makes no sense for a primary care physician to initiate an antidepressant regime without at the same time exposing the patient to behavioral strategies for managing depression and preventing relapse. An integrated service delivery approach, focused on helping the primary care provider select the appropriate medication at the appropriate dose as well as exposing the patient to key relapse prevention principles, can have a major impact in stopping the revolving door for depressed patients in primary care.

A final area where integrated primary care behavioral health services may make a major impact is in the prevention of iatrogenic conditions: health or behavioral health problems that arise as a result of the treatment delivered for another problem. An excellent example is the patient experiencing intense anxieties related to family, marital, or career issues who is started on an unrestricted course of tranquilizers. This patient's anxiety will probably respond to the tranquilizer, but drug addiction could develop as the patient begins to believe that anxiety cannot be managed without the continued assistance of medicines. Another example is the patient with a fresh back-injury who is placed on temporary work disability and then started on pain medications with the instruction to take them until the pain goes away. This patient is at high risk for developing a chronic pain functional disability cycle, as the patient learns to expect that treatment should eliminate pain and returning to work is impossible as long as pain persists. Primary care is replete with health care dilemmas such as these. Integrated services can deter the iatrogenic and reinforcing effects of the short-term relief strategies that primary care providers feel pressured to give, which nonetheless may lead to negative long-term outcomes.

Controlling Chronic Medical Utilization

Primary care medicine has its own population of chronic utilizers of services as a result of medical condition, mental disorders, psychosocial concerns, or their combination. This group of patients is frustrating to primary care providers because they generally do not profit from medical interventions, but are very demanding of them at the same time. As a group, they disrupt daily practice routines because of recurrent "emergency" phone calls, walk-in health care requests, or frequent, unplanned return visits because of treatment or self-management noncompliance. In some cases, visits are made strictly to obtain social support unavailable from the patient's natural environment. In other cases, the patient is seeking a miracle cure for a chronic condition, such as low back pain. On other occasions, psychological factors are clearly implicated in physical dysfunction, but the patient only wants more medical tests and treatments. The common element of this group of patients is that expensive health services are being used without much in the way of a demonstrable health or mental health outcome. In general, primary care providers have trouble working constructively with high-utilizing patients. Integrated behavioral health can address and control excessive medical utilization by shifting the patient to more frequent, lower-cost services such as brief one-to-one consultations, in-house psychoeducational classes, and so forth. Even more "arms length" treatment strategies seem to work, if practiced from an integrated care perspective. Robinson (1996) studied the effects of a brief phone-based behavioral intervention for high utilizers of medical services. The intervention emphasized behavioral activation, problem solving, and the use of acceptance strategies. Compared to a control group of high utilizers of health care, patients in the intervention group reported significantly improved self-perceived health status, reduced depression, and a greater attitude of acceptance toward their physical health limitations.

THE CRUX OF THE INTEGRATION PROBLEM

The Epidemiological Catchment Area study (Narrow et al., 1993) of nearly 20,000 randomly selected households in the United States has dramatically altered the course of health and mental health care policy formation. In addition to revealing an astoundingly high annual onset rate of mental disorders (17.9%), this study also demonstrated that 50% of all care for patients with mental disorders is delivered solely by general medical practitioners, and that 50% of all patients seek no formal care at all. The dilemma is complicated by the fact that 80% of a primary care population will make at least one health care visit annually. The conclusion is that approximately 65–70% of potentially treatable patients are cycling through the general medical sector, whether they are recognized and treated or not. This is probably the most single important factor promoting the need to integrate services. Without some type of system for detecting and intervening with this huge cohort of patients, there is very little chance of controlling the use of health care services at the system level.

The same facts that promote the need for integration also suggest that delivering specialty mental health services to this patient population would require at least a 100% increase in the supply of mental health providers, something that is highly unlikely to occur. Simply locating mental health specialists in primary care practices and asking them to deliver traditional specialty mental health care would completely outstrip the available behavioral health resources in this country. This system design problem has been largely ignored in the discussions about integration, probably because the popularity of the topic is relatively new and system planners have not yet faced the realities involved in building an integrated delivery system that works. From a population-based care perspective, what is needed is a model of care that can accommodate a tremendous unmet demand for services, without an appreciable expansion in required mental health resources.

PRIMARY MENTAL HEALTH CARE: A NEW INTEGRATED SERVICES PARADIGM

A *primary mental health care* model of integrated primary health care involves a consultative, time limited approach to the provision of behavioral health services in primary care (Quirk et al., 1995; Strosahl, 1994b, 1996a, 1996b). The goal is not to take over responsibility for providing behavioral health care to the (literally) hundreds of thousands of primary care patients in need, but to provide consultative support to primary care providers to increase the impact of their ongoing psychosocial interventions. In its emphasis on behavioral health as a consultative primary care service, the primary mental health approach is consistent with the goals and philosophies of primary care medicine. Interestingly, the mental health industry never evolved as a "primary care discipline." Perhaps in an attempt to legitimize mental health as a health care service, the industry has always defined itself as a "specialty." The notion of specialist has a particular significance in the world of primary health care and it has helped foster the philosophical and turf schism that exists between behavioral health and primary care providers. A specialist takes over care of the patient from the referring primary care provider, treats, and stabilizes the patient. This distinction carries with it an inherent tension regarding who is "in charge" of the patient's care. This dynamic is not unique to behavioral health but occurs just as readily in interactions between primary care providers and medical subspecialists. In all likelihood, integrated behavioral health services will remain a pipe dream as along as the behavioral health industry approaches integration from a specialty care model. Most supporters of integration continue to articulate a solution that simply involves placing a mental health therapist on site in primary care to provide specialty mental health services. An alternative is to develop a model of behavioral health care that is not specialty oriented, but rather is consistent with the goals, strategies, and culture of primary care.

The primary mental health care model involves providing direct consultative services to primary care providers and, where appropriate, engaging in temporary comanagement (with the primary care provider) of patients who require more concentrated services. Like primary medical care, consultative and/or condensed treatment services are delivered as a "first line" intervention. If a patient fails to respond to this level of intervention (or is obviously in need of highly specialized services), the patient is transferred into the specialty mental health system.

The primary mental health care model is unique both in terms of its goals and in the structure of care. As can be seen in Table 6.1, the primary mission of integrative services is to enhance the effectiveness of primary care providers who are delivering behavioral health interventions to their patients. A notable characteristic of the primary mental health model is that it is based in an intervention philosophy that is consistent with the mission of primary care. This involves detecting and addressing a wide range of health and mental health concerns with the aims of early identification, quick resolution, long-term prevention, and wellness. Most importantly, primary mental health is based in a consultation-liaison model, in which the consultant supports the behavioral health interventions of the primary care provider. The focus of consultation is on resolving problems within the normal primary care service structure, as well as to engage in health promotion and monitoring for at-risk patients. Typically, consultation visits are brief (15 to 30 minutes), limited in number (1 to 3 visits), and provided in the primary care practice area as a form of primary care service. The referring primary care provider is the chief "customer" of the service and, at all times, remains in charge of the patient's care.

From the patient's point of view, the behavioral health consultant is in a frontline position, on a par with other primary care team members. Like other members of the team, the behavioral health specialist brings specialized knowledge to bear on problems that require additional expertise and may even engage in limited and strategic follow-up with selected

TABLE 6.1
Key Goals and Structural Characteristics of
Primary Mental Health Care

GOALS	SERVICE DELIVERY STRUCTURE
Improve clinical outcomes through enhanced detection, treatment, and follow-up strategies used by primary care providers.	Uses limited brief consultation visits to build upon existing interventions and to suggest new ones; primary health care provider is "in charge" of the patient's care.
Manage at-risk patients to prevent the onset recurrence of a mental disorder.	"See all comers" service philosophy encourages a broad-spectrum referral pattern, and utilizes the physician-patient relationship to detect at-risk situations, such as life stresses, transitions, etc.
Educate primary care providers in the use of appropriate medication and psychosocial treatments.	Primary product of consultation is the consultation report and face-to-face feedback; consultation strategies are tailored to the "15-minute hour."
Manage high-utilizing patients with chronic health and behavioral health concerns to reduce inappropriate medical utilization and to promote better functional outcomes.	Longer-term consultative follow-up is reserved for the small number of patients with numerous medical and/or psychosocial concerns; consultative comanagement over time.
Deliver integrated programs of care for high-frequency mental and addictive disorders (i.e., depression, anxiety, alcohol abuse) and psychosocial stresses.	Service has "pathway-driven" consultative intervention programs, which use a temporary comanagement model to manage and resolve a particular condition within the context of primary care services.
Accurately identify and place patients who require specialized mental health treatment.	Service is organized to triage patients to specialty care and to function as a liaison between the specialty provider and the health care provider.

(continued)

TABLE 6.1
Continued

GOALS	SERVICE DELIVERY STRUCTURE
Address the behavioral health needs of the entire primary care population.	Service is provided in a population-based care framework, using both horizontal and vertical service delivery methods.
Deliver service in a way that is consistent with the goals and mission of primary care.	Consultant is part of the "primary care team"; health care provider is the primary customer of consultative services.
Deliver service in a manner that is "acceptable" to all consumers of health services.	Service functions as part of primary care, located in same practice area, used as an ancillary element of routine medical visits.

patients. In all cases these activities are designed to support the effectiveness of the primary care provider in responding to the patient's behavioral health needs. Referrals for behavioral health consultation can come from any member of the primary care team, including physicians, midlevel providers, or nursing staff.

LEVELS OF PRIMARY MENTAL HEALTH CARE

As is illustrated in Table 6.2, primary mental health services also exist on a level of care continuum to respond to different levels of need within the primary care population. Generally, levels of primary mental health care are built to correspond to (a) the level of complexity of the problem and (b) the proportion of the primary care population that will "penetrate" the service. At the most basic level of care, the service delivery model is almost exclusively founded in a horizontal integration perspective. At the highest levels of care, the vertical integration approach is more dominant.

Behavioral Health Consultation

The foundation of an integrative primary care service is the general consultation visit. In general, this service is available to any primary care

TABLE 6.2
Levels of Primary Mental Health Care

LEVEL OF CARE	% OF PRIMARY CARE POPULATION	KEY SERVICE CHARACTERISTICS
Behavioral health consultation	60%	Brief, general in focus; oriented around a specific referral issue from health care provider. Visit interval (15–30 minutes) matches pace of primary care. Designed to enhance effectiveness of psychosocial and medication interventions by health care provider. Exclusively consultative in nature.
Integrated care programs	30%	Usually focused on high-cost and/or high-frequency conditions. Employs temporary comanagement approach; ultimate goal is to return care *in toto* back to health care provider. Program structure is manualized, with condensed treatment strategies; emphasis is on patient education and self-management strategies.
Specialty consultation	10%	Reserved for high utilizers and multiproblem patients. Emphasis is on containing excessive medical utilization, giving providers effective behavioral management strategies and community resource case management. Goal is to maximize daily functioning of patient, not necessarily symptom elimination. Service is consultative in nature; visits are brief (15–30 minutes), infrequent, and predictable over time.

patient who is referred for any reason. The "see all comers" philosophy is also consistent with the general medicine approach of primary care. The goal of the 30-minute consultation visit is to help the primary care provider and patient work more effectively to target the psychosocial concerns that emerge. The consultation model is very flexible in that it may involve the consultant, patient, and primary care provider in any combination. Normally, the behavioral health specialist will see the patient and, less frequently, the patient and primary care provider together. The aim of the consultation is to increase the impact of the physician's medication and psychosocial interventions. In order to achieve this objective, suggested interventions must be tailored to fit the demands of the "15-minute hour." Practically speaking, this means an acceptable behavioral health intervention can only take two to three minutes of a typical health care visit, or it likely will not be implemented by the primary care provider. Typical interventions recommended by the consultant are limited behavioral activation, psychoeducational readings, or initiating a medication and working briefly with the patient concerning compliance and side effects. If one or two follow-up visits with the consultant will help build "positive momentum," the consultant may elect this option as long as it is clear that the primary care provider remains in charge of the patient's care. Viewed from a horizontal integration perspective, the behavioral health consultation service model addresses the two important service delivery criteria of *capacity* and *turnover*. The limited visit span and compressed session length results in greatly expanded impact in the primary care population. At Group Health, a consultant can see six to eight patients in a half-day of practice, and still have time to provide face-to-face feedback to referring providers.

A secondary goal of an effective consultation service is to raise the skill level of the referring providers so that routine problems are handled successfully within the forum of the medical visit. A consultation approach allows in vivo training to occur based upon shared casework. With feedback regarding hundreds of patients seen by the consultant, primary care providers begin to see the same themes recur in their panel of patients and also gain firsthand experience using effective intervention strategies while being supported by the behavioral health consultant. Eventually, the provider integrates the skills and implements both psychological and pharmacological interventions more effectively. Clinical experience as well as research to be discussed subsequently suggest that consultative behavioral health services improve the process of care for behavioral health issues, including both medication practices and the more frequent and appropriate use of psychosocial intervention strategies.

Specialty Consultation

The specialty consultation level of primary mental health care is for patients with chronic psychosocial and/or physical problems that need to be managed over time within the primary care setting. This may involve any number of subgroups of patients, including those with chronic, progressive diseases, personality disorders, long-term evolving stress factors (e.g., care giving for a parent with Alzheimer's disease) or high utilizers of medical services. Providing consultative support over longer periods of time is generally necessary to manage these patients. Since this approach involves targeting specific groups of patients for more aggressive management, it carries elements of the vertical integration approach. The consultative visit structure is consistent with the behavioral health consultation level of care, but the consultation regime is less concentrated (i.e., once quarterly) and may be continued over months or years. Consultations are focused on care management or community resource needs, managing excessive medical utilization, and helping the patient cope better with the demands of everyday living. The activities of the consultant are designed to help the primary care team efficiently manage the patient's health and behavioral health care needs.

Integrated Care Programs

The integrated care level is designed for high-frequency and/or high-cost primary care populations, such as major depression or panic disorder, and is based in a vertical integration approach. It involves using highly condensed, specialized treatment packages that are tailored for the fast work pace of primary care. The intent is to treat and resolve the index condition within primary care, as well as to prevent relapse in the case of recurrent disorders. To achieve this end, the consultant and primary care provider "choreograph" their respective interventions, so that each is supporting the work of the other. More behavioral health visits may be delivered, although the emphasis remains on patient education, self management skills, and feedback to the primary care provider regarding 2- to 3-minute interventions to use during medical visits. Although it is tempting to label this as "therapy," it more accurately can be described as *temporary comanagement*, where the aim is to return total responsibility for care to the primary care provider once the acute mental health concern is stabilized. An excellent example is the Integrated Care Program For Depression (Robinson, Wischman, & Del Vento, 1996), in which a primary care provider and behavioral health consultant work together to combine medication and cognitive behavioral treatment for patients with major or minor depression This program employed a structured intervention involving 2.5 to 3.5 hours of contact with a behavioral health consultant and 1 to 2 hours visit time with a primary care provider. The focus of the intervention was on helping patients learn practical depression management strategies, managing medication side effects and compliance issues, and helping primary care providers implement appropriate antidepressant therapy regimes. A randomized clinical trial comparing this model of care to "usual care" showed that the integrated model produced superior clinical outcomes, better medication compliance, better management of side effects, more satisfied patients, and more satisfied primary health care providers (Katon et al., 1996; Robinson, Katon, et al., 1996). The remission rates among patients with major depression treated in the integrated care model were comparable to those obtained in many clinical psychotherapy studies using highly specialized treatments for depression. These comparable remission rates were obtained using only a fraction of the behavioral health resources that are used in many specialty treatments for depression (2.5 to 3.5 hours versus 16 to 20 hours). An equally intriguing finding was a less robust but clear indication of better clinical outcomes among patients with minor and subthreshold depressions, a group that has been notoriously refractory to medication and/or specialty psychotherapies.

COLOCATION, COLLABORATION, AND INTEGRATION: THE MAGIC TRIAD OF INTEGRATIVE CARE

While the opportunities involved in integrated care are endless, there are many potential barriers to achieving the best system architecture in this rapidly growing area. The popularity of the integration theme in contemporary behavioral health systems has led to a plethora of different initiatives that are advertised as reflecting an integrated care philosophy. Programs as diverse as providing problem solving and coping skills classes to high utilizers of health care or conducting conjoint therapy visits with physicians and their patients are equally likely to be portrayed as examples of integration. The point here is not to belittle these efforts or the individual creativity that breeds them, but rather to illustrate a bigger problem that needs to be solved before integrative models can move into the mainstream of health care. Specifically, current initiatives lack a consistent philosophical and system design basis and tend to either ignore or underemphasize three critical and interrelated themes: colocation of services, collaboration between providers, and adopting an integrated health care mission.

Colocation of Services: On Site, Not On Call

Colocation of services is a necessary, but not sufficient, condition for an effective integrated care system. Many types of behavioral health services can, and have been, delivered within the primary care office setting. It is standard practice for fee-for-service mental health providers to station their offices close to primary care physician practice groups. This leads to more referrals and more opportunities to provide specialty mental health care to primary care referred patients. However, providing services in an office separate from the physician's practice area is conceptually different from practicing on site within the health care cluster in the context of routine medical care. There is a world of difference between the office practice and medical practice gestalt, and integrated care begins with a conscious attempt to position behavioral health within the service delivery context of routine medical care. Complete integration of services can occur only when the behavioral health specialist is on site, practicing in the medical cluster as a part of the primary care team. Many network model behavioral health systems respond to the demand for integrated services by offering on-demand, phone-based consultation for health care providers who have a behavioral health emergency.

While on-demand consultative services are a nice gesture, they generally are used by physicians only during infrequent psychiatric emergencies and have little impact on overall integration of routine behavioral health and primary care services. Most importantly, they have little chance to raise the skill level of primary care health providers with respect to the thousands of routine psychosocial interventions that are employed in daily practice of primary health care. The only effective vehicle for touching the lives of thousands of primary care patients is the in-house consultant with a continuous and predictable presence. This requires a commitment to on-site staffing at a level that guarantees acceptable access for newly referred patients. Generally, maintaining two to four hours' weekly consultation availability for every 1000 lives covered by a health care practice is the bare minimum for maintaining adequate access and follow-up capacity. The presence of colocated services does not in itself guarantee an integrated service philosophy, but it is a critical first step.

Collaborative Care: How Different Is it Really?

Many proponents of integration espouse a "collaborative family health care" philosophy, which, stated simply, involves having the mental health provider function on site as a specialty mental health therapist in close coordination with the patient's physician or health care provider (Pace, Chaney, Mullins, & Olson, 1995). Conjoint visits with the physician and patient are sometimes employed to address issues in the physician-patient working relationship. This approach has originated largely from behavioral scientists practicing in university-based family practice and general internal medicine residency settings and promotes a family systems philosophy of case conceptualization and intervention. There is an assumed overlap between the goals and strategies of family practice medicine and family psychology/family systems interventions that makes this approach outwardly appealing.

There are, however, many reasons to question whether the collaborative family health care model provides a strong foundation for integrated care. First and foremost, collaborative care essentially involves relocating the specialty mental health model within the primary care setting. Many mental health providers share this definition: conducting psychotherapy with physician-referred patients, sometimes in partnership with the physician or other members of the health care team. Employing a "retread" of the specialty mental health service delivery model may inadvertently promote the continued separation of health and mental health care, even if the services are colocated and provided by members of the same health care team (Quirk et al., 1995). The "house shrink" role reinforces an age-old stereotype held by many health care providers that mental conditions are treated in a specialty service delivery model and are not a legitimate part of routine health care.

Second, it is no accident that many individuals prefer to have their behavioral health issues addressed by their primary care physician. It is perceived by many patients to be less stigmatizing and more convenient to do so. Because of this, many primary care patients are reluctant to accept specialty mental health care, even if it is provided in close proximity to the doctor's office. Consumer focus groups at Group Health Cooperative have suggested that most patients prefer to have their mental health issues managed in the primary care setting and in a style that is similar to how health care services are delivered, that is, visits are short, infrequent, simple, and action-oriented.

Another concern is that specialty mental health care tends to require more time and therefore has a limited capacity. It would require an enormous expenditure of health care resources to staff such a model so that all willing primary care patients would have appropriate access to services. It is highly doubtful that the necessary resources will be available to support this type of service delivery structure.

Finally, there is increasing evidence to support the notion that general medicine practitioners are unlikely to use family systems interventions in their medical practices outside the confines of residency training. Robinson et al. (1995) have shown that family practice physicians actually employ quite pragmatic cognitive behavioral interventions in their interactions with depressed patients. The vast majority of medical care is provided in a one-to-one visit context, a factor that directly militates against systems interventions. When systems interventions are employed, they are cumbersome and often require more follow-up visits as well as longer visit times. In my experience, few general practitioners have the time or the patience to make this model work and instead gravitate to individual interventions that are pragmatic and fit the two to three minutes that typically are available to address psychosocial issues during a routine medical visit. In settings which are outside the heavily structured context of residency training, the family health model has given way to a much more pragmatic, time-effective form of general medicine. This is not meant to imply that physicians have no interest in family health. Indeed they do, but the demands of contemporary medical practice and managed care have elevated time-effective strategies to a position of primacy.

The Mission of Integrative Behavioral Health Care: To Think and Act Like a Primary Care Provider

It is clearly desirable to have effective collaboration between behavioral health and primary care providers. However, good collaboration can be achieved without a meaningful integration of the primary care and behavioral health "missions." Many systems that have attempted to provide on-site collaborative care have quickly discovered that it simply reintroduces the problems inherent in the specialty mental health model. Experience at Group Health suggests that, when mental health specialists practice on site as psychotherapists, they can quickly become swamped with referrals for specialty care, have problems with access, and regrettably have very little overall impact on the behavioral health of their population of primary care patients. As a consultant to other behavioral health systems who have attempted to integrate services, I have repeatedly observed the same difficulty with the "house shrink" model of integration. All of these adverse impacts will occur in a context in which both health and behavioral health providers will readily admit that the process of care is far more collaborative than it has ever been. This is not an insignificant achievement, but the integrated care system of the future must be both feasible and consistent with the requirements of a population-based care framework.

As is presented in Table 6.3, there are a variety of features that distinguish integrated care from collaborative care. The most important philosophical shift is that behavioral health is seen as a form of routine primary care. It is no longer viewed as a specialty service, but as a front-line feature of primary care medical visits. A patient is just as likely to see a behavioral health consultant as he or she is to see a registered nurse during a routine medical visit. The behavioral health provider is part of the primary care team, not part of a specialty mental health group located in the same professional office complex. The cost of primary mental health care is built into the cost of primary care medical services. Accordingly, it is billed as a medical service, similar to laboratory, pharmacy, or nursing support services.

This has profound implication for the position behavioral health occupies in routine medical practice algorithms. Following are some examples.

- Rather than referring a patient with recurrent tachycardia to a cardiologist after trying other medical interventions, the patient is referred to a behavioral health consultant for evaluation of possible panic disorder.
- The patient who is about to encounter a major life stress such as divorce or death of a parent, or whose child has been recently diagnosed with a chronic illness, is sent to the behavioral health consultant for prophylactic stress management and coping skills planning. These activities become part of the patient's general medical record, so that stress management/coping strategies are reinforced during all routine health care visits.
- The patient with recurrent major depressions, once stabilized by the combined clinical activities of the consultant and health care provider using an integrated program approach, makes a protocol-triggered visit to the behavioral health provider to form a relapse prevention plan. This plan is discussed during the primary care team meeting and becomes a part of the patient's priority health care objectives.
- The patient who presents with an on-the-job back injury, prior to

TABLE 6.3
Distinguishing Characteristics of Integrated
and Collaborative Care Models

DIMENSION	COLLABORATIVE CARE	INTEGRATED CARE
Mission	Provide specialty mental health care while keeping health care providers "in the loop"	Provide a primary care service focused on behavioral health issues
Location	In separate location or colocated in "mental health wing"	In medical practice area
Primary provider	Therapist	Health care provider
Service modality	Therapy session, conjoint visits with primary care provider more likely	Consultation session; conjoint visits with primary care provider less likely
Team identification	"One of them"	"One of us"
Professional moniker	Therapist or mental health specialist	Behavioral health consultant
Referral statement	"Go see a specialist I work with in the mental health wing."	"Go see one of our primary care team who helps out with these kind of issues."
Philosophy of care	Behavioral health is a specialty service done outside the context of routine health care	Behavioral health is part of the process of general health care
Patient's perception	Receive a separate service from a specialist who is in close collaboration with a health care provider	Looks like, feels like a routine aspect of health care

being started on a pain cocktail, is sent to the behavioral health consultant for a chronic pain and disability risk assessment. Consultant and physician then support each other in emphasizing that time off from work will be limited, pain medications will only be used for a specific period of time, and the patient will need to learn practical pain management strategies from the consultant as part of the return-to-work plan.

- The patient with depressive symptoms is started on an antidepressant by the primary care provider and, as part of standard protocol, is sent to the behavioral health consultant for assistance with goal setting, personal problem solving, and behavioral activation. The consultant determines that the patient is suffering from minor depression or dysthymia. The consultant recommends, and the physician agrees, that medications are probably not indicated and should be discontinued while the consultant teaches the patient skills for self-management of depressive symptoms.

- A patient with unstable diabetes is not complying with dietary restraints and blood glucose monitoring requirements and is sent to a behavioral health consultant to work on compliance enhancement. The consultant discovers the patient is depressed and feels hopeless about life since developing the disease and begins to work with the patient to initiate "do-able" social, leisure, and recreational pursuits as well as a written daily diabetes self-management plan which is placed in the medical chart. In follow-up medical visits, the physician reinforces the importance of planning and following through on pleasant activities and reviews success with the written daily self-management plan generated by the consultant.

There are many other examples, far too numerous to elaborate here, of how the daily practice of primary care medicine and behavioral health can be "seamlessly" integrated. Notice that in each of these examples, the behavioral health provider functions as part of a system of medical care. The advantages of such a system are obvious: better coordination of care, better clinical outcomes, reduced medical practice costs, increased customer satisfaction, and a more satisfying practice environment for primary care and behavioral health providers.

SUMMARY

Building integrative primary care behavioral health systems that work will require an extraordinary amount of vision and courage. The vision will carry us through the cacophony of the managed care "shakedown" with all of the associated fears regarding cost containment and professional survival. Taking a myopic view of this transition is likely to squelch innovation, while maintaining a vision of the future can inform us of when and where radical innovation is needed. This era is not so much a reshaping of health care as it is the re-engineering of the health care system. The final product may bear scant resemblance to what we have become accustomed to. Courage is always at a premium in troubled times such as the era of health care reform. Courage is easier to come by when there is a destination and set of directions that holds promise of not just survival, but also prosperity and a win-win situation for key stakeholders in the future. Hopefully, the primary mental health care model will be a major part of the foundation of what promises to be an exciting and complex solution.

REFERENCES

Beardsley, R., Gardocki, G., Larson, D., & Hidalgo, J. (1988). Prescribing of psychotropic medication by primary care physicians and psychiatrists. *Archives of General Psychiatry, 45,* 1117–1119.

Bolestrian, S., Williams, P., & Wilkinson, G. (1988). Specialist mental health treatment in general practice: A meta-analysis. *Psychological Medicine, 18,* 711–717.

Cummings, N. (1995). Impact of managed care on employment and training: A primer for survival. *Professional Psychology: Research and Practice, 26,* 10–15.

Frasure-Smith, N. (1991). In-hospital symptoms of psychological stress as predictors of long-term outcome after acute myocardial infarction in men. *American Journal of Cardiology, 67,* 121–127.

Friedman, R., Sobel, D., Myers, P., Caudill, M., & Benson, H. (1995). Behavioral medicine, clinical health psychology and cost offset. *Health Psychology, 14,* 509–518.

Katon, W., Robinson, P., Von Korff, M., Lin, E., Bush, T., Ludman, E., Simon, G., & Walker, E. (1996). A multifaceted intervention to improve treatment of depression in primary care. *Archives of General Psychiatry, 53,* 924–932.

Kroenke, K., & Mangelsdorf, A. (1989). Common symptoms in primary care: Incidence, evaluation, therapy and outcome. *American Journal of Medicine, 86,* 262–266.

Narrow, W., Reiger, D., Rae, D., Manderscheid, R., & Locke, B. (1993). Use of services by persons with mental and addictive disorders: Findings from the National Institute of Mental Health Epidemiologic Catchment Area Program. *Archives of General Psychiatry, 50,* 95–107.

Pace, T., Chaney, J., Mullins, L., & Olson, R. (1995). Psychological consultation with primary care physicians: Obstacles and opportunities in the medical setting. *Professional Psychology: Research and Practice, 26,* 123–131.

Quirk, M., Strosahl, K., Todd, J., Fitzpatrick, W., Casey, M., Hennessey, S., & Simon, G. (1995). Quality and customers: Type 2 change in mental health delivery within health care reform. *Journal of Mental Health Administration, 22,* 414–425.

Reiger, D., Narrow, W., Rae, D., Manderschied, R., Locke, B., & Goodwin, F. (1993). The de facto U.S. mental and addictive disorders service system: Epidemiologic Catchment Area prospective 1 year prevalence rates of disorders and services. *Archives of General Psychiatry, 50,* 85–94.

Robinson, P. (1995). New territory for the behavior therapist: Hello depressed patients in primary care! *The Behavior Therapist, 18*, 111–123.

Robinson, P. (1996, November). *Acceptance and commitment strategies among older primary care patients.* Paper presented at the 29th annual meeting of the Association for the Advancement of Behavior Therapy. New York.

Robinson, P., Bush, T., Von Korff, M., Katon, W., Lin, E., Simon, G., & Walker, E. (1995). Primary care physician use of cognitive behavioral techniques with depressed patients. *Journal of Family Practice, 40*, 352–357.

Robinson, P., Katon, W., Von Korff, M., Bush, T., Ludman, E., Simon, G., Lin, E., & Walker, E. (1996). *Effects of a combined treatment for depressed primary care patients on behavioral change and process of care variables.* Manuscript submitted for publication.

Robinson, P., Wischman, C., & Del Vento, A. (1996). *Treating depression in primary care: A manual for physicians and therapists.* Reno: Context.

Shea, T., Elkin, I., Imber, S., Sotsky, S., Watkins, J., Collins, J., Pilkonis, P., Beckham, E., Glass, D., Dolan, R., & Parloff, M. (1992). Course of depressive symptoms over follow-up: Findings from the National Institute of Mental Health Treatment of Depression Collaborative Research Program. *Archives Of General Psychiatry, 49*, 782–787.

Simon, G., VonKorff, M., & Barlow, W. (1995). Health care costs of primary care patients with recognized depression. *Archives of General Psychiatry, 52*, 850–856.

Smith, G., Rost, K., & Kashner, T. (1995). A trial of the effect of a standardized psychiatric consultation on health outcomes and costs in somaticizing patients. *Archives of General Psychiatry, 52*, 238–243.

Sobel, D. (1995). Rethinking medicine: Improving health outcomes with cost-effective psychosocial interventions. *Psychosomatic Medicine, 57*, 234–244.

Strosahl, K. (1994a). Entering the new frontier of managed mental health care: Gold mines and land mines. *Cognitive and Behavioral Practice, 1*, 5–23.

Strosahl, K. (1994b). New dimensions in behavioral health primary care integration. *HMO Practice, 8*, 176–179.

Strosahl, K. (1995). Behavior therapy 2000: A perilous journey. *The Behavior Therapist, 18*, 130–133.

Strosahl, K. (1996a). Confessions of a behavior therapist in primary care: The odyssey and the ecstasy. *Cognitive and Behavioral Practice, 3*, 1–28.

Strosahl, K. (1996b). Primary mental health care: A new paradigm for achieving health and behavioral health integration. *Behavioral Health Care Tomorrow, 5*, 93–96.

Strosahl, K., & Quirk, M. (1994, July). The trouble with carve outs. *Business & Health.*

Strosahl, K., & Sobel, D. (1996). Behavioral health and the medical cost offset effect: Current status, key concepts and future applications. *HMO Practice, 10*, 156–162.

Wells, K., Stewart, A., Hays, R., Burnam, A., Rogers, W., Daniels, M., Berry, S., Greenfield, S., & Ware, J. (1989). The functioning and well being of depressed patients: Results of the Medical Outcomes Study. *Journal of the American Medical Association, 262*, 914–919.

7

Integrating Primary Care and Mental Health in a Health Care Organization: From Pilot to Mainstream

C. J. Peek   Richard L. Heinrich

C. J. Peek and Robert Simpson have the longest continuous experience in integrated care in medical settings of the authors in this volume. While authors like Margaret Heldring, Tillman Farley, Thomson Davis and George Biltz, and Patrician Robinson and her collaborators describe the practical improvements that can be made by instituting integrated primary care in a particular setting, C. J. Peek and Richard Heinrich describe cultural changes that occur over significant periods of time in an organization where integrated primary care is practiced. They have seen the different disciplines work together long enough to begin to distinguish the similarities about their work. Their concept of "generic problems" in health care provision, such as overserviced and underserved patients, and their delineation of generic standards of good health care practice are, in my opinion, our first look into the new world that develops when the learning that is part of integrated primary care begins to be translated into the routines of practice and organization of social roles of an entire health system.

Peek and Heinrich speak from the point of view of one of the most highly evolved health care markets in the country. In the 13 years since Peek started working on an integrated team, all of the health reform stages that have happened anywhere in the country have happened in Minneapolis. From their advanced position there is a sense of their seeing the basics of health care in a new way. Maybe their perspective should be called "forward to the basics."

This chapter should be of special interest to the highest levels of management in health care delivery systems. It focuses directly on the contingencies that exist in a large organization and on the issues that managers will have to face in the implementation of integrated primary care. By explaining the approach to take with each primary care unit that may be a pilot for a broader implementation, the authors help managers understand both the unique and the generic ways of approach that will need to be used throughout the entire process.

The authors' emphasis on the uniqueness of approach of each primary care practice or clinic is an important reminder for how all of the chapters in this book should be approached. Each chapter represents an example of good practice in integrated primary care. The summary chapters are descriptive of patterns that are developing throughout the country. These are not prescriptive, not stock programs to be implemented "by the numbers" in any setting. Of all the chapters, this is the one that most directly tells you what to do and yet, what they tell you to do is to be flexible, to listen, to meet people where they are, to understand that development takes time, and to be patient.

THIS CHAPTER IS THE result of an extended conversation between the authors and Alexander Blount. It is meant to bring out the general principles we have learned about developing integrated primary care, first in pilot programs and then in the mainstream of a large, complex managed health care system. We have tried to tell the story of what we have done at HealthPartners in a way that highlights what we have learned and how we learned it. Because the chapter began as a conversation rooted in our everyday experience, it retains that conversational style. We hope that style will make it easier for readers to connect the ideas with their own everyday experience.

REASONS TO INTEGRATE BEHAVIORAL HEALTH AND PRIMARY CARE

Our experience with collaborative care began 10 to 12 years ago at what was then called Group Health Inc., a nonprofit, member-governed, staff model health maintenance organization (now part of HealthPartners).

All clinicians were salaried by the organization, and health plan members prepaid, usually through employers, for a comprehensive package of health care. It was founded in 1957 as a product of the cooperative movement and grew to approximately 300,000 members by 1990. It developed from a single clinic in 1957 to a multisite, multispecialty clinic system* staffed by 350 physicians and over 100 mental health clinicians practicing in 19 medical clinics.

In the turbulent Minnesota and Twin Cities managed care environment, Group Health merged in 1991with a health plan (MedCenters) and in 1994 with an academic physician-hospital group (Ramsey Clinic Associates and St. Paul Ramsey Hospital) to become HealthPartners.

The HealthPartners mental health benefit and care delivery department is a relative newcomer to the organization, having been established in the mid-seventies, at about the same time as legislative mandate for specifically designated HMO mental health coverage. Before that time, mental health care was done as a normal part of primary care medicine with some outside specialty mental health or chemical dependency consultation and referral. Most subscribers to the health plan had unformed views and expectations of mental health care at that time. At the department's beginning, referral to mental health was done only by physicians who detected mental health conditions in need of evaluation. Physicians served a specialty "gatekeeping," evaluation, and agenda-setting function. Mental health visits were entered in medical charts like any other patient visit.

As a large freestanding mental health department emerged, the gatekeeping function of primary care physicians was lifted, and direct patient access to mental health appointments was established. Patient conception of the mental health benefit and services changed accordingly. By 1983 concern about confidentiality and logistical problems with medical chart traffic to mental health clinics resulted in the creation of a separate and confidential mental health chart and a confidentiality statement that formalized the separation of mental health and medical records. The view that medical and mental health care are fundamentally different

---

1. The term "clinic" can have several meanings and usages. In this chapter "clinic" refers to individual clinics that comprise the HealthPartners Medical Group and Clinics. Most of these clinics provide adult medicine, pediatrics, medical and surgical subspecialty, and dental services. The collaborative care project has involved adult medicine and pediatric care units in specific clinics. Each clinic is composed of anywhere from 5 to 15 physicians and the nurses and receptionists with whom they work. Health psychology collaborative care placements have also included oncology, endocrinology, pediatric nephrology, and an internal medicine pain clinic.

and should be kept apart became widespread not only among patients but also among clinicians and managers. Medical staff rarely ordered and read mental health charts (and were often under the impression that they were not allowed to do so). Mental health providers rarely read medical charts. "Phone tag" (this was pre–e-mail and voice-mail) between medical and mental health clinics made routine coordination of care less practical.

Gradually, medical and mental health staff became strangers. Mutual stereotypes between physicians and psychotherapists flourished, often confirmed by experience as misunderstandings lingered, there being little opportunity to routinely discuss and resolve the problems. The reputation of the mental health department with physicians and medical clinics dropped as frustration built and compounded.

The mental health department drifted away from physicians and medical clinics, taking the path of a traditional freestanding mental health clinic. The mental health benefit was more or less independent of the medical benefit, and as time went on, the department became less and less well adapted for the task of serving medical patients with disguised mental health problems and serving physicians treating mental health problems disguised as medical complaints. At the same time, tremendous member demand and expectation for freestanding mental health and counseling services had developed. Handling this became the main challenge for the department. A great deal of high quality, and often inspired, mental health work went on behind the closed doors of the department, invisible to and unappreciated by medical providers, who increasingly experienced the doors being closed on *them*. Physicians often characterized referral to mental health as sending their patients to "a black hole." This kind of story is not at all unusual. We have heard similar stories all across the country. Parallel and distant medical and mental health services have been the rule, not the exception.

It was in this setting that we and the mental health department began piloting the integration of behavioral health clinicians in primary care and specialty clinics 10 or 12 years ago. Collaborative care in our setting is a set of responses to the problems in *taking care of patients* and *the delivery of health care services*. The basic problem is that the traditional separation of biomedical and psychosocial health care services has offered patients and their caregivers a forced choice: organic or functional, biomedical or mental health; two kinds of problems, two kinds of providers, two kinds of clinics, and two kinds of covered benefits. This tradition continues even though it is clear that many, if not most, clinical presentations result from the interplay of biomedical and psychosocial factors. The result of superimposing this either-or structure on a continuous reality creates clinical fragmentation, poor service, operational inefficiencies, and financial waste.

Every clinic, medical group, integrated service delivery system, network, or other health care organization has its own particular difficulties stemming from this general problem. We believe the general principles and practices of collaborative care, implemented structurally in a program of integrated primary care, will play an important role in relieving this general problem and its specific manifestations.

Keep in mind that in our particular organization, the earliest interest and leadership for primary care/behavioral health integration was mostly from the mental health side of the house, and consequently our story is told by us from the perspective of mental health people reaching out to medical clinics. That's not *necessary*; it's just how it was here. Once the early pilots began, more and more people from the medical side of the house joined the effort. The commitment to bringing mental health services into medical settings came from the experience of the authors and from those physicians and medical leaders who saw the potential in it. It was based both on the practical need to solve problems that had developed in a parallel system and on an intellectual commitment to finding a model that transcends the artificial mind/body dichotomy for addressing human problems.

THE FIRST PILOT

Our first demonstration project began in 1984, with one health psychologist (CJP), one dentist, one physical therapist, one dental assistant, and one receptionist who built up an integrated team within a dental clinic for patients with TMD (temporomandibular disorder) referred by physicians and dentists from the entire care system. TMD is a common cause of jaw pain, ear pain, headache, and problems with jaw function. TMD patients often clench or grind their teeth and have other habits of muscle bracing. Prior to our project, these patients often received disconnected trials of dental therapy, physical therapy, and sometimes mental health therapies, but often enough did not really get better or stay better. Their care was usually *sequential and independent* rather than *simultaneous and integrated*. This patient group appeared to complain about their care and ask for referrals to outside specialists much more than the average group of patients with a particular disease. These complaints and requests tended to find their way to the desks of the dental director and the member services director, where good solutions were not easy to find. After we formed the TMD team, and began to take care of chronic TMD patients from all across the system, the complaints and requests for trips "to the Mayo clinic to find out what's *really* wrong" dried up for both the dental director and the member services department.

Over a six-year period, CJP hand-picked a small group of health psychologists to do similar work in the primary care and specialty clinics of the care system. The written mission for this separated-from-the-mainstream group was:

> To create within HealthPartners an innovation in the provision of health care services. This innovation shall be marked by:
>
> - A biopsychosocial model of human health
> - Paradigm shifting methods for synergizing the work of psychological and medical professionals
> - The integration of medical and mental health care at clinics with health psychologists
> - The appearance of seamless care systems for complex patients for whom separate medical and mental health care leads to unsatisfactory clinical, systems, and financial outcomes.

The goals were to formulate and demonstrate within HealthPartners clinics much improved clinical, operational, and financial practices for integrating the psychosocial dimension of health care.

From 1984 to about 1991 this group gradually established "beach-heads" in about 14 primary care and specialty clinics. What characterized this very early stage was hand-picked and trained health psychologists for hand-picked clinics. Nonstandard clinical, operational, and financial methods were specifically designed for integrated work as a normal part of medical clinics. Of the many possible primary care and specialty clinics, only the most interested and ready ("ripest") ones became pilot sites with a psychologist on staff, on site. During this stage, CJP exerted a great deal of control on choice of staff and clinics, and how the clinics would incorporate the psychologist. It was a series of consistently designed and supervised experiments across the care system, loaded for success, using a highly dedicated and mutually supportive group of health psychologists. Salaries and leadership energies for this small group were funded, and tracked separately, by the mental health department as part of its contribution to the organization's overall effort to build a better care system.

These experiments were considered successful: valuable to physicians, patients, and the care system. Clinical, operational, and financial paradigms for integrated care were demonstrated well enough and broadly enough that by 1991 it was time to begin moving the experiments into the mainstream. By this time, RLH had joined the organization and together we set out to bring the experience from the 1984–91 pilot to the mainstream.

By 1996 the pilots had evolved considerably from what they looked like in 1991. RLH's current challenge is to pilot behavioral health integration in several new clinics (the old experiments continue in several of the original clinics), but with regular staff, mainstream systems and "rules," no "experimental" resource budget, no protection from greatly intensified market pressures clinics are experiencing, and an increased expectation for hard data on results. This means running pilots with far less control over staffing, resources, goals, methods, and style than during the era of the early health psychology pilots. We now subject our pilot projects to mainstream forces and conditions, with much less of the "hand-built" attention and control of the early days. But since they are for practical reasons to operate only in a portion of the total care system, we still call them pilots.

THE JOB OF A PILOT PROJECT

A pilot is a *demonstration* of value and feasibility. The pilot must demonstrate and test all key design concepts you intend to use later in the mainstream. That means a pilot project should be designed to work *clinically*, *operationally*, and *financially*. These are the three key perspectives, or "three simultaneous worlds of the health care system" required for real-world success (Peek & Heinrich, 1995). Without demonstrating feasibility from all three perspectives or "worlds," the pilot will be neither convincing to skeptics nor enough of a learning experience for the "champions" trying to bring it to fruition. It will go nowhere in the mainstream. The principle is, "If an action fails in one of the worlds, it will eventually fail in all three." Everyone has seen what happens when a program is worked out in one of the worlds, but not in the others. It is easy to elicit examples where clinicians presented great ideas only to have them shot down for lack of an operations or resource plan. Or where insurance ideas or benefits decisions were shot down because they made no clinical sense. Or where operational systems were designed without a basic understanding of the clinical process they were to support. Everyone knows the personal and organizational tension created when the clinical, operational, and financial perspectives clash rather than collaborate with each other.

Since a pilot is a *demonstration* of all these key design elements, the goal is to find out if it *can* effectively work all these elements together.

At this stage the goal isn't to demonstrate that it can work in *any* clinic, with *any* set of staff, or at *any* pace. As our colleague Thom Davis says, "First you make it *work*, then you make it work *right*, then you make it work *efficiently*" (personal communication, 1991). Pick the best persons you can find to staff it, the clinic where the medical people are most ready. The very first pilot is to show that it *can* work well, in at least one spot. In this very beginning pilot stage, hand-pick the people and the clinic. Load the pilot for success.

Moving to the mainstream can be thought of as going from a "hand-built bench model" to a "repeatable production model." Experience from the pilot project is used to design things to work in the "standard ordinary clinic" with "standard ordinary clinicians. But in reality, there is no sharp distinction between the pilot and the mainstream. Over time, things get less "pilot-like" and more "mainstream-like."

Other Functions of a Pilot

A pilot project should also open up alternatives to prevailing mental models and stimulate organizational change. As the pilot evolves, let people know about it. Feed the imagination of people across the system. Make sure leadership is in the loop; use the pilot to cultivate the understandings needed for the next step. Don't wait until the pilot is "done" and then engage people "cold" for the next step. Warm people up all along, because if the larger system is completely cut off from what you're doing while you get more and more excited and more and more *different*, you end up greatly hurting your chances for broader implementation.

You must do more than make sure people know what's going on; you must also export the intellectual capital or "harvest the learnings" as you go along. The pilot should become a source of new "popular wisdom" and "interest in change" circulating in the culture. Compact nuggets learned along the way are especially helpful. Here is one example. The health psychology group began to put what it learned from the school of hard knocks in the form of "mottos" they could quote to each other and use to teach new health psychologists. One of the early ones says, "Most *difficult* patients started out as merely *complex*." Another is "The right kind of time at the *front* of a case saves time over the *life* of the case." Mottos like these were catchy, humorous, and appealed to things everyone already recognized but often ignored. Things like that circulating in the culture help create a sort of intellectual readiness ahead of you. It's very important to project as much "intellectual capital" and "inspiration" into your future as you can.

CHARACTERISTICS OF A CLINIC READY FOR A PILOT

Look for a small group of physicians willing to meet and talk about what they would like to see, what they want different in their lives in the clinic. Look for more than "I want a mental health person down the hall," as if it were a new part to be bolted on because "you ought to have one." One sign of clinic "ripeness" is the physicians' willingness to meet with you to seriously talk about why they want to do this, why they want to do it now, and why they want to complicate their lives with behavioral health integration.

Engage clinic physicians and staff by asking, "What do you think you could gain from this? What made you think about this now? What's the problem with the way things are now? What kind of outcomes would make it worthwhile? What do you envision as a 'better way'? What are the top five patient-care 'headaches' in your practice? What do you see as your particular obstacles to successful and rewarding practice?" Start with that kind of a dialogue right from the get-go; the kind of questions any good consultant might open with.

Use your own ideas as a springboard, but do it in a way that opens, rather than closes, the dialogue. Leave an invitation and plenty of room for *their* ideas of what the essential features of the pilot need to be. Even though you are going in with some experience and well-formed ideas of what things need to be like in the pilot, this is a mutual creation rather than, "Here it is—this is exactly what you need." You want to reach agreement on what problems the pilot is going to solve and what consciousness the pilot is going to develop. Since the clinic and its physicians need to be your partners in taking care of patients, start by treating them as partners in the creation of the program. You can't achieve a collaborative end with noncollaborative means. It will work better in the long run if the clinic puts its own mark on the plan, rather than letting you tack onto their operation an off-the-shelf product with just *your* mark on it.

It is important to work like a consultant. Commence discussions with different ways of being helpful in mind and be ready with a variety of clinical methods, tools, questions, experience, ways of looking at things. But start discussions where the clinic wants to start them and let the clinic draw from you whatever it needs. Regardless of what *you* think should be important to a clinic, you must start by understanding what the clinic is really struggling with and its own "prescriptions" for itself. Sometimes all the physicians have is their own frustrations to reflect on until someone helps them find new ways of looking at things and practical ways of reducing those frustrations.

Be open to new options that appeal to the clinic. For example, one clinic identified its most important need as improving nursing triage of mental health issues. We never thought of this ourselves, but this clinic's need pointed us toward helping them improve their own clinical assessment of mental health complaints. This help was best provided by a psychiatric nurse working alongside the clinic's medical triage nurses, not by a health psychologist in the usual role alongside the physicians. This has resulted in improved service to patients and more effective collaborative care staffing than we would have thought of by ourselves. Perhaps a clinic feels a need to do better with a particular population or problem such as families dealing with ADHD kids, education and self-care for patients with physical symptoms, or women's health issues.

Articulating Clinic Needs

In years past, physicians often assumed there's a right and wrong way to do things, and asked us to tell them what the right way is, and we usually recommended the highly integrated clinical and relationship model we had been using in health psychology, targeted at chronic illnesses and unfocused utilization. At that time, it was a good "off-the-shelf" answer. But today, competitive pressures have led physicians and clinics to more actively determine their top needs. With today's pilots more subject to mainstream currents and conditions, it is more and more important to elicit physician thinking about what they *really do* need, by way of help and partnership from behavioral health.

Helping the clinic articulate its needs requires a personal appeal to what already matters to providers in their working lives. For example, you can ask, "Has anybody here ever come to work, seen a particular name on the schedule, and wanted to go home?" When the smiles and nods come, you can follow with, "Well, what is it about those patients?" Someone will start, "Well, you know they're not really sick, but they keep coming back mad at me even though I've done all I can do. I end up feeling impotent, helpless, and angry. Sometimes I actually feel like telling them to stop wasting my time, or getting myself fired from the case, but I know I can't do that. I probably know mental health issues are behind the symptoms but I can't for the life of me bring that up successfully. Whenever I try to get them to see that they are depressed, they intensify their *physical* complaints, and they just won't leave me alone." At this point, you have an opening to inquire about how physicians would really like to have these cases unfold in a better way.

Someone else may say, "Yes, but even when my patients *ask* me for a good referral to mental health, I don't know who to refer to. I don't know any of your people over there, and I feel like I'm sending them over to a black hole." This is an opening to talk about the alternatives to mental health referrals.

Another person might say, "We have certain patients in this clinic that end up making us all mad at each other. Our team gets divided somehow. Half of us want to get really tough and the other half want to take the person home and take care of him in our family. This is the stuff that drives us crazy and makes us feel incompetent and sometimes ashamed." There is an opportunity to talk about better teamwork for difficult personalities coming to the clinic.

Someone else might say, "Better appointment availability is what we need here. If we could just reduce the number of unnecessary physician visits, things would be much better for everyone." This is a chance to talk about what wastes appointment time, commonplace clinical challenges that affect appointment availability, or clinic utilization data.

As you talk about the common things that already matter to people, emphasize systemic solutions to difficult areas of clinic life, not isolated techniques or a program. Draw out and legitimize how physicians and other staff feel, in their heart of hearts, about some of their work, and then go on to help them paint a picture of how mental health teamwork could improve clinic life. Most primary care physicians *want* to keep difficult or challenging patients in their practice. It's just that without the right kind of help to do so, they often clench their teeth or entertain escape fantasies. Emphasize that you're not there to take their patients away, either by "off-loading" patients they don't want to see or by "saving" patients from the medical model. The purpose is to prevent clinician frustration, isolation, and emotional reactivity that can lead to inadequate care planning for such complex patients, and to make working with these patients a more effective *normal* part of the clinic.

Patient "ownership" is actually *increased* by behavioral health integration. For example, you can ask a group of physicians, "Have you ever had things you'd like to ask a patient, but are nervous about asking the next question because you might not have a way of dealing with the answer?" Most physicians will smile knowingly at this one. You can then ask, "If you had someone next door to work with, would you be more comfortable asking the next question?" Most physicians will nod to that. Patient ownership increases when you have an immediate and trusted way of handling whatever you might uncover.

Understanding the Clinical, Operational, and Financial World Views

After finding out about the clinic's felt needs, add structure to later conversations by saying that a program should be able to demonstrate and test key clinical, operational, and financial elements of behavioral health/primary care integration. This weaves together two essential concepts: the idea that a pilot is a demonstration of key working elements needed later in the mainstream, and that the pilot must not only test the *clinical* elements, but the *operational* and *financial* elements as well. You've already said a lot, but you have merely opened another stage of discussion.

Since physicians' language or dominant perspective is clinical (rather than operational or financial), this is a great place to engage them first. Once we have a shared view of what the goals are and what the relationships should look like clinically and professionally, then we go on to address the operational and financial worlds.

The Clinical World

A view of what the pilot is to achieve clinically can be achieved with a conversation like the one just described for helping the clinic articulate its needs. But before leaving the clinical world, help the clinic think through its needs and options for "bridging professional cultures" and building relationships with the behavioral health provider.

Explore how the behavioral health professional or therapist could indeed become a "citizen" of the medical clinic. This could mean many things, such as understanding, accepting, and working with medical patients in a medical frame of reference and learning about the top diseases and care management challenges that face primary care physicians. It could mean learning medical customs, language, work style, and ethic, appreciating the different sense of time and scheduling, getting comfortable with stirrups and other paraphernalia in the exam rooms, white coats, walk-in patients, quick "curb-side" consults, and the generally unpredictable nature of a primary care practice.

Ask what kind of relationship the clinic physicians would like to have with their mental health clinician. They may assume there is a specific one-size-fits-all relationship required, or they just haven't thought about anything different than having an on-site referral provider. Explore what kind of citizen they want in their midst. What kind of understandings, technical knowledge, and ready-to-go capabilities are they counting on their therapist to have?

What role do the physicians want their behavioral health clinician to play in their practice? For example, do they want the person to disappear into a corner of the building with the clinic's difficult patients? Do they want someone to *send* patients to with *instructions*, but not to participate prominently in overall care planning? Do they want someone to help their *patients*, but stay outside the physician group and its struggles with patient care? Or do the physicians want someone to help their patients, and, even more, to help *them* with these patients too? Do they want a *team member* who can eventually become a fully trusted "one of us"?

In the same way you bring out the clinic's ideas for better patient care, bring out the clinic's ideas for the professional relationships needed to accomplish those goals. Create a neutral, accepting moment for the clinic physicians to put into words what they really want, might dare to want, or have merely *assumed* they want by way of professional relationship with a behavioral health clinician. If they draw a blank, saying, "We don't know anything about this. Tell us what *you* think would work best; that's why you're here today," go ahead and paint a picture of a clinician well-integrated as a normal part of a medical clinic. But link elements of that picture to what you know *already matters* to them. Include branching options in the picture, where it isn't clear what kind of patient outcomes, professional relationships, or "team intimacy" matters to them.

The Operational World
Ask about what the pilot would mean to operational systems like space, transcription, chart flow. How and where should the scheduling be done? Would the behavioral health person work in the medical clinic, but depend on a call to a distant mental health clinic for scheduling or message support? Imagine the medical transcriptionists doing chart notes from a mental health provider. Imagine the behavioral health provider working out of clinic space. Do people envision a big office with a couch and a fern? If so, they either draw a blank ("we don't have the space") or envision it in some far off corner of the building. Engage people in imagining the behavioral health person working out of an exam room, right in the traffic pattern like everyone else. Have them imagine the effects of space and scheduling on communication and the feeling patients will get as a result. Ask people to test such ideas, first in their imaginations and later in practice.

Don't dwell on the details at this point or try to solve them operationally. The goal at this stage is to *touch* things like this just enough to help them achieve a picture of their preferred future. Do not make the project seem like a big new load on an already stretched clinic. As for actually making it work later, "the devil is in the details," but the attitude for now is "clear away the brush as you go."

The Financial World
When you get to the financial world, you will face questions such as, "When a diabetic person sees his or her mental health person in the clinic, is the visit a medical visit or a mental health visit for financial purposes?" In a managed care context, "What co-pay is charged? Is the visit checked off the remaining mental health visits to which they may

use? Or is this visit just another medical visit, like visits to the diabetes nurse, the nutritionist, the nurse practitioner, the endocrinologist, or the primary care physician?"

What logic governs this? The "three worlds" paradigm says that all action must make sense in all three worlds in order to succeed. That means not only that there must be clinical, operational, and financial plans, but also that these plans must *cooperate* rather than *clash* with each other. The three worlds of health care are like the three engineering drawings of a machine part: the front view, the top view, and the side view. A coherent notion of the *whole* is needed before sketching in the clinical, operational, and financial views of it. Just as an engineer can't go down to the production floor with a front view and top view, but no side view, we can't go to health system management with a great clinical idea unspecified operationally and financially. Even if health system managers let the project slip by with a clinical view of one thing, an operational view of a different thing, and a financial view of an entirely different thing, the project will certainly unravel later at the full-scale "production" stage.

Our own answer to whether a diabetic patient's visits to the clinic's behavioral health clinician are medical visits or mental health visits has been clear, especially in our earliest pilot stage. Everything pointed to building a new way of doing *medicine*, where the behavioral health provider is a long-missing team member bringing a long-missing set of skills to medical care. Therefore, the visits are medical visits. They are to be counted as part of total medical costs, subject to whatever co-pays apply to medical visits, and are not checked off against mental health visit allotment. We have always considered this a key element of our model, and have worked from it in all the early pilots since 1984. This is written up as a "four-sector model" of integrated health care in the same article containing the "three worlds" paradigm (Peek & Heinrich, 1995).

It is worth saying a little more here about the financial models used in the pilots. We have operated in a mostly capitated environment. That means most of our patients (and their employers) pay a flat rate for a comprehensive package of care. It is up to the care system to field the right team in the clinics to effectively take care of the patients, wisely using the resources these "customers" contribute up front for the care. Hence, clinic finances are driven mostly by clinic membership and fixed budgets, not fees. Designated mental health and medical benefits correspond to portions of the overall flat rate that employers and members pay. Even with the advent of "self-insured" employers, the overall system behaves as capitated.

In the beginning, the mental health department sponsored the health psychology demonstrations by supplying leadership and health psychologist salaries. This was a very small portion of the overall mental health capitation, and was tracked separately as a contribution to the overall goal of building a better care system. (All managers across the care system are to be engaged in "building a better mousetrap," and this was one way the mental health department was fulfilling that obligation). The clinics received their health psychologists "free," courtesy of the mental health department, although health psychology visits for medical problems were counted as *medical*, rather than *mental health*, visits for co-pays, support staff, space, and other local expense, and in utilization figures.

As we moved further into the mainstream, the clinics themselves began to pick up the behavioral health expense (at least that portion dedicated to the medical care of medical patients). They are building this expense into their budgets the same way they build in nursing, nurse practitioner, and physician expense. But clinics were not *told* to do so. Medical and mental health leadership jointly asked clinics to choose whether to incorporate the health psychology component as a normal part of their budgets (as well as their clinical and operational worlds), or let it go. All the clinics with the original health psychology pilots elected to budget for and retain their health psychologists, and those funds (original pilot "seed money") were to be moved to the medical care budget. The process of accomplishing all this is still underway.

Several new pilot sites are now working with a blend of medical and mental health goals and a blend of medical and mental health budgeting. Earlier we said there is no sharp line dividing pilot from mainstream; it is more like a gradual transition. With that gradual transition comes a mixture of old and new paradigms and methods that leads to a certain amount of unavoidable "mess" in the operational and financial worlds. This is a normal part of making practical transitions. A new financial model able to support integrated clinical models must at the same time be made intelligible to existing systems in the old paradigm such as insurance companies and government payers. It takes continuing work to develop new financial models while remaining intelligible within the old models. The "final" financial model is yet to arrive. There is little controversy about the clinical ideas, goals, and methods. They have been around for a long time and make a lot of sense to anyone practicing in the real world. The controversy usually comes in drawing the operational and financial views to match!

Nursing and Clinic Management Readiness

When we look for pilot sites, we are not only looking for *physician* readiness. We may start with the physicians, but there are other important "customers" for a pilot like this, especially nursing and clinic management.

In many of our clinics, nurses are key players who are not always present in the initial discussions. Clinics may employ triage nurses, consulting nurses, rooming nurses, or specialty nurses, for example, who care for diabetic patients. Nurses are often interested, already involved, and have a day-to-day perspective on patients moving through the clinic. In some clinics it's a nurse who knows the most about patients, their families, and psychosocial factors. Nurses often help patients and families engage in their care, including referrals to specialists or other caregivers. Nurses often provide physicians and patients with very helpful follow-through and preparation, and are often informal or formal leaders in the clinic. So bring nurses aboard!

Clinic administrators and managers are also very important. If the pilot is to function in the clinical, operational, and financial worlds, it's hopeless to think the physicians alone will carry it off. The pilot will affect operational systems like space, schedules, dictation, accounting, etc., as we mentioned earlier. You need to have key operations managers, whatever their particular titles, in the discussions as soon as you realize the physician group is interested in pursuing the idea further. Clinic managers need to understand the clinical vision, and then help craft the operational and financial world methods to help carry it off. They have to be brought in as full partners in the pilot or it will fail.

All formal and informal leaders in the clinic should be involved. It helps if individuals playing key roles in the whole clinic develop an interest in dealing more effectively with mental health issues in primary care. This is another sign of "ripeness" for the pilot. Bring key people along, whatever their profession or role in the clinic. Help the physicians understand how it helps to bring the nurses, managers, receptionists, informal leaders, and other key players into the picture, even though at the core, the pilot is a clinical thing. It's frustrating to fight uphill battles later on, merely because someone with a key role or with misgivings about mental health was overlooked during the planning. All who exert leadership in the clinic have the potential to be helpful (or unhelpful) in the pilot, and later on during mainstreaming.

WHAT A CLINIC NEEDS TO KNOW
BEFORE PROCEEDING

Patient Case Mix

While helping a clinic assess its readiness for a behavioral health integration pilot, it is good to ask if the information systems in place can show the patient case mix of the clinic. We have found it useful to look together at information about the clinic's current patients in useful statistical terms. This is important nowadays because the assignment for health systems is to take care of *populations* as well as *individuals*, and to do so with good stewardship of (usually fixed) resources. Therefore, it helps to characterize the population in terms of risk factors, utilization patterns, distribution of patient stage of life (child, adult, elderly, families), and presenting problems. Then, if you can, look at clinic performance with prevention and management of certain diseases measured against guidelines or benchmarks. There is a great deal of development effort going on in this area right now. In Minnesota, entire care systems and clinics are publicly compared to one another on standard measures of satisfaction, cost, and quality.

Here is one small example in the area of service utilization. RLH once plotted the distribution of patients and utilization for four large primary care clinics that took care of a total of 60,000 patients in about 300,000 visits for one year. In these four clinics combined, 23% of the patients used about 53% of the visits, and 2% of the patients used about 10% of the visits. This proportion was about the same across all four clinics. Also, each clinic had patients who visited more than 100 times per year, and all four had at least one patient who came in over 140 times! This distribution was startling to us and to clinic leaders. The burning question was, "What is going on in those top 2% or 10% of cases?" We had no answer then, but showing the data and posing the question itself generated clinic interest in better understanding its high-utilizing patients, a group we believe behavioral health/primary care integration is particularly helpful for. Our family practice department head, Steve Lucas, calls this group the "overserviced and underserved." Early data suggests that physician utilization is reduced and better focused with an integrated approach to these patients.

Even in the pilot stage it is important to be thinking about what mainstream effects you eventually want. Raise consciousness about desired goals (e.g., the overserviced and underserved), and corresponding measurements. Sketch possible measurements and the information systems that could be used to evaluate the pilot. Include something, even if it's very basic, about clinic case mix and potential clinical targets for collaborative care interventions. Create at least "placeholder" outcome measurements so they remain part of the picture, even if unsophisticated. Using patient case mix information, as sophisticated or crude as it is, helps the clinic decide which patients the pilot should focus on.

The point is to build an evaluation and measurement mindset into the pilot, and keep it there, even if your measures are initially crude. After all, you may not get a high-class evaluation function in a pilot demonstration project. The pilot is there to demonstrate all the essential features, including evaluation, but is unlikely to have the kind of sophistication or academic credibility that your mainstream evaluation function may require.

Realistic Time Frames

Help the clinic to be realistic about when to expect things to change by seeding the discussion with questions about how long it takes to develop effective working relationships of the kind it is shooting for. Help the group to keep a realistic view of their readiness to collaborate and what it takes to develop collaborative relationships, to the extent their goals require them. Contrast the time it takes to "tack on a new technique" versus the time to build an effective care team. This should be part of early discussions about when to start, how much time to allow for getting it up and running, and a realistic time frame for seeing changes and results for patients and providers.

The choice of mental health professional for the role affects the realistic time frame. Will it be someone with well-developed behavioral medicine and collaboration skills and cultural adaptation in this area, or will it be an interested therapist whom we train in medical clinic practice from scratch? What level of seasoned clinical skill and ready-to-go capability is the clinic looking for in its behavioral health provider? (Hopefully you already have had these discussions before selecting a person for the role).

Choosing the Mental Health Provider

We've come to appreciate the clinic that wants to interview prospective team members rather than take whoever comes. It tells us something about the interest and readiness to assimilate a team member as "one of us." The group that says they want to interview candidates already has a sense that the person chosen is to be someone important to the clinic, is going to be part of the team, and wants to be sure it is someone with whom they can live. Their interviewing makes it easier for them to choose how "seasoned" a person they are comfortable taking on. This affects *their* lives and time frame.

By interview time, it's important for the clinic to recall what they are trying to build in the first place. Without a clear picture of what they are trying to do, and how the behavioral health clinician needs to fit this, the clinic will have little to interview *from*. Help the interviewers remember what they are hoping to accomplish in partnership with this prospective behavioral health provider.

PREPARING THE MENTAL HEALTH CLINICIANS FOR ROLES IN MEDICAL CLINICS

In our experience, behavioral health clinicians do not need a particular "school of therapy" orientation to work in medical clinics. One particular background, such as cognitive-behavioral, short-term, or solution-focused, does not necessarily make a clinician better suited for primary care.

I (RLH) spend time in our oncology clinic with two health psychologists. Several months ago one of them and I interviewed a cancer patient together. I am trained as a psychiatrist with background in behavioral and family systems medicine, psychobiology, and cognitive-behavior therapy. The psychologist came from a counseling psychology training program and a pharmacy background before that. Her orientation is broadly humanistic, cognitive-behavioral, and she is a skilled practitioner of mind-body approaches including hypnosis and visualization. During the interview, sometimes she took the lead and sometimes I took the lead, but either way, the timing and things we focused on were almost identical. It was striking how the pacing, timing, focus, and way of relating to patients had to do with a way of working that is learned over time. The approach isn't cognitive-behavioral or family systems or solution-oriented; it's a melding of all of these approaches and more, shaped by the demands of this kind of work. Over time in this work, we become much more alike than different.

In selecting a behavioral health professional to work in primary care, we want to know what the person knows how to do, and something about their general grasp and know-how with the generic challenges in this kind of work. While interviewing someone, we often ask how he or she describes his or her profession. Many will automatically say, "I'm a psychotherapist" or "I'm a family therapist" or "I do therapy and biofeedback." But sometimes a person says something like, "I am a health care clinician, with training and credentials in [whatever] area." He or she is identifying with the generic profession of *health care clinician* (the team), rather than identifying only with the specific techniques that belong to his or her profession (the "guild"). We find that the more seasoned in this work a person becomes, the more he or she identifies with the generic skills and responsibilities of *health care clinician* as well as with his or her specific credentialed skills and techniques.

Generic Care Management Challenges

Experience has taught us to value systematic development of the care system and *generic* clinician skills and responsibilities needed in the overall process of taking care of patients. But physicians on the interviewing team may initially approach this with a *specialty* mindset. They may say to a mental health provider, "We need help with certain diseases" or "We want you to provide us with certain referral therapies or techniques." This difference between a generalist and specialist approach is worth discussing further.

Clinicians tend to think in diagnostic categories or about *techniques*. They tend to think first about *diseases* with which they have difficulty and the *techniques* that they might want to have available, not the *generic care management challenges* across diseases. There are common generic challenges around many specific diseases, for headache, chronic pain, diabetes, asthma, gastrointestinal problems, and so on. Clinicians must understand specific issues relative to the organ systems or disease processes involved *and* recognize and master the generic care management challenges for achieving recovery or care across all those diagnoses. For example:

- Disability management is not itself a disease, but a generic care management challenge that crosses all chronic illnesses and injuries. It has to do with helping patients resume life, rather than seeing them gradually become disabled. Sometimes managing the *disability* is a much bigger challenge than managing the *disease*.
- Another generic challenge is helping the suffering patient who has a very different understanding of her illness from that of her physician, is mad at her doctor for "not getting it," and wants a trip to the Mayo Clinic "where they know what they're doing." When confidence and health care relationships are on the skids, technically appropriate care is unlikely to "take."
- A similar challenge is treating the patient whose emotional life is intertwined with his physical problems but insists on a purely physiological explanation and cure. Learning to care for patients who do not yet make the connections between physical symptoms and personal realities is needed for many diseases.
- It is not uncommon to find yourself serving a patient whose family chaos or social poverty is really much more threatening to recovery than the illness itself. For example, patients living in actively abusive situations often appear to be swimming upstream when it comes to managing their symptoms and illnesses.
- Everyone has had "difficult patients" or, more properly, "difficult

patient-clinician relationships" (Keller & Carroll, 1994). Yet clinicians and the care system are capable of turning ordinary *complex* cases into *difficult* patients if the complexity is not dealt with well early on. Hence the care management motto, "Most *difficult* patients started out merely as *complex*."

- This generic issue faces everyone: "How do I know when I need a team and when I don't?" Specifically: "When do I just proceed on my own? When do I just make a referral to some specialty medical or mental health care that I don't really need to be part of? When do I need consultation to do it right? When do I need to integrate the care in a tight team approach, well-orchestrated with a "jointly owned" care plan? When and how do I recognize and address the complex interplay of both biomedical and psychosocial agendas?"

Most clinicians recognize these generic challenges, but often they do not think to design a project with the generic issues (rather than specific diseases and techniques) in mind. Clinicians as a broad group could benefit from shared repertoire for meeting these challenges.

Much of this clinical repertoire is generic, suitable for use by any health care professional, not just the behavioral health person. We use the concept of "ecology of care" (Peek & Heinrich, 1995) to help people see beyond their own interests and niche into the broader arena in which care must be managed and collaboration must take place. We hope to see a common culture of care delivery gradually emerge, based on what it means to be a health care clinician (not just an internist, family practitioner, or psychotherapist), and what it means to collaborate. This broader umbrella of challenges that face all of us is the key to long-range, mainstream success. This is a different focus for physicians and other clinicians everywhere, who are oriented primarily to *their* professions, techniques, and target diseases.

Profession versus Technique

Distinguishing between profession and technique stimulates people to think more broadly about what they do. For example, psychotherapy can be viewed as a *profession* or as a *set of techniques*. Techniques include hypnosis (and there are hypnotists), acupuncture (and there are acupuncturists), biofeedback (and there are certified biofeedback practitioners), and the list goes on. But is a profession any more than a technique or set of techniques? We like to think of a profession as having not only its exclusive techniques, but also *general* capabilities and obligations.

The psychotherapy example is especially relevant here. We have been talking about patients with significant mental health or behavioral issues factored into their overall health concerns, whether they know it or not. It is common for patients to hold their entire suffering in a medical frame of reference, even when a purely medical approach has little or nothing to offer them. These patients are unlikely to seek psychotherapy on their own and are often quite reluctant to accept psychotherapy referrals. Only when they glimpse that the way they are living or feeling may have something to do with their suffering, will they consider a mental health referral.

However, there exists a common pejorative stereotype that psychotherapists often do not engage these patients, describing them as "not good therapy candidates." The therapist may probe for a "personal or psychotherapy agenda" then complain that all the patient could think about was his headaches and fatigue. The root phenomenon giving rise to these stories is the psychotherapist who is so identified with doing traditional psychotherapy (the techniques) that he or she does not realize that the situation calls for something besides traditional application of these techniques. In this case, the situation calls for the therapist to help a patient distill a personal agenda out of a whole pot of physical suffering and anger at life or medical people, while allowing the patient to retain the medical frame of reference for the suffering. This does not necessarily look or sound like psychotherapy to the patient or to the therapist. We suggest that mental health clinicians who have developed this part of their professional repertoire have expanded their profession beyond the techniques of psychotherapy into the profession of health care. The *profession* has exceeded its exclusive *techniques*.

I (CJP) am reminded (Peek & Heinrich, 1995) of a music teacher I once knew, who distinguished between *instrument* lessons and *music* lessons. He always said, "Your first instrument is the hardest, because you have to learn *music* along with it." He sensitized his students to fundamental skills and sensibilities that transcend any one instrument but unite them all under the umbrella of music. He emphasized things like timing, harmony, reading music, intonation, communication with the ensemble, improvising, recovering from mistakes, controlling anxiety, rehearsing, learning your own strengths and weaknesses. For him, this was *musicianship* and was more fundamental than any one instrument. He said you can later learn other *instruments* much more easily because you don't have to learn *music* again. But he also said, with great sorrow, that some people learn an instrument but never learn music. From him I learned that music is more fundamental than any of its instruments. I also learned that what unites musicians is not so much their chosen instrument but their shared musicianship. Ensembles are governed by their common understanding of music: good musicianship. This makes for good ensemble playing.

I think this is an apt metaphor for health care professionals who want to operate in the larger collaborative context we have been talking about. As a particular kind of professional, a physician, social worker, psychiatrist, nurse, psychologist, whatever, you play an instrument in the ensemble of health care professions. We, as health care professionals, must speak meaningfully about *good providership* just as musicians speak of *good musicianship*. Even musicians who have never played together can often sit down and play together quite well, united by their shared musicianship. Clinicians need shared "good providership" if they are going to work with expanded roles in large contexts where they aren't necessarily going to know each other personally. We need more than ever to share a common ground of good providership regardless of our particular "professional ethnicity."

We usually think of our profession in the broadest terms as *health care clinician*. As physicians or behavioral health professionals, our *specific* profession is a *species* of health care clinician, one voice in the chorus of health care providers. We find that emphasizing this distinction helps people develop the common culture across disciplines needed for collaboration. A literature has been building on principles and models for collaboration between mental health and medical practitioners, for example, Cummings, Cummings, and Johnson (1997), Doherty and Baird (1983, 1986, 1987), McDaniel, Campbell, and Seaburn (1995), and Seaburn, Lorenz, Gunn, Gawinski, and Mauksch (1996), to name just a few.

Care Plan versus Technique

A care plan is the agreement between the clinicians, the patient, and the family for the entire care of a specified problem. It contains diagnoses, contributing factors, participants, roles, goals, treatments, structure, timing, and anything else needed to convey what the whole case is about and how the care is supposed to go. Techniques are chosen for their combined ability to serve the care plan. For example, the care plan for chronic headaches might involve diet change, medication, muscle relaxation, and improved understanding, recognition, and control of behavioral and emotional headache triggers. Various techniques such as biofeedback, relaxation exercises, physical therapy exercises, and psychotherapy might be brought forward in combination, using a team, to help the patient manage headaches.

Sometimes clinicians think of their own techniques as *the* care plan, rather than as *ingredients* to an overall care plan that includes, but goes beyond them. Thinking of *your* own techniques as *the* care plan can lead to an unconnected series of providers applying a series of techniques, rather than a coordinated effort. The mindset we try to cultivate is captured by the following pair of care management mottos:

- Evaluation of the *case* informs the evaluation of *today's problem.*
- Care plans precede technique application, and techniques are always subordinated to care plans.

Training

At the beginning of our health psychology program in 1985, there was only one health psychologist, and training was done via individual mentorships. Each new psychologist was hired because he or she indicated a strong interest in medical clinic work and collaborative care and had suitable credentials as a psychologist. Each new person was assigned a health psychologist mentor and "acculturated" by spending the first couple of weeks traveling with the mentor, getting to know clinic people, and sitting in on the mentor's sessions in the medical clinics. As the new person began to see patients, the mentor sat in on many of the sessions. (It is common practice in medical settings for medical students, residents, and other health care professionals to shadow and be shadowed by the regular providers.) For a few weeks, the schedule was set slower than usual to allow time for debriefing and coaching. Gradually, the pace was increased and the sitting-in and debriefing time was decreased according to the mutual comfort of the mentor and mentee.

All new health psychologists participated in such an acculturating mentorship for six months as one of the terms for joining the group. By that time it would be clear whether the skills and "fit" would be right for continuing in that role. A formal review and group celebration occurred when this six-month marker was successfully passed. The most recently trained person generally became a mentor for the next new person in the spirit of "see one, do one, teach one."

However, that does not mean the end of supervision, training, and consultation. All health psychologists attend a weekly 90-minute case rounds group, and have done so for 10 years. Discussion of challenging cases brings out the accumulated knowledge and wisdom of the group. Not only do new health psychologists have the opportunity and obligation to put their tough cases on the table, they also learn from everyone else's tough cases. Case rounds is not only about the care of the patient, but also about the therapist's own relationship to the work and the care system. Case rounds still is the primary ongoing training modality for the health psychology group. No one "graduates" from case rounds.

Case rounds starts with a check-in: "Here are the cases that are on my mind." Criteria for putting a case on the table include when *you* have symptoms about the case, not just when the *patient* presents with a challenging picture. The goal is that everyone with a case that puzzles them or gives them cold hands goes out of the room with a next step to take. The other, equally important function of case rounds is to build common culture and best practices among the group going out to medical clinics. The health psychology group began to capture the wisdom that experience had been teaching them in the form of the care management mottos we have quoted here. This set of about 40 mottos expresses the basic intellectual capital of the group, built up over years of practice.

As the project moved into RLH's hands and more into the mainstream, RLH and others developed a mentoring program for mental health clinicians already on staff in the mental health department but not working in the medical clinics. It was a pilot training program that drew heavily from the individual mentorship program for the health psychologists, but was designed to appeal to what matters to all established mental health clinicians with interest in learning to do what we called "integrated care." This mentorship program included a series of classes, time shadowing a health psychologist, and a version of case rounds.

Four introductory classes were given, a month apart, building on the idea of adapting what mental health clinicians *already know*, such as how to do comprehensive evaluations. They were taught how to do a basic evaluation from a psychobiological, behavioral medicine, health psychology, or mind-body perspective. The four lectures focus on four clinical areas: variations of pain complaints, headaches (because headaches are so common everywhere in primary care), managing chronic illness (with a focus on terminal illness as well as other kinds of chronic illnesses), and assessing children and families with medical illness.

People also shadowed a seasoned health psychologist for a day or two in the clinic. They experienced the pace and feel of the clinic, the kinds of people working and getting care in medical clinics, what medical charts look like, how scheduling works, how to greet a patient and discuss medical concerns, and how to talk about life and mental health factors in the context of physical complaints.

As mentioned, we also established case rounds for these mental health clinicians and their mental health cases, hoping that it would help them recognize and gain comfort in addressing mind-body or medical-mental health interactions in the complaints or in the treatments. We have found that it does not work as well for mental health clinicians to bring their current *mental health* cases to case rounds as it does for the health psychologists to bring their current *medical* clinic cases. We recommend getting people in the medical situation and training them with cases that arise from that context.

Supporting both Teams and Guilds

Clinicians of a given stripe organize themselves into departments, or what we sometimes call "guilds," representing a single discipline or closely related cluster of disciplines. These define quality, community standards, and scope of practice for that discipline. Clinicians also tend to organize themselves into teams in order to divide the labor and expertise needed to treat a population of patients. We believe that clinicians need to be members of both teams (which deliver the goods to patients) *and* guilds (which deliver high-quality "position players" to the teams). Team members need to understand what is common good practice among *all* clinicians in order to formulate common goals and follow-through. Without team membership, you are a soloist (or paired with someone just like yourself, which is probably not much of a team). At the same time, if you are to be any good to a team, you will have to be a competent, disciplined master of your craft, a fine position player. So you also need membership in your guild to stay sharp, to get feedback on your own special repertoire, and to face colleagues who let you know good craft from poor craft.

At an organizational level, health care systems employing health care professionals need to cultivate interdisciplinary care teams in clinics to take care of patients. They also need to nourish departments (made up of the members of a discipline) in order to maintain quality control and keep a good supply of sharp players for those teams. Organizations need managers whose job is to build, mentor, and maintain teams. They also need managers whose job is to build, mentor, and maintain the guilds. They also need upper managers to maintain a balance between the resources and influence belonging to both teams and guilds. (Unless steps are specifically taken to prevent it, guilds and teams tend to begin jockeying for influence). Guilds and teams need each other to stay healthy. Therefore, we try to build professional communities among clinicians within both guilds and teams.

Guild Support

Even seasoned mental health professionals piloting integrated care in medical clinics should not be sent out there as "lone rangers." They are likely to be the only mental health professional in the entire clinic, unlike the physicians who have peers to talk to about cases. Everyone needs colleagues to bounce things off of. This is especially true in the early stages, when the clinic often focuses its new health psychologist on its "worst" cases.

At HealthPartners, we have established a professional community of behavioral health providers who go out to medical clinics. These behavioral health providers are not themselves a team; they are position players for the teams out in the medical clinics. This group of health psychologists and other clinicians in the same role meets 90 minutes weekly at the same time and place for the case rounds meeting described earlier. The purpose is for each person to get help with challenging casework so he or she can go back the next week with the benefit of peer coaching and good ideas (and without "white knuckles").

Nourishing such a professional community has to be an explicit part of your management practices. For example, the health psychologists not only are *allowed* to meet weekly in case rounds, but they also *expect* each other to. Performance expectations apply to participation in this meeting. Support the professional community of behavioral health clinicians who establish pilots at medical clinics because it also plays a vital role in the mainstream stage. We operate from the proposition that "an organization is a community with a mission" (Putman, 1990). Explicit methods such as case rounds are required if this is to be anything more than a slogan.

Team Support

How the medical clinic supports its team is less under our control than how we support our behavioral health clinicians. Clinics often have clinician meetings, although they are frequently administrative in nature. The behavioral health clinicians participate in clinic meetings if held on their day in the clinic. We encourage clinics to coordinate their scheduled meetings with the schedule of the behavioral health clinician. We seed the idea of group meetings with *clinical* purpose and content, and this occurs to various degrees in various ways. In what we sometimes call a "mature" clinic, this kind of professional community development takes place as a normal part of clinician relationships, and some teams build up recognized standards and community practices about how to handle casework. A functional equivalent of case rounds may develop, and we have certainly seen high degrees of interdependency, trust, mutual accountability, and "intellectual capital" build up in the more mature clinic teams (Lucas & Peek, 1997).

However, at the pilot stage of development, most medical clinics are not able to support the professional-community needs of a behavioral health provider. Not only because there may be only one or two behavioral health providers there (hence no guild group), but also because medical clinics rarely come with a culture that emphasizes peer consultation, some functional equivalent of case rounds, or the development of increasing group competence and "common property" among their various clinicians. Some clinics are modeling teamwork and development of cross-disciplinary understandings in the organization, but this is a very gradual change in medical culture.

LAUNCHING A PILOT

There will come a day to start the pilot.

1. Be sure the shared vision is sufficiently operationalized to actually work on the first day. Where exactly will the behavioral health provider work? Is there a mailbox and a phone number? Do the receptionists know how to schedule the person, forward messages? Has his or her name and provider number been entered in the computer? How will his or her time be used during the first week?

2. Set up some checkpoints at the clinic over the first few months: a time and place to look at what has been happening, how things are going, and jointly make course corrections as needed. Don't launch a pilot and then immediately put it on "autopilot." If you and the clinic leaders don't learn what's working and what's not working and make course corrections as you go along, there is a good chance the project will become marginalized in the clinic and then dropped.

3. If possible, start with a psychological professional who already knows how to work in the medical culture and who is trained broadly in health psychology or behavioral medicine — but don't leave even a seasoned behavioral health care provider, sophisticated as he or she may be, alone in the process of becoming a new provider in a primary care clinic. The early phases of working in a clinic, no matter how well the professional is trained, involve entering a unique culture with its own practices, decision-making principles, and ways of doing things. It's particularly stressful during the first four to six months, especially for people new to this role.

4. Establish a supportive professional community in the background; people who have been through this and who will help the therapist solve problems as they come up. This professional community of

support needs to understand, model, and teach the basic challenges and paradigms of collaborative care in the context of daily work. In our setting, this takes place primarily through case rounds, as described earlier.

5. Reinforce all the principles and distinctions for preparing behavioral health providers for roles in medical clinics; they will be turned from theory to practice during the pilot. For example, one of the first and most common situations that behavioral health clinicians will face in a new clinic is a patient who begins the session with, "I have terrible headaches. My life is fine, the headaches are not emotional, and I'm real upset that the doctors haven't figured out what's wrong." One of the mottos we teach our behavioral health clinicians is, "Play the ball where it lies." We teach therapists early how to do mental health work without forcing the patient to give up their medical conception of the problem. It's really not that hard once you have ways to approach headaches that don't require you to deal with "underlying" mental health problems in order to go on. Make use of such principles and distinctions from the very beginning of your pilot.

THE DECISION TO TAKE A STEP
TOWARD THE MAINSTREAM

Evaluate the Pilot

Wherever information systems make it possible, we evaluate the pilot by looking for the impact on patient satisfaction, provider satisfaction, access to physician appointments, and utilization of services such as referrals to consultants, hospital admits, and bed days. A look at treatment outcomes, especially for chronic illness and disability management, somatizing, or other "difficult" patients is also important. Scientific data on much of this is difficult to obtain at the pilot stage. Existing information systems often do not capture everything we would eventually like to look at. But in our experience, enough information can be gathered in the pilot stage to make a reasonable decision about whether to move forward.

Once the pilot is considered successful according to its original goals or whatever data or impressions emerge, it is time to move it toward the mainstream. In our case, this moment came after about five years of the health psychology demonstrations in primary care and specialty clinics.

At that time, CJP made a hand-off to RLH, who took it from there. We eventually said, "Here's what we've all learned from the pilot phase. How has it gone? It's now time to fish or cut bait. What do you want to do?"

We looked at several kinds of data from the pilot:

- the "anecdote bank"
- management outcomes
- appeal to community standard
- overall medical utilization

The Anecdote Bank

The "anecdote bank" is what people say, based on what they can see *by just looking*. Some kinds of firsthand experience require no further data to be convincing, at least for purposes of making local management decisions. For many people, the good reputation enjoyed by the health psychology pilots was enough to conclude that the idea, in some form, should continue. Enough physicians and staff, including clinic chiefs, department heads, or clinic managers, had seen benefits. Testimonials were easy to get, and a number of physicians publicly said things like, "I would never want to go back. Don't take my health psychologist away!"

The reasons given to continue varied across clinics. Some felt that certain patient groups, for example, chronic pain or somatically focused patients, did much better. Some felt that the physicians themselves did much better, and felt much better, about patients with strong mental health factors in their medical complaints. Some felt physician appointment access was improved. Others felt that patient service was improved because the clinic wasn't always sending patients away to a distant mental health clinic or "black hole." Others felt that the physicians and staff were much better at keeping their patients in the clinic, in their practice, rather than having them drift away unhappy. Others felt like their team was more complete or that "this is what family medicine was supposed to be like all along." We collect these anecdotes and have them to share with other clinics who are considering integrating care.

Management Outcomes

For us, a management outcome is a beneficial effect on someone in management. For example, we already mentioned how establishing the temporomandibular disorder (TMD) clinic caused complaints to the dental director and member services director to dry up.

Here's another example of a management outcome. There was once a physician in a primary care clinic who had many chronically ill patients with significant psychosocial factors. This physician was empathic, patient, and popular with these patients. However, the physician was over-whelmed with the neediness of these patients, and was not the best at managing it. The manager of this clinic used to go around publicly saying that the health psychologist "kept one of our doctors from quit-ting" by helping out with the psychosocial factors and teaching the physi-cian about constructively setting limits and successfully finishing out the workday.

Appeal to Community Standard

A variation on a management outcome is setting or conforming to a "community standard." For example, at one point during the 1980s, public concern about insurance benefits for TMD erupted. Hearings took place at the state legislature. People from the university (from whom we patterned our TMD clinic) testified with data about the value of an integrated clinical approach that required an integrated benefits approach. Our organization was mentioned as one of the few that had achieved a good level of care and a matching benefits solution in this area. This helped consolidate the legitimacy of our TMD clinic and was part of the reason it was mainstreamed within the dental division, through a cooperative arrangement with the medical division.

Our experience is that management outcomes and a robust anecdote bank are important, and are often the first "data" to show up. If the principle is "appeal to what already matters," then it is hard to imagine a successful pilot without a favorable anecdote bank, management out-comes, and a growing sense that you are setting a good standard of care. But that is just the beginning. Pilots will need to show more systematic data before mainstreaming.

Overall Medical Utilization

Recall that a pilot has to demonstrate the essential elements of the de-sign, including evaluation. But the evaluation will probably be a pilot-scale project too, not likely a full-blown rigorous study. To begin, a survey of the effect of the health psychologists on utilization was done (Davis, Leary, & Heinrich, 1994). It was not a rigorous study at all, but confirmed people's impressions. It was a simple database review of total medical utilization one year pre- and post–health psychology intervention for about 1,000 continuously enrolled patients in medical clinics. For the whole group, there was about a 9% drop in physician visits (hopefully translating into increased appointment availability), and about a 50% increase in mental health visits, not including the health psychology visits (hopefully focusing the care more sharply where it belongs). There was a big increase in referrals to hospice (perhaps coming from increased atten-tion to personal and family issues in chronic illness). For about 250 patients who were hospitalized at some point during the two-year period, there were about 27% fewer hospital admissions and bed days in the "post" group. It looked like any savings that resulted were most likely coming from the inpatient area. Simplistic financial estimates suggested the whole program might pay for itself based on reduced hospital days.

This was especially noteworthy: Hospital admissions were fewer in an *already* highly managed environment. Despite the fact that we're pretty good at reducing unnecessary hospital stays, there is plenty of room to improve the overall process of taking care of patients, especially those with complex problems.For example, every care system has its "overserviced and underserved" patients, typically somatically focused and high-utilizing patients still unhappy with their care.

Clinicians and clinics often have become habituated to the traditional inefficiencies and fragmentation along the mind-body split in health care. Many of the costs a collaborative care pilot may have a chance of reducing have been accepted as a "normal cost of doing business." People often don't realize that there could be a better way. Sometimes we try to help physicians and clinics see that what they accept and budget as normal cost in dollars and frustration doesn't have to be that way. We try to cultivate a "new normal," in which frustrations and inefficiencies are seen as hidden system costs, not really "normal" costs.

As encouraging as these numbers are, bear in mind that the methodology and resource expenditure for this utilization survey was at the *pilot* level. This isn't the kind of evaluation you try to publish in a scholarly journal, but one that has been persuasive in the context of deciding whether to move forward. One reason this little survey has been persuasive is that it merely confirms with numbers much of what the anecdote bank and management outcomes have been.

Apply the Data to the Broader Organization's Agenda

Sometimes a little bit of luck can go a long way in moving pilots to the mainstream. By 1995, we had the right kinds of management outcomes to interest the top medical leadership, the right kind of anecdote bank to interest clinic leadership, and some data on probable cost offset to reassure them, but we didn't have an organizational "executive champion" in primary care. About the time RLH was pounding on doors to expand mental health practice into the medical clinics, HealthPartners recruited a new associate medical director for primary care, Macaran Baird, a family physician and family systems therapist who has worked in, supported, and published about integrated care delivery and collaboration between primary care and mental health (Baird, 1995; Doherty & Baird, 1983, 1986, 1987, 1990).

Baird and RLH began a dialogue on how the health psychology pilot could be a platform for further development at HealthPartners. Primary care had already been defined as including mental health and obstetrics and gynecology for purposes of managing and developing the care system, based on the answer to the question, "Who needs to be at the table in order to get things done properly in primary care?" By the fall of 1995, Baird went further and charged the primary care leadership group with defining the role of the primary care physician at HealthPartners and developing an empirically derived list of the most common problems or care management challenges primary care clinics would have to be able to handle well.

The primary care leadership group (which included leaders from family practice, internal medicine, pediatrics, mental health, obstetrics and gynecology, and several centralized clinical functions) reviewed actual data on the most common problems presenting in HealthPartners' primary care clinics. Mental health problems was the third most frequent cluster of reasons for seeking care, just below general medical exams and upper respiratory infections. Pregnancy care was the fourth most frequent cluster. Based upon this data, and the previous positive experience with health psychologists, the primary care leadership supported further expansion of the existing health psychology pilots into the mainstream by integrating mental health services into an additional five primary care clinics. This decision fit well with other publicly declared priorities in primary care, such as building care teams, bonding patients to physicians, and improving physician-patient communication.

Long-term success requires the project to appear in the larger organizational agenda. Without a formal place in the larger scheme of things, demonstration projects, even good ones, remain isolated pockets of progress, insulated from a mainstream that doesn't really change.

We have begun to make pilot evaluation and study more visible. To do that, we were fortunate to be able to formalize an evaluation and research component for this project through a proposal funded by Bristol-Myers Squibb, "The Over-serviced and Under-served: The Mental Health/Primary Care Collaboration Project." The HealthPartners Primary Care and Behavioral Health Divisions, the HealthPartners Research Foundation, and Bristol-Myers Squibb are collaborating to support the project and disseminate its findings. The project will allow us to study the process of integrating the mental health services and evaluating the impact on the clinics, staff, and patients.

The project has four phases. The first phase (now complete) collected baseline data and "harvested the wisdom" from the demonstrations of primary care/mental health integration that began in 1987 with the health psychology program (the early pilots we have been talking about here) (Fischer, Heinrich, Davis, Peak, & Lucas, in press). We also developed a methodology to identify the "over-serviced and under-served" patients and further developed the tools to characterize clinic patient populations.

The second stage (now in progress) builds integrated mental health capability into five primary care medical clinics not part of the previous demonstrations (most of the original pilots continue). The development process is being tracked and studied descriptively and through program evaluation methods. In this phase, pilot and control clinic functioning is compared while training and redesign processes are being recorded for study and dissemination. Evaluation involves provider and patient surveys, qualitative process analysis, and analyses of outcomes, utilization, and cost.

Subsequent phases will focus on training, dissemination of what has been learned, and formal evaluation of the impact and effectiveness of collaborative efforts, especially "disease management" interventions using controlled, randomized trials. We hope to coordinate these latter stages of the project with other centers of primary care mental health research.

CONCLUSION

To those interested in integrating behavioral health and primary care, we offer a caution and a reminder: Collaborative care and the integration of mental health and primary care are solutions to a set of general problems in health care delivery that we call "fragmented care." Don't expect any off-the-shelf model to apply in all organizations or in all corners of any one large health care delivery system. *Every new clinic interested in developing integrated care needs to examine for itself the considerations we discussed here.* Instead of recommending a one-size-fits-all approach, ask the clinic or care system about the specific problems with fragmented care or other health care delivery problems they find most troublesome. What problems in health care delivery do *they* want to improve, and how do these problems play out in the kind of health care system *they* are working in? Proceed with what already matters to people within that clinic. You can also keep the consultant hat on and ask similar questions of an entire *care system*.

Remember that successful implementation is not just a one-time technical installation to a clinic or care system. Take a developmental view of it. New principles and practices of collaboration are gradually mastered by the people working in clinics, and new operational and financial systems gradually drawn to match. Expect things to grow rather than to appear fully mature. Expect to have to *help* them grow. Expect growing pains. Expect different growth patterns from clinic to clinic. Expect improved clinical, operational, and financial results, but don't expect to see them full-blown from day one.

Many care systems are experimenting with mental health providers in primary care clinics, and we are probably all in the early phases of these experiments. Mental health/medical integration in health systems as we see it today is probably an early version of something. There are no standard designs. Health care systems are in the midst of turmoil and change, so the best solutions are yet to be invented and the final stories yet to be written. But the goal of better integrating biomedical and psychosocial care would not persist if the demonstrations did not show great promise in meeting very important quality, service, and efficiency needs of patients and care systems. We think the picture in the mainstream will be a lot clearer five or ten years from now. In the meantime, we will continue to emphasize generic principles, practices, and design issues that we think can guide the search for specific solutions for diverse care systems, and it is very exciting to be doing so.

REFERENCES

Baird, M. A. (1995). Building the ship as we sail it. *Family Systems Medicine, 13*(3/4), 269–273.

Cummings, N. A., Cummings, J. L., & Johnson, J. N. (Eds.). (1997). *Behavioral health in primary care: A guide for clinical integration*. Madison, CT: Psychosocial Press.

Davis, T. F., Leary, D., & Heinrich, R. L. (1994). Unpublished survey. Data also appears in (1996, May) *The over-serviced and under-served: The mental health/primary care collaboration project, profile analysis report, phase I*. Unpublished manuscript, Health-Partners.

Doherty, W. J., & Baird, M. A. (1983). *Family therapy and family medicine*. Guilford.

Doherty, W. J., & Baird, M. A. (1986). Developmental levels in family-centered medical care. *Family Medicine, 18*, 153–156.

Doherty, W. J., & Baird, M. A. (Eds.). (1987). *Family-centered medical care: A clinical casebook*. New York: Guilford.

Doherty, W. J., & Baird, M. A. (1990). Risks and benefits of a family systems approach to medical care. *Family Medicine, 22*, 396–403.

Fischer, L. R., Heinrich, R. L., Davis, T. F., Peek, C. J., & Lucas, S. F. (in press). Mental health and primary care in an HMO. *Families, Systems, and Health*.

Keller, V. F., & Carroll, J. G. (1994). *A new model for physician-patient communication*. West Haven, CT: Miles Institute for Health Care Communication.

Lucas, S. F., & Peek, C. J. (1997). A primary care physician's experience with integrated behavioral healthcare: What difference has it made? In N. A. Cummings, J. L. Cummings, & J. N. Johnson (Eds.), *Behavioral health in primary care: A guide for clinical integration* (pp. 371–398). Madison, CT: Psychosocial Press.

McDaniel, S., Campbell, T., & Seaburn, D. (1995). Principles for collaboration between health and mental health providers in primary care. *Family Systems Medicine, 13*(3/4), 283–298.

Peek, C. J., & Heinrich, R. L. (1995). Building a collaborative healthcare organization: From idea to invention to innovation. *Family Systems Medicine, 13*(3/4), 327–342.

Putman, A. O. (1990). Organizations. In A. O. Putman, & K. E. Davis (Eds.), *Advances in descriptive psychology* (Vol. 5, pp. 11-46). Ann Arbor, MI: Descriptive Psychology.

Seaburn, D. B., Lorenz, A. D., Gunn, W. B., Gawinski, B. A., & Mauksch, L. B. (1996). *Models of collaboration: A guide for mental health professionals working with health care practitioners*. New York: Basic.

8

Integrated Care for the Frail Elderly: The Group Care Clinic

Patricia Robinson   Alison Del Vento

Charles Wischman

I find this chapter intellectually compelling and touching at the same time. It is compelling because it is a very creative integration of medical and psychological services that fits the needs of an important population of patients particularly well. It is a program that is easily adaptable to other settings. It should be a model for programs in primary care in many areas, since the population it serves is growing in every medical practice.

The chapter is touching because the commitment and creativity of the staff are so clear, as are the respect and affection for the patient. The authors deserve credit for being highly caring and committed health professionals and for finding a program model that tends to promote this sort of behavior in any staff member.

Providers in integrated primary care settings often report that they feel they can involve more sides of themselves in their work without blurring boundaries or becoming inappropriately personally involved with patients. The relationship they have with team members who are peers working with the same patients is very different than the relationship they have with colleagues who treat different patients in the same practice or with lower level staff who are performing less complex parts of the same treatment with the same patients. The team structure and the involvement and discussion between team members form a natural boundary that allows providers to be much more open and comfortable with patients without beginning to use patients for approval or personal support.

THIS CHAPTER REVIEWS literature concerning delivery of health care services to older adults and describes an innovative, integrated program for older medical patients who need consistent health care monitoring and treatment services. After reviewing studies pertinent to design of medical programs for older adults, we describe our meeting as primary care and behavioral health professionals and the frustrations that led us to create the Group Care Clinic. We will present our initial program objectives, as well as the goals our patients suggested to us as we evolved a new system of care. In an effort to pave a road for professionals wanting to follow our trail, we offer examples from our curriculum. We present modest data suggesting that this integrated program influenced health care service utilization and patient satisfaction in positive directions. We conclude with suggestions to readers that may help them improve upon our pioneer efforts.

THE OLDER ADULT AND HEALTH CARE

Numerous researchers have focused on health care utilization among elderly persons (Huka & Wheat, 1985; Patterson, Crescenzi, & Stell, 1984; Wan, 1989; Wolinsky, Mosely, & Coe, 1986). Patient decisions concerning use of health care services are complex (Robinson & Hayes, in press), and a patient is influenced by a myriad of factors when deciding to use a medical service. While poor health status is a major factor in medical utilization (Branch et al., 1981; Wan & Odell, 1981; Wolinsky & Coe, 1984), other factors may figure prominently. Specific sociodemographic factors are related to increased utilization. These include having fewer social supports, facing more stressful life events, being out of the work force, being married, and being older (Wan, 1982; Wan & Odell). Other factors influencing utilization include those related to personality and interpersonal style. These include the patient's ability to monitor bodily states, his or her personal theories of illness causation, the sociocultural context influencing illness beliefs (Mechanic, 1978), and the patient's confidence in the health care provider and service. Social and psychological factors interact with patient health status and figure prominently in health care utilization. For example, patients with higher levels of body awareness are more likely to initiate illness visits to medical clinics and to hospital emergency rooms in a health maintenance organization (Hansell, Sherman, & Mechanic, 1991). As a patient population, elderly adults appear to use more medical services and to contribute disproportionately to medical expenditures.

Psychological distress is associated with medical care utilization (Leaf et al., 1985; Wan & Arling, 1983). As with younger adults, physical and psychological health are closely related in the elderly. Older adults may express psychological distress in terms of physical illness symptoms (Mechanic, 1978). Further, an older person's mental health problem may interfere with his or her ability to manage coexisting medical problems skillfully and in this way contribute to a decline in health and use of more intensive medical services (Broadhead, Blazer, George, & Tse, 1990; Johnson, Weissman, & Klerman, 1992). When troubled by a combination of anxiety and depression, patients may suffer particularly severe difficulties in functioning in day-to-day living (Fifer et al., 1994; Reynolds, 1994). Older depressed patients make more frequent visits to primary care physicians than nondepressed elderly (Waxman, Carner, & Blum, 1983) and have significantly more days of both inpatient care and follow-up treatment than nondepressed elderly inpatients (Koenig, Shelp, Goli, Cohen, & Blazer, 1989).

When older patients who have psychological problems seek care, 92.5% go to a general medical doctor (Phillips & Murrel, 1994). These care-seekers are quite different from their cohorts. They have poorer psychological well-being, more physical health problems, higher levels of unpleasant stressful events (e.g., bereavement, social and economic loss), and greater deficits in social support (Phillips & Murrel). Unfortunately, they often present with complaints, such as headaches, insomnia, or foot pain. Understandably, their doctors discuss psychological coping strategies with them less often than with younger patients, who are more willing to admit to psychological problems (Robinson et al., 1994).

When older primary care patients have a mental problem, it is most likely to be depression. Depression is the most frequent psychiatric diagnosis among persons over 59 years of age and the fifth most common of all diagnoses made by physicians (Richter, Barsky, & Hupp, 1983). Physicians appear to treat depression in older adults differently from depression in younger adults. For example, older patients are less likely than younger patients to receive antidepressant prescriptions (Richter et al.). Also, primary care physicians are less likely to refer older depressed patients for counseling services, even when services are available within the health care system (Robinson, 1994). These age-related differences in treatment are understandable in that older adults are more likely to be taking medications that make antidepressant therapy a more complex method of treatment and older adults are less likely to use counseling services, even when referred by a physician (Robinson, Wischman, & Del Vento, 1996).

For many reasons, older adults are an excellent target for programs that integrate medical and behavioral health care. Programs that combine physical and psychological care may help patients acknowledge psychological problems and involve health care providers in designing interventions that address the problems. Unnecessary medical utilization may also decrease when patients learn to monitor specific health indicators, understand theories of illness causation, and apply effective treatments that combine medical and psychological strategies to quality of life issues. Medical and psychological providers of care may learn a great deal from working together. Their collaboration will support development of new models of care.

THE BEGINNING OF COLLABORATION

We began working together seven years ago. We had worked for the same staff model health maintenance organization for many years and had strong interests in gerontology. Dr. Wischman, a primary care physician, and Ms. Del Vento, a primary care nurse, had shared responsibility for a panel of patients for several decades. They met Dr. Robinson, a psychologist, when a research project brought her to their primary care clinic to provide a six-session, cognitive-behavioral group treatment program for stressed, demoralized older adults referred by primary care providers. During the course of this project, we began a collaboration. While many older patients were initially suspicious about referral to Dr. Robinson's group, many were successfully supported in giving the behavioral health service a try. Slowly, patients began to see the group as an acceptable health care service. Of those who started the group, most completed the six-session curriculum. The group protocol included devising a written plan that suggested follow-up activities by the primary care nurse or physician. The relapse prevention document supported patient and primary care provider interactions about the content of the sessions. Dr. Wischman and Ms. Del Vento were impressed by the fact that patients would accept and use a behavioral health care program delivered in the primary care setting. Dr. Robinson was impressed by the fact that primary care providers were working diligently to meet the needs of such a large group of older patients who were troubled by significant psychological problems, concurrent with multiple medical problems.

When the research project ended, we were reluctant to end our new primary care and behavioral health partnership. Dr. Wischman and Ms. Del Vento learned of a pilot project involving integrated care to older primary care patients that was being evaluated by a sister health care organization (Kaiser-Permanente of Northern Colorado). They shared this information with Dr. Robinson and invited her to join them in developing a similar program for their panel of patients. She obtained the support of the supervisors in the staff model mental health department, and the three began to develop the Group Care Clinic.

We had numerous frustrations with the prevailing model of care, and these energized our work to create a model. Over 20% of the panel that Dr. Wishman and Ms. Del Vento served were 65 years of age or older. Many of these patients suffered from medical and psychological problems and needed frequent medical contacts. The accepted model of care was to serve them individually through a combination of contacts, including physician and nurse visits and nurse telephone calls. Because there were so many patients to serve, providers sometimes felt visits were rushed. Many patients were socially isolated and contact with a primary care provider was a highly significant social event. Patients often tried to prolong the medical contact through listing out numerous vague symptoms when their most pressing needs were social and psychological. The medical providers felt obliged to investigate all symptom complaints, and, of course, such investigatory efforts impacted cost. Both patient and provider sometimes experienced disappointment in the results of such medical contacts. At times, Dr. Wischman or Ms. Del Vento suggested that the patient see a specialist in the staff model mental health clinic. The mental health service was only a 10-minute walk from the primary care clinic. However, most patients who were referred to the mental health service did not follow through with the referral. Of those who overcame the initial obstacles (e.g., accepting that they had a "mental" problem, making one or more calls to schedule an appointment with a new provider in a new location), many did not keep the initial appointment or did not continue with treatment after the initial visit to mental health. The delivery of mental health services to this group of patients was problematic in the existing system of care. We were prepared to change, and our first step was to develop a method for selecting patients for participation in a new model.

SELECTING PATIENTS FOR THE GROUP CARE CLINIC

We developed several criteria for selecting patients, and Ms. Del Vento took the primary responsibility for this, implementing the agreed upon process. Selection criteria included the following:

1. aged 65 years or older
2. experiencing multiple chronic medical problems which required regular clinic visits, hospital visits, multiple prescriptions, etc., and described as "frail" by their providers
3. experiencing no cognitive impairments that significantly impaired ability to learn new information and to follow through with health care plans
4. willing to participate in a group model of care

We limited participation to patients aged 65 and older in order to minimize diversity in life circumstances. We knew that patients would have a variety of medical problems. We wanted to maximize similarity of experience to facilitate development of early cohesion in the group. Our criteria for inclusion concerning chronic medical problems was to select patients who required at least one medical contact per month in order to receive adequate monitoring and treatment of chronic medical illnesses. Of course, patient participation in the group care clinic model was completely voluntary, and patients were recruited by invitation.

Our invitation to patients offered the following explanations concerning our suggestions that they participate in the Group Care Clinic.

You were chosen to participate in this clinic because:

1. You are special and need special health care.
2. We want to see you every month.
3. You and others invited to participate share commonalities in age and health challenges and may be resources for each other.
4. We feel this program will improve your satisfaction with health care services.

The invitation to patients also explained that patients needed to make several commitments as a part of planning to participate in the new model of care. These included committing to regular participation in the group, to spending 30 minutes on assigned activities between monthly group meetings, and to providing support to one or more members of the group on at least one occasion between group meetings.

Nineteen of 24 (79%) of the invited patients agreed to participate. These patients ranged in age from 71 to 89 and included 7 males and 12 females. To prepare for the start of the group program, the nurse conducted a chart review of all patients agreeing to participate. Chart review information was summarized in individual patient medical records.

The chart review included evaluation of patients' immunization status (including flu shots), most current radiology procedures (e.g., mammogram, chest film), pharmacological treatment risks (e.g., taking Coumadin or Pravastatin), and other health care issues (including most recent EKG, complete physical examination, eye exam, and whether the patient was diabetic). Additionally, the nurse evaluated necessary lab tests and recommended schedules for follow-up testing. She also evaluated specialty referrals and noted whether follow-up was requested and whether resolution was reached concerning specialty referrals. Finally, the chart review evaluated patient status regarding physician directives, living wills, etc. Table 8.1 provides a summary of the most common of the 126 medical problems noted in the medical charts. Table 8.2 summarizes participants' use of specialists in the past year. Almost 70% had seen multiple specialty physicians in the past year. Table 8.3 summarizes the prevalence of psychological problems identified by chart reviews. Over 40% of the agreeing participants had depression or dysthymia noted in their medical chart problem list. Thirty percent had no advance physician directive concerning end-of-life issues recorded in the medical chart.

The group care clinic nurse prepared individualized health care materials for all consenting participants. These materials were organized into Patient Medical Diaries. Each patient received her or his health care diary at the first Group Care Clinic meeting. The diaries included chart review information, current health problems and recommended treatments, and protocols for controlling specific disease processes. The nurse asked that participants bring their diaries to group care meetings and file materials from Group Care Clinic meetings in their diaries for future reference. The psychologist agreed to prepare outlines and handouts for all behavioral health lectures, exercises, and assignments.

GROUP CARE CLINIC OBJECTIVES

As a team of providers, we designed the following objectives for our group:

TABLE 8.1

The Most Common Medical Conditions Noted in Medical
Charts of Initial Participants

CONDITION	FREQUENCY (n = 19)	%
Angina	8	42%
Depression/dysthymia	8	42%
Cataracts or other visual impairment disease	8	42%
Asthma	7	37%
Hernia repair	7	37%
Allergy	6	32%
Congestive heart failure	6	32%
PUD/ulcers	6	32%
Hypothyroid	6	32%
Skin problems	6	32%
Appendectomy	5	26%
Diverticulosis	5	26%
Glaucoma	5	26%
Osteoarthritis	5	26%
Smoker or past smoker	5	26%
COPD	4	21%
Gastritis	4	21%
Hypertension	4	21%
HTN	4	21%
Orthopedic problem	4	21%
Varicose vein stripping	4	21%

TABLE 8.2
Use of Specialty in Past Year by Initial Participants

SPECIALTY USED	FREQUENCY (n = 19)	%
Cardiology	4	21%
Neurology	4	21%
Ophthalmology	4	21%
Urology	4	21%
Gastrointestinal	3	16%
Orthopedics	2	10%
Rheumatology	2	10%
Endocrinology	1	5%
Dermatology	1	5%
Surgery	1	5%

TABLE 8.3
The Most Common Psychological Problems Noted
in Medical Charts of Initial Participants

PSYCHOLOGICAL DIAGNOSIS	FREQUENCY (n = 19)	%
Depression	7	37%
Insomnia	3	16%
Neurodermatitis	3	16%
Panic attacks	2	10%
Anxiety	2	10%
Bereavement	1	5%
Caregiver stress	1	5%
Dysthymia	1	5%
Stress reaction	1	5%

1. Provide phone and clinic visits needed to address the care needs of chronically ill older patients.
2. Make interventions in the group care context prior to escalations in health problems that would result in delivery of more intensive services.
3. Build cohesion among group participants and facilitate planning among members in an effort to improve quality of daily life.
4. Teach specific skills for coping with medical and behavioral health challenges confronting patients.
5. Enlist patients as partners in updating medical diaries and determining Group Care Clinic norms.
6. Increase provider satisfaction in working on a monthly basis with complex patients for whom there are no predictable pathways for resolving illness.

These goals were shared with patients in the initial meeting.

Medical Health Objectives

Our medical health objectives included teaching patients to actively monitor and plan appropriate interventions to maximize health in daily living. We hoped to teach patients to accurately monitor health care indicators associated with specific disease processes confronting them. Additionally, we planned to increase patient skillfulness and confidence in coping with specific illnesses. We planned to accomplish these objectives by providing patients with written educational materials and brief lectures at Group Care Clinic meetings. We planned to supplement the expertise of core staff in the Group Care Clinic by inviting guest speakers. Core staff included Dr. Wischman, Ms. Del Vento, Dr. Robinson, and Mr. Burt Swendt, a pharmacist. We sought to improve patient adherence to prescribed medications and recommended laboratory procedures by reviewing pharmacy and laboratory data on each patient prior to each monthly meeting. We intended to make recommendations concerning medications and laboratory procedures at the Group Care Clinic meeting so that patients could visit the pharmacy or laboratory during or after the meeting. We also planned to structure meetings so that adequate time was available for the physician to provide any necessary individual physical exams or procedures during the group meeting or shortly after the meeting. We also planned to focus on prevention by addressing wellness issues on an ongoing basis.

Behavioral Health Objectives

We hoped to help patients identify strategic methods for coping with life circumstance problems. We anticipated that formal problem solving techniques and acceptance-based strategies would be helpful to this population. We also reasoned that we could help patients prevent the development of depression or demoralization by teaching them warning signs and potential triggers and ways to buffer the stresses of aging. We knew that promoting affiliation among group members would be our first objective.

As the group developed and formed a personality of its own, we discovered new objectives. Specifically, patients lead us to focus on refining communication skills between patients and providers. They asked us to evaluate the role of patient self-confidence in coping, as well as the contribution of actual coping skills to improvement of individual health care outcomes. Other emerging objectives included integrating sociocultural issues into health care plans and building a community that would grow and change, facing life and death together for years to come.

THE CURRICULUM FOR THE GROUP CARE CLINIC

We began with a structure for group meetings that accommodated our need to have more than one activity in process during several periods of the group meeting and a flow between more serious and playful activities. Our agenda usually included the following:

1. Partner check-ins, monitoring, chart and diary updates
2. Dr. Wischman speaks out
3. Questions and answers
4. Tea, presentations by patients
5. Behavioral health hour with Dr. Robinson
6. Follow-up and future plans from Nurse Del Vento

We decided to begin with a less formal preclass period. This first 10–15 minute section was designed to accomplish a number of maintenance activities, including individual physical exams by the physician as they were needed and monitoring of vital signs by the nurse. The nurse updated patients concerning needed lab tests and other procedures. She also reviewed patient's questions and triaged them to the appropriate provider. Ms. Del Vento sent a question form to participants along with the planned agenda two weeks prior to every Group Care Clinic meeting. See Figure 8.1 for an example of the types of questions patients brought to the Group Care Clinic. Ms. Del Vento also helped patients with medical diary updates. Our pharmacist usually made an appearance during this preclass time and talked with patients individually or in small groups concerning medication issues. Every participant had a partner and this preclass time allowed time for the partners to visit with each other.

Dr. Wischman usually updated patients on changes within the local health care system, national health care issues, and recent medical discoveries of interest to the elderly. Additionally, he presented brief lectures on topics suggested by patients. These included topics such as vitamins, foot care, dry skin, cancer, genetics, youth, crime, television, diet, etc. He addressed questions posed by participants in writing during the preclass section or prior to the meeting. Other group care staff members participated in the question-and-answer discussions as well. Midway through the two-hour group, we served tea and a snack. One or more participants made a brief presentation during the tea. Their presentations included sharing poems and other intellectual and artistic pursuits.

As tea was finished, we moved to a presentation by Dr. Robinson. The behavioral health hour was always supported by a written handout. The agenda for this section included follow-up of the previous behavioral health assignment, a brief lecture on a new topic, an exercise designed to provide practice of the new skill, and assignment of a new behavioral health experiment. We often included a game or performed a community ceremony of some type (e.g., celebrating a participant's birthday) during this hour.

Our agenda was enriched by outside speakers every three months. We invited specialists from speech and hearing, physical therapy, podiatry, mental health, ophthalmology, other specialty departments, and local political figures. Participants were polled on a regular basis regarding their preferences for guest speakers and topics of interests. Our pharmacists also provided quarterly updates on new medicines for participants.

Behavioral Health Curriculum

The theoretical basis of our behavioral health curriculum is derived from acceptance and commitment therapy (ACT) (Hayes, 1987; Hayes & Strosahl, in press; Hayes, Wilson, Gifford, Follette, & Strosahl, 1996; Robinson & Hayes, 1996). This theory describes a contextual approach to change that relies heavily on a person's ability to embrace suffering. Aging presents more and more difficult circumstances (e.g., failing health, loss of friends and loved ones), and optimal responding requires

Today's date: _____January 17, 1994_____

My question is for: _____*_____ Charles Wischman, M. D.

                                  _____ Alison Del Vento, R. N.

                                  _____ Burt Swendt, R. Ph.

                                  _____ Patti Robinson, Ph. D.

My questions: 1. Shortness of breath seems to be an increasing problem. Anything we can do?

                     2. Headaches are a problem. I am resorting to Tylenol with codeine more often than I want to. What can I do?

                     3. My wife is having more difficulty walking. Is that due to a physical problem or because her brain doesn't tell her how?

I want this question answered: _____*_____ Privately

                                  _____ In front of the group

                                  _____ Today

                                _____*_____ In a phone call later this week

Sincerely,

John Smith

(your name)

Figure 8.1. Example of question form used by patients. This form was mailed to Group Care Clinic participants two weeks prior to the monthly meeting.

graceful acceptance of these unwanted and painful events. ACT defines a combination of psychological acceptance and behavioral change strategies that empower a person to experience the challenges of aging while committing to a day-to-day life that reflects his or her highest values (e.g., having loving relationships, being generous or forgiving, taking risks, learning, etc.). ACT emphasizes personal responsibility, the wisdom of direct experience, and choice (Robinson, 1996).

Our group began in the late summer of 1992 and continued until late winter of 1996. During this 41-month period, we passed through several recognized stages of growth as a community of providers and patients seeking to evolve a new system of care. We developed a love for each other and for the time we shared together. The following are examples of the behavioral health curriculum that ripened within each of the three stages. These are outlined in Table 8.4.

The Early Stage: Relaxing into a Community

We were all nervous in the beginning. Our experiences with health care had prepared us for brief, one-on-one, formal encounters about specific problems. We were experimenting with a system of care that required us to meet for several hours in a large group. The job of the psychologist was to help us find connections with each other and to relax into being a community.

1. *Psychological neoteny: Play and curiosity are lifelong states of being.* One of our very first meetings concerned the assessment of qualities of psychological neoteny among participants in the clinic. Ashley Montagu (1990) introduced the concept of psychological neoteny and defined it as the presence of desirable childlike qualities in an adult. These include laughter, spontaneity, curiosity, and asking questions forthrightly. Dr. Montagu's research suggested that people who were high in these qualities lived longer and enjoyed life more. Further, Dr. Montagu's findings suggested that these qualities could be relearned in adulthood. Participants selected one or more qualities that they wanted to increase in their daily lives and designed plans to support development of the targeted qualities.

2. *Breathing: Take in what is; let go of what was.* Diaphragmatic breathing was introduced as a relaxation and concentration exercise. We also discussed posture and its relationship to breathing. We practiced belly breathes while seated slouching, seated with a straight back, standing against a wall, and walking. Partners worked with each other to help develop open chests for breathing. Participants planned morning and evening practice of belly breaths. Breathing exercises became a regular part of behavioral health hour during the first year of the clinic.

TABLE 8.4

Examples of Behavioral Health Curriculum from Three Stages
of Development in the Group Care Clinic

TOPIC	*MESSAGE*
Early Stage: Relaxing into a Community	
Psychological neoteny	Play and curiosity are lifelong states of being.
Breathing	Take in what is; let go of what was.
Middle Stage: Becoming Skillful and Proud of It	
Behavioral health	Let's lower blood pressures.
Concentration and critical thinking	Use language accurately and effectively.
Improvisation	We are a healing team.
Control	I'm driving this bus . . . whatever happens
Acceptance and accommodation	Use it or lose it . . . line dance, drum, or just hum.
First death	Rituals help a community change.
Later Stage: Wow! Was that a Meteor?	
States of consciousness	We live until we die.
Meditation	Glide through the last wild ride.
Dreams	Understand and use all perspectives.
Group care resource book	What and who has worked for you?

Middle Stage: Becoming Skillful and Proud of It

During the second phase of our development, we focused on mastery of
a variety of coping strategies to improve health and quality of life. We
taught relaxation skills, concentration techniques, improvisation acting
strategies, personal assertion skills, problem-solving strategies, and psychological acceptance methods. Our participants insisted that mastery of
skills involved "know-how" and confidence. Personal assessment scale
data (which will be discussed later) suggested that participants began to
experience considerable self-efficacy.

1. *Behavioral health: Let's lower blood pressures.* Participants learned
several approaches to relaxation. The psychologist introduced systematic
relaxation (Jacobson, 1974), cue-controlled relaxation, and visualization
strategies. Patients were encouraged to select the strategy that matched

their individual strengths and to practice it daily. After a month of practice, we conducted an experiment during the group care clinic meeting. Several nurses took blood pressure readings. Then, participants practiced their selected method of relaxation for five minutes. Blood pressure readings were taken at the end of the brief relaxation practice; readings decreased for all participants. Dramatic reductions occurred for several participants. We also provided information and support concerning other methods of preventing and reducing hypertension, including weight reduction, sodium and alcohol restriction, and increased physical activity (Dubbert, 1995).

2. *Concentration and critical thinking: Use language accurately and effectively.* One of the topics suggested by participants concerned memory. Several clinic meetings concerned development of memory strategies. The literature about memory and aging was reviewed and summarized for participants. They were particularly fond of strategies involving use of colorful language to maximize concentration and attention and use of rhythm for supporting memorization of long passages. Further, they were encouraged to learn that older people often have better long-term memory than young people.

3. *Improvisation: We are a healing team.* Participants were quite interested in the foundations of improvisation. Once learned, they formed a context for play for the group. When we needed to connect as a community, we could return to our improvisation skills. Foundations for improvisation exercises in the group included: (1) always say yes; (2) accept what is given and add to it, and (3) we are growing something together and what is not the issue, only how and now. One of our first improvisational exercises involved becoming a big healing machine. The psychologist started her healing sound and arm movement, and, one-by-one, participants joined in with their own individual sounds and movements. It was quite a scene.

4. *Control: I'm driving this bus . . . whatever happens.* The more time we shared together, the more losses we shared. One participant lost his wife. One had a son sent to prison. One lost use of an arm. As we faced these heartbreaking events, we shared our values. We asked each other what mattered the most. Our goal was clear: Live everyday according to our values. We discussed and implemented strategies for keeping our values before us. Participants wrote notes to themselves and to each other to support courageous action.

5. *Acceptance and accommodation: Use it or lose it . . . line dance, drum, or just hum.* One of Dr. Wischman's favorite expressions was "Use it or lose it." It was a sound principle for maintaining health and

was applied over and over again. To balance out difficult times in the group, we often planned a meeting to play or share recipes and eat together. One participant related that she'd once loved square-dancing. She'd outlived her husband and all of her long-term friends and had no children. To celebrate her ninety-first birthday, the psychologist taught participants a line dance routine. Those who could stand, stood and danced. Those who couldn't stand, drummed or sang. One or two just hummed. Participants received support from staff and each other for using all abilities, expressing all interests, giving away all gifts.

6. *First death: Rituals help a community change.* In our seventeenth month, we experienced our first death. This prompted more sharing about death, spirituality, and our individual preferences concerning experience of our own death. We also developed ceremonies for our group to use in observing the loss of a participant. Our rituals were quite simple: the physician and nurse would share information about the death; all of us would offer a remembrance of the person we lost; we would have our tea in silence; we would wait three months before adding another member to our community.

Later Stage: Wow! Was that a Meteor?

As we became a skillful community with a history, we addressed future issues that were personal and difficult. Discussions of death were initiated with ease. Participants were quick to volunteer to reach out to clinic participants who missed a meeting. We began to share practical information that helped individuals interface successfully with the larger community. We developed a resource book. We noticed when an 85-year-old participant picked up a prescription for a 90-year-old participant he planned to meet for lunch. With really very little effort, we had become a community.

1. *States of consciousness: We live until we die.* Participants became quite fascinated with the psychobiology of mental control. We discussed Hypocrites, the founder of Western medicine, and his suggestion that disease resulted from disharmony of the mind, body, and environment. We discussed lifestyles and life contexts and made plans to change unhealthy coping styles and living situations. Participants were interested in the human nervous system and the general adaptation syndrome. We discussed the emergency response system, resistance, and exhaustion. We discussed self-efficacy theory (Bandura, 1986, 1991) and applied it to daily living issues as well as dying.

2. *Meditation: Glide through the last wild ride.* The Group Care Clinic participants enjoyed telling and hearing stories. We did this often.

They particularly enjoyed metaphors. Charlotte Zoko Beck (Beck & Smith, 1993) developed one of our favorite metaphors. She described the experience of a pilot who flies into a hurricane and takes a terrible pounding before landing temporarily in the eye of the hurricane. She explains how the pilot may obsess with the control panel in an effort to stay in the eye. Of course, the pilot might as well be flying a glider, as there is no way to stay in the eye. When we accept a fundamental lack of control, we are free to experience the eye, the hurricane, and the in-between. This metaphor was experienced as descriptive and useful by participants with near-death encounters. Other materials concerning the effectiveness of meditation were presented to patients (e.g., Kabat-Zinn et al., 1992).

3. *Dreams: Understand and use all perspectives.* Many participants woke during the night, and they benefitted from learning to enjoy returning to sleep. It was in this context that we began to discuss dreams. We studied different methods for understanding dreams. In one exercise, partners took turns asking each other a list of specific questions about a recent specific dream.

4. *Group care resource book: What and who has worked for you?* One of our participants struggled with income tax preparation and reported a negative experience with an accountant. This lead to our start of a Group Care Resource Book. This book included several sections (e.g., Professionals that Provide Good Services to Seniors; Best Places for Lunch). Participants provided information concerning a recommended resource and identified themselves as the person recommending the resource. This was another step toward looking after each other.

QUALITY OF CARE: GROUP CARE CLINIC OUTCOMES

Our effort is best described as an unevaluated pilot conducted in a thoughtful manner. Our present results are limited to basic program evaluation information and chart review data. We also have information about participant satisfaction and quality of life, and we can also describe our satisfaction as providers.

Utilization of Health Care Services

The Group Care Clinic visit replaced monthly individual appointments for many participants. Most patients would have required, at minimum, 15 minutes of physician and 15 minutes of nurse time in individual clinic visits on a monthly basis. These visits were replaced by the 2-hour Group

Care Clinic monthly meeting. Also, our nurse spent 4 hours per month preparing for Group Care Clinic meetings and following up with patients. Her preparation time included reviewing patient charts, sending out reminders to patients, and locating guest speakers.

In an effort to assess trends in health care utilization behavior among individual participants, we completed a review of medical charts one year after the Group Care Clinic ended. We evaluated patient utilization of medical services during three time periods: (1) pre–Group Clinic; (2) Group Care Clinic, and (3) post–Group Care Clinic. The pre- and post–Group Care Clinic reviews covered 12-month periods. The Group Care Clinic period involved 41 months. We reviewed the following variables: phone calls, primary care visits with physicians and physician assistants (including Group Care Clinic visits), primary care nursing visits, visits with providers other than primary care (including physical therapy, ophthalmology, and all specialty physicians), emergency room visits, and episodes of care from the home health/community nursing program. Patients who died during the course of the Group Care Clinic were excluded from the review.

Several case examples demonstrate the types of changes in utilization associated with participation in the Group Care Clinic. Figure 8.2 presents graphs of utilization data on three participants in the Group Care Clinic during the three periods of chart review. Graphed data are averaged utilization rates (concerning emergency room visits, primary care physician visits, and telephone contacts) per month for each of the three periods reviewed in the charts. Post–Group Care Clinic data are not presented for the third participant, as he died two months after the Group Care Clinic program ended. As can be seen from the graphs, Group Care Clinic participation tends to be associated with increases in phone contacts between health care providers and patients and decreases in use of emergency room visits and primary care visits. We plan to extend our chart review to an 18-month period in the future.

Consumer Satisfaction with Care

Patients were surveyed by the mental health service six months after the start of the Group Care Clinic. The survey was conducted so that participant responses were confidential and not identified with individual participants. We asked participants to compare the Group Care Clinic with their previous method of care. Figure 8.3 summarizes the data resulting from the question, "How does the Group Care Clinic compare with your previous method of care?" We also wanted to know if participants felt they were learning new information in group care clinic meet-

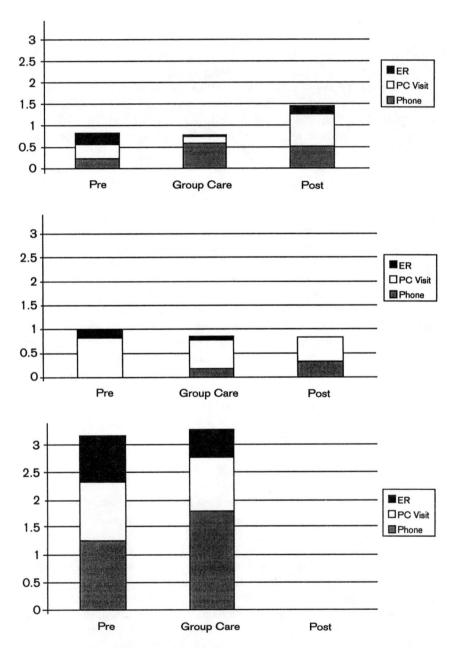

Figure 8.2. Utilization data for three Group Care participants pre-, during, and post-Group Care Clinic participation. Graphed data are mean number of emergency room visits, primary care physician visits, and phone calls per month.

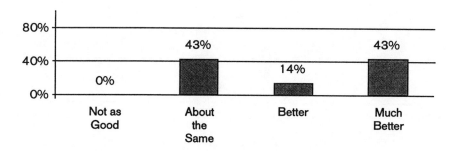

Figure 8.3. Graph of participant evaluations of the Group Care Clinic in comparison with previous method of care six months after start-up

ings. Eighty-six percent indicated that they were learning ways to maintain or improve their health.

Empowerment: Personal Assessment Scale Data

The Personal Assessment Scale (PAS) is a self-report instrument suggested by Birkedahl (1991). We suggested this instrument to participants at the beginning our second year because we believed results would help us plan pertinent behavioral health programs. Table 8.5 presents the score range and mean for each of the eight areas on the PAS. Participants expressed strong self-images, a high level of serenity, rewarding interpersonal relationships, and a neutral world outlook.

Provider Satisfaction

Early in our first year of working in the Group Care Clinic, our nurse evaluated the social and familial networks of participants. She determined that we, as providers of health care, were functionally the closest relatives for almost 40% of the participants. We were jarred by this statistic. We ranged in age from 45 to 55, and we had numerous living relatives and friends. The Group Care Clinic gave us a format that supported our delivery of care in the context that reflected the reality of our relationship with these patients. We developed a sense of honor and reverence for these relationships and were more prepared as we became the closest relative for more of our Group Care Clinic patients.

We noticed that our interactions with patients became more and more personally meaningful to us. Dr. Wischman noted a drastic decline in vague complaints of mild symptoms. Ms. Del Vento noticed a stronger link in phone communications with patients, which she used to intensify

TABLE 8.5
Participant Ratings on the Personal Assessment Scale
at the Conclusion of Year One

ASSESSMENT AREA	RATING CRITERIA	RANGE	MEAN RATING
Physical strength and wellness	1 = excellent; 7 = poor	3–6	4.1
Self-image	1 = good; 7 = poor	1–4	2.3
Wants and needs are satisfied	1 = good; 7 = rarely	2–5	3.0
Most of the time I feel:			
anxiety	1 = secure; 7 = frightened	2–4	3.1
sadness	1 = happy; 7 = sad	2–6	3.1
anger	1 = serene; 7 = angry	1–3	1.8
Expect future to be	1 = bright; 7 = cloudy	1–4	2.1
Relationships with others are	1 = rewarding; 7 = conflicted	1–4	1.3
Stresses in my life are	1 = manageable; 7 = overwhelming	2–4	3
World outlook	1 = good; 7 = grim	2–6	3.4

treatment when needed. We were all inspired to work a little harder to be well-read and ready for substantial discussions on a wide range of health care and relationship issues. We became more comfortable with saying, "I don't know but I will study up on this for you." We were challenged to be creative and playful and to apply the skills we suggested to patients more tenaciously in our own lives.

SUGGESTIONS FOR THE FUTURE

We encourage other health care providers to develop integrated care programs for older adults. Integrated programs need to be housed in the primary care clinic. The leadership needs to be shared and the presence of an on-site behavioral health professional is ideal. This approach provides continuity for patients and flexibility for providers, who need vacations and have sick days now and then. We hope that the practical details presented in this chapter help you make a start in your setting. We offer the following ideas in an effort to help you improve upon our initial efforts.

1. *Evaluate patient health status on a yearly basis.* The Duke Health Profile (Parkerson, 1996) is brief, yields helpful information, and can easily be administered over the phone on a yearly basis.
2. *Evaluate utilization.* Patients may use less specialty and hospital care when they are supported by strong primary care programs that address medical, psychological, and social needs.
3. *Evaluate patient retention.* Patients have choices about health care, and patient retention is an important health care outcome measure. We never had a patient decide to leave the Group Care Clinic or the health maintenance organization because of dissatisfaction with care.
4. *Let the health care team decide whether or not to implement an integrated health care program for the elderly.* This method of care requires a great deal of openness and commitment from providers. Providers need to be willing to rethink the traditional structure of the doctor-patient visit. Voluntary participation will allow providers to assess their readiness to make this commitment.
5. *Focus educational programs about integrated care for older adults on older providers.* Older doctors often have a higher proportion of older patients. They are more ready to see the need for a change in the model of care.
6. *Say yes to all the obstacles that greet you in starting an integrated care project for older adults.* Study the obstacles and plan temporary solutions that will suggest a next step in solving the many problems associated with changing a health care system.

Most of all, enjoy your work. Learn from your mistakes and from your patients. There is tremendous potential for developing efficacious, integrated programs for older adults that are satisfying to patients and providers.

REFERENCES

Bandura, A. (1986). *Social foundations of thought and action: A social cognitive theory.* Englewood Cliffs, NJ: Prentice-Hall.

Bandura, A. (1991). Self-efficacy mechanism in physiological activation and health-promoting behavior. In J. Madden (Ed.), *Neurobiology of learning, emotion, and affect.* New York: Raven.

Beck, C. H., & Smith, S. (1993). *Nothing special: Living Zen.* New York: Harper Collins.

Birkedahl, N. (1991). *Older & wiser: A workbook for coping with aging.* Oakland, CA: New Harbinger.

Branch, L., Jette, A., Evashwick, C., Polansky, M. Rowe, G., & Dichr, P. (1981). Toward understanding elders health services utilization. *Journal of Community Health, 7,* 80–91.

Broadhead, W. E., Blazer, D. G., George, L. K., & Tse, C. K. (1990). Depression, disability days, and days lost from work in a prospective epidemiologic survey. *Journal of the American Medical Association, 264*, 2624–2528.

Dubbert, P. M. (1995). Behavioral (life-style) modification in the prevention and treatment of hypertension. *Clinical Psychology Review, 15*(3), 187–216.

Fifer, S. K., Mathias, S. D., Patrick, D. L., Mazonson, P. E., Lubeck, D. P., & Buesching, D. P. (1994). Untreated anxiety among adult primary care patients in a health maintenance organization. *Archives of General Psychiatry, 51*, 740–750.

Hansell, S., Sherman, G., & Mechanic, D. (1991). Body awareness and medical care utilization among older adults in an HMO. *Journal of Gerontology, 46*(3), S151–S159.

Hayes, S. C. (1987). A contextual approach to therapeutic change. In N. Jacobson (Ed.), *Psychotherapists in clinical practice: Cognitive and behavioral perspectives* (pp. 327–387). New York: Guilford.

Hayes, S., & Strosahl, K. (in press). *Acceptance and commitment therapy: Understanding and treating human suffering.* New York: Guilford.

Hayes, S. C., Wilson, K. G., Gifford, E. V., Follette, V. M., & Strosahl, K. (1996). Experiential avoidance and behavioral disorders: A functional dimensional approach to diagnosis and treatment. *Journal of Consulting and Clinical Psychology, 64*(6), 1152–1168.

Huka, B. S., & Wheat, J. R. (1985). Patterns of utilization: The patient perspective *Medical Care, 23*, 438–460.

Jacobson, E. (1974). *Progressive relaxation.* Chicago: The University of Chicago Press, Midway Reprint.

Johnson, J., Weissman, M. M., & Klerman, G. L. (1992). Service utilization and social morbidity associated with depressive symptoms in the community. *Journal of the American Medical Association, 267*, 1478–1473.

Kabat-Zinn, J., Massion, A. O., Kristeller, J., Peterson, L. G., Fletcher, K. E., Pbert, L., Lenderking, W. R., & Santorelli, S. F. (1992). Effectiveness of a meditation-based stress reduction program in the treatment of anxiety disorders. *American Journal of Psychiatry, 149*(7), 936–943.

Koenig, H. G., Shelp, F., Goli, V., Cohen, H. J., & Blazer, D. G. (1989). Survival and health care utilization in elderly medical inpatients with major depression. *Journal of the American Geriatric Society, 37*(7), 599–606.

Leaf, P. J., Livingston, M. M., Tischler, G. E., Weissman, M. M., Holzer, C. E., & Myers, J. K. (1985). Contact with health professionals for the treatment of psychiatric and emotional problems. *Medical Care, 23*, 1322–1337.

Mechanic, D. (1978). *Medical sociology* (2nd ed.). New York: Free.

Montagu, A. (1990, February). Psychological neoteny. *Longevity*, pp. 47–53.

Parkerson, G. (1996). *User's guide for the Duke Health Profile.* Durham, NC: Duke University Medical Center.

Patterson, C., Crescenzi, C., & Stell, K. (1984). Hospital use by the extremely elderly (nonagenarians): A two-year study. *Journal of the American Geriatric Society, 32*, 350–352.

Phillips, M. A., & Murrel, S. (1994). Impact of psychological and physical health, stressful events, and social support on subsequent mental health help seeking among older adults. *Journal of Consulting and Clinical Psychology, 62*, 270–275.

Reynolds, C. F. (1994). Treatment of depression in late life. *The American Journal of Medicine, 97*(suppl 6A), 6A-39S–6A-46S.

Richter, J. M., Barsky, A. J., & Hupp, J. A. (1983). The treatment of depression in elderly patients. *Journal of Family Practice, 17*(1), 43–47.

Robinson, P. (1994, September). *Treating depressed primary care patients: New models.* A presentation to the HMO Group, Minneapolis, Minnesota.

Robinson, P. (1996). *Living life well: New strategies for hard times.* Reno: Context.

Robinson, P., Bush, T., VonKorff , M., Katon, W., Lin, E., Simon, G. E., & Walker, E.

(1994). Primary care physician use of cognitive behavioral techniques with depressed patients. *Journal of Family Practice, 40*(4), 352-357.

Robinson, P., & Hayes, S. (1996). Acceptance and commitment: A model for integration. In N. Cummings, J. Cummings, & J. Johnson (Eds.), *Behavioral health in primary care: A guide for clinical integration.* Madison, CT: Psychosocial.

Robinson, P., Wischman, C. & Del Vento, A. (1996). *Treating depression in primary care: A manual for primary care and mental health providers.* Reno: Context Press.

Wan, T. T. H. (1982). *Stressful life events, social support networks, and gerontological health: A prospective study.* Lexington, MA: Lexington.

Wan, T. T. H. (1989). The behavioral model of health care utilization by older people. In M. G. Ory, & K. Bond (Eds.), *Aging and health care: Social science and policy perspective.* London: Tavistock.

Wan, T. T. H., & Arling, G. (1983). Differential use of health services among disabled elders. *Research on Aging, 5,* 411-431.

Wan, T. T. H., & Odell, B. G. (1981). Factors affecting the use of social and health services among the elderly. *Aging and Society, 1,* 95-115.

Waxman, H. M., Carner, E. A., & Blum, A. (1983). Depressive symptoms and health service utilization among the community elderly. *Journal of the American Geriatric Society, 31*(7), 417-420.

Wolinsky, F. D., & Coe, R. M. (1984). Physician and hospital utilization among noninstitutionalized elderly adults: An analysis of the health interview survey. *Journal of Gerontology, 39,* 334-341.

Wolinsky, F. D., Mosely, R. R., & Coe, R. M. (1986). A cohort analysis of the use of health services by elderly Americans. *Journal of Health and Social Behavior, 27,* 209-219.

9

Forming a Multidisciplinary Team

Thomson F. Davis   George R. Biltz

Chapters 8 and 9 represent the farthest point on the continuum of integration. Both are written by teams that work together regularly in a primary care environment to address the needs of a particular population. They illustrate primary care–based vertically-integrated care (see Chapter 6). Both teams exhibit a passion for the care of their population of patients, which is a feature of good teamwork.

Davis and Biltz highlight the uniqueness of a team that has worked together so much that each team member carries the patterns of the team as a whole. In practice, it means that if one team member cannot conduct the intake interview, another team member is fully capable of doing the intake from the point of view of his or her colleague, whether it be medical, psychological, or nutritional. In such teams, each team member is a resource to the other team members.

In settings such as Davis and Biltz describe, where each team member has learned the language and logic of the other skill sets represented by the other team members, a foundation has been laid for new and different ways of thinking about serving the population.

Perhaps the most compelling reason to form multidisciplinary teams within primary care is simply that certain patient problems require it. Whenever the patient asks, "What should be done, Doctor?" and the physician has an effective answer, there is no need for a team. Often, the complexity of the problems and the needs of the patient are not this simple or straightforward. Faced with limited time and multiple demands, primary care physicians may respond solely to the acute biomedical needs of their patients while underdiagnosing and undertreating the psychosocial factors that contribute to their patients' problems (Ford, 1994; Wagner, Austin, & Von Korff, 1996). Developing a multidisciplinary team is one response to clinical problems that do not fit neatly into the biomedical frame of reference.

This chapter is a story about the evolution of a multidisciplinary team: the pediatric Center for Exercise and Nutrition Therapy (CENT). CENT started with a single physician, Dr. George Biltz, a pediatrician practicing within a large HMO in the Twin Cities of Minnesota. The story will be told in narrative form — at first in the voice of Dr. Biltz, later in the voice of the team — to capture the historical sequence of events and to provide the clinical context. We expect that many of the scenarios within the story will be familiar to most readers despite differences in setting and specifics of the presenting problems. The patients, their families, the symptoms and problems, the context of care: This is the territory all providers must survey.

Woven into the story is an analysis of the narrative. What was going on in the situation described? What was learned from the encounter? What decisions were made and what evolved out of the experience? The "patient-to-principle" process provides a clinical framework. It is our hope that the analysis will help the reader to learn what we took from our experience. Readers still may come to alternate conclusions from the narrative provided.

The chapter closes with a description of the concepts and principles that we learned over the course of developing our team. These concepts and principles support the formation of integrated health care teams and provide criteria for evaluation and planning.

DR. BILTZ'S STORY

CENT began at the convergence of my clinical observations about obesity and fitness. These clinical observations revealed two very distinct populations. On one hand, I was seeing some very athletic children and adolescents because of acute and overuse injuries they had sustained on the playing field or during athletic training. These children were highly motivated to be active, they were goal-oriented in their training, and they were supported by a large set of resources and rewards from family and community. On the other hand were the patients with striking obesity. These children were highly sedentary, they often preferred "screen time" and watching to physical activity, and most demonstrated diminished capacity for sustained physical exertion. Most of these children were neither supported nor rewarded for participation in community athletic or active recreational programs. Typical of obese children (Sheslow, Hassink, Wallace, & DeLancey, 1993), many were discouraged. A common cultural message was: If you're not good at something, don't do it at all. These two groups of children were different not only in level of activity but also in their daily lifestyles and social experiences.

Coincidentally, I was coordinating an adult seminar on fitness. Fitness was defined as the dynamic interplay between physical condition, mental attitude, and nutritional state. This seminar was presented with two colleagues with similar interests and complimentary expertise. I had also given a pediatric grand rounds on fitness testing in the office setting. This preparation further defined fitness for me and clarified the principles of physiologic adaptation to task environment. At the same time, I gained insight into the practical means to measure components of fitness in my medical practice.

In these two activities were the seeds of CENT: fitness as an operational definition of health and team effort as a problem approach and practice style.

I began to work with obese patients in my practice. I provided an individualized approach to becoming fit based on a training or conditioning approach, including pep talks — "coaching" to motivate behavioral change. The message emphasized the need to increase physical activity and to reduce total caloric intake. Balancing the energy equation was relatively straightforward: Increase calories expended, decrease the caloric intake, and weight reduction would theoretically follow. The physiology was predictable. Fitness was culturally desirable. The expectation was fair and the requirements practical.

I gave patients sample diets deemed calorically appropriate. These were based on diets developed for diabetic patients: 1,200 to 1,500 calories per day. At first the exercise goal was just to get more activity along the recommended guidelines of the American College of Sports Medicine (1978): 30 minutes, three times per week.

Although no formal data were collected, I had a growing sense of being ineffective in changing obesity trends. My frustration grew with the persistence of the complaint "Something needs to be done, Doctor" and the question, "What else can we do, Doctor?"

Mrs. Golden has three daughters who are periodically seen in the general pediatric clinic. Of the three daughters, the youngest, seven-year-old Terri, has the most problems with weight control (obesity). There is desperation in Mrs. Golden's voice when she talks about the weight problem and the teasing at school. School refusal is becoming an unexpected problem. General eating and activity recommendations aren't being implemented. The plan is appropriate but the approach obviously needs to be modified, but how? What is reasonable to expect in terms of compliance with the recommended care plan? Mrs. Golden says, "Since gym time at school is a source of embarrassment, could she be excused? Would you write a note?"

Terri continues to gain weight and to refuse the activity participation that seems essential to her weight control. Issues of patient compliance, parental control, and provider expectations begin to collide. Something needs to be done.

Mrs. Sandler's daughter, Rose, is gaining excessively, and although there is compliance at home — Mrs. Sandler has been controlling snacks and portion sizes — Rose is eating the other children's lunches and snacks at school. Mrs. Sandler is concerned, "What should be done to control her weight, Doctor?"

Fourteen-year-old Nadine Cotton is seen for parental and personal concerns about obesity. She is 5'10" and 244 pounds. She has been overweight since age five. Previous recommendations about weight control appear to be unheeded or not generalized. There is increasing clinical concern after detection of cholesterol greater than 240, triglycerides at 420, and HDL (good cholesterol) at 29. All values are abnormal. Nadine and her mother attended the clinic's class on managing cholesterol and they are trying to change their eating habits. Nadine is passive and makes poor eye contact. She and her mother live alone in a trailer court where they know few people. Mrs. Cotton is too tired after her work to commit to a walking program with her daughter. In the summer, Nadine works at Burger King five days per week and eats there before walking home to the trailer court about one mile away. This after-work walk occurs only before it gets too dark outside. Nadine thinks her ideal weight should be about 100 pounds. What else can be done?

What is common to all of these cases? Clearly it was neither the patient data nor the environmental circumstances. It was a level of clinical complexity beyond a 15-minute regular office visit; a level of complexity outside the usual medical arena and beyond the provider's belief that the recommendations will work at all. Therein rises the specter of noncompliance. A 1989 national survey of pediatricians revealed that only 22% felt competent in prescribing a weight loss program for children and only 11% agreed that such efforts were professionally gratifying (Price, Desmond, Ruppert, & Stelzar, 1989). The label of noncompliance becomes more likely as the level of complexity exceeds the resources of the patient and the provider.

I felt it was necessary to redefine the problem, to search for organizational allies, people to help internally. I also looked for experts and models that worked, that could be emulated, refined, modified, and adapted. For me, the model for a this new approach was developed by Dr. Oded Bar-Or, an internationally recognized expert in the field of pediatric exercise science. He had established the Children's Exercise and Nutrition Centre at McMaster University in Hamilton, Ontario, Canada. I visited there in the summer of 1988 and borrowed liberally from his approach. At the core of the team was a nutritionist, psychologist, physical educator, and a nurse-manager. The center had supporting grant money in a university environment. I needed to establish a center in an HMO environment.

Ten years ago, fitness was primarily understood within the context of exercise physiology, physical education, and athletics. Traditional medical management did not appreciate fitness as a medical concept, much less as a service priority. There were commercial weight control programs and school-based physical education programs for that. But obesity was clearly associated with significant physical and psychological morbidity, and obesity as a medical problem has multiple etiologies, different risks, and different responses to treatment (Rosenbaum & Leibel, 1989). CENT as a project was sold to HMO management as a multidisciplinary approach to the diseases of hypoactivity: heart disease, diabetes mellitus, and obesity. The pediatric intervention CENT advocated would be a way to save medical resources in the long term.

I envisioned a multidisciplinary center that would consolidate expertise in one place, an approach that would focus more information on the problem. Each participant could contribute his or her slice of expertise toward the solution of the problem. I recruited a licensed practical nurse who understood the personal side of obesity. She had struggled with her weight in childhood and adolescence and had found physical activity a key to successful weight control. She also had firsthand knowledge of nutrition and caloric reduction. She was able and willing to work with families on behavioral issues. CENT was launched on one half-day per week, staffed by the nurse and me, and equipped with a basic treadmill, plastic skin fold calipers, charts to estimate body fat from skin fold data, a homemade "sit and reach" box for flexibility testing, a mat for testing abdominal strength by doing graded sit-ups, handouts recommending walking programs, American Dietetic Association diets, and handouts listing the caloric content estimates for a variety of popular fast foods and snacks. To justify the costs at a time when any addtional program was vulnerable unless it had high utiliztion, the clinic was opened to both adult and pediatric patients.

The problems caught in this broadly cast net were unexpectedly complicated, and the demand for services greatly exceeded clinic capacity. CENT needed to narrow its focus, so the clinic was restructured to be strictly a pediatric center. In a 1989 business plan I requested the services of a health psychologist and dedicated nutritionist, but only the nutritionist was available at the time. In those days, health psychologists and nutritionists were among a group of service providers who worked in several different sites or programs. They were paid out of a central budget and "donated" their time wherever they were welcomed. When they became a regular part of a program, that site might pick up a portion of their salary out of the site's budget. This allowed collaboration to develop that never would have occurred if sites had been required to know exactly how to use these providers and had to pay for them in order to start their involvement.

Nutrition services were an easy interface to medical practice. Both the nutritionist and the physician have similar scientific backgrounds, beliefs, and expectations. Their worldview is shaped by biomedical science, the so-called "medical model," and traditional patient expectations. Patients come with problems to be solved. If one can carefully determine the key components to the problem, a plan for resolution between patient and provider can be conceived and communicated. The plan is made actionable and compliance is expected. Despite these apparently reasonable assumptions, the patients continued to present new challenges that required new insights.

Marie Vale is the 12-year-old daughter of two physicians. Her parents have noted a progressive increase in her weight over two years, along with an increasing difficulty in keeping up with her soccer team. She also has some patellofemoral (knee) pain that disproportionately limits activity. A point system has been tried to limit desserts, but initial weight losses have been regained. Power struggles are increasing. Marie's parents are concerned about her lack of peer relationships. Mr. Vale sees sports participation as a needed source of friendships; Mrs. Vale is reluctant to push weight control because her mother made it an issue throughout Mrs. Vale's childhood. While Mrs. Vale continues to struggle with weight concerns and multiple diets, Mr. Vale has always been successful at weight control and expects Marie to be the same.

The nutritionist and I realized that the Vales were "informationally rich" parents. The power struggle was the focal point. It was easy to name the problem. However, the problem wasn't simply knowing *what* needed to be done about weight control, it was also how to replace the power struggles with shared responsibility for weight control.

Power struggles surfaced as a recurring theme in our patient families. Often there was a great sense of unfairness felt by the obese child with skinny siblings or superfit parents. There was predictable anger related to issues of autonomy with the obese teen. In many cases there was a history of psychological loss (Maine, 1991). The obese child may eat to soothe these feelings or exert her autonomy, and thereby increase her obesity. Frequently the obese child was not concerned about his weight — clearly not as concerned as his parents. The fact that the child was not concerned became another concern of the parents. Parents often had their own story of childhood obesity and the teasing that left scars. Some parents continued to struggle with obesity and wanted to spare their children the suffering. Others appeared to have controlled their weight but their methods remained secret: Some of these parents didn't want to share their past difficulties; others had probably lost weight by starving or vomiting and did not want their children to take these paths. What we thought was common ground of weight control appeared far more complicated. There were layers of the past leading up to the present. For each patient there was a story buried in these convoluted layers, but who was prepared to unfold it? Both the nutritionist and physician felt limited in coping with the feelings that fueled these problems. We needed help entangling these behavioral road blocks.

A health psychologist became available to join our team. The health psychologist came from a different culture, with different expectations about patient behavior. The simplistic assumption from medicine is that authoritative information exchange will result in behavioral change. The physician seeks to know *what* changes in eating and activity habits will result in the desired outcome, while the health psychologist seeks to know *why* the patient would want to change at all. Feelings, expectations, and relationships are as fundamental as information about diet, exercise, and physiology. All health care providers must learn to cope with the feelings as well as the facts to facilitate behavior change. In our patient population, behavior change was prerequisite to physiologic improvements.

The initial role of the health psychologist was directed more at provider consultation than direct patient service. The health psychologist didn't have previous experience with obesity management. The critical goal was to facilitate the work and broaden the skills of the nutritionist and physician as they coped with the power struggles and other behavioral entanglements. The health psychologist sat in with me primarily to learn about the patient population and my "moves" in trying to help. Simultaneously, I was listening to the questions the psychologist was asking the patient and family. I simplistically assumed that health psychology, like medicine, was fundamentally about information exchange. The health psychologist could hopefully answer the question "How do we get them to change their eating and activity habits?" Instead, the psychologist asked, "Why would you want to change? Would anything be better for you if you made any changes? Is it worth the effort?"

We established a noon lunch meeting to review the morning patients and preview the afternoon patients. This facilitated an easy exchange of professional viewpoints and the planning of patient care. For the biomedically grounded nutritionist and physician, the health psychologist offered new interpretations of the problems presented by our patients.

Thirteen-year-old Steve lives in a single-parent household. He openly resents being at a "fat clinic." From his perspective, his excessive weight is not a problem. The family history of maturity onset diabetes mellitus isn't of immediate concern to him — this is several lifetimes away.

From a traditional medical perspective, there is little to negotiate when someone announces no interest. The lack of an acceptable agreed-upon outcome suggests either more complicated problems than first realized or patient noncompliance. The patient either has a problem and is willing to work on it, or the patient becomes the problem, blocking or limiting the solution. Noncompliance with recommendations seems inevitable. To disengage seems logical. The health psychologist offers another approach (Lipchik, 1988). Patients are not always immediate "customers" of health services. In fact, it may be acceptable to be a "visitor" for awhile, to shop around at the clinic before buying into the program and its recommendations. This visitor-customer classification allows contact and exchange of perspectives and information without feeling the loss of autonomy that is often paramount in teenagers. The visitor status permits participation without doing what someone else expects or demands. From the provider perspective there was one major expectation: After several visits, you must clarify your status. Are you a customer? If not, then we will help you clarify the indicators for returning when you feel ready to be a customer.

The Harper family has three obese children. During the intake, Mrs. Harper cries about her children's weight problems. The physician offers her a tissue. The health psychologist asks her to tell us more. She acknowledges a personal history of struggles with eating and repeated weight loss and regain. She also speaks of being overwhelmed with work and too tired to exercise. Mr. Harper, a truck driver, acknowledges that he looks to his wife to take care of things at home while he is on the road. They ate at a fast food restaurant on the way to this appointment since they were rushed. The mother seems to be the emotional "barometer" of the family. The daughters seem attached and sensitized to the mother's mood. How much do we need to know from the mother about herself? What are we prepared to "unpack" in this first interview?

The health psychologist was able to ask questions that helped the nutritionist and physician learn the level of inquiry appropriate to the circumstances and their own counseling skills. Focusing on the mother's probable eating disorder too soon might unfairly shift the burden of family obesity to her. All members needed to share in the family's lifestyle choices and to take appropriate levels of responsibility for improved eating and activity habits.

For the behaviorally grounded psychologist, the physiology of fitness provided new insights. The physician distinguished three aspects of the fitness concept: (1) fitness may be seen as an adaptation to tasks, that is, fitness as a process; (2) fitness may be defined as a level of performance in an athletic event or fitness test; (3) fitness may be seen as a dynamic state that prevents the diseases of hypoactivity and premature loss of physical capacity and promotes participation in life's activities. The latter is fitness as prevention and participation, fitness as an operational definition of health. These conceptual descriptions of fitness melded with the psychologist's family systems thinking. Fitness was a reflection of the total context in which the individual is functioning. In order to have an impact on an individual's level of fitness, the broad psychosocial context must be evaluated and changed, as needed and where possible.

THE TEAM'S STORY

A true multidisciplinary team had come together. We had our shared patients, shared space in which to practice, and we were developing our skills at working efficiently and effectively together. We knew that families with one or more obese family members present with a full spectrum of emotions and relationships: sadness, loss, anger, enmeshment, etc. Family resources for coping with problems also range across the socioeconomic and psychological spectrum. Our challenge was to develop a program or approach that could adjust to the context of each case, that could be responsive to our shared pool of patients. The team needed a clear sense of the overarching goals, accepted methods, and measures of success. We needed to articulate a shared voice. Practically, we needed to organize how we delivered services to support the team and to deliver truly integrated care.

We knew we needed joint provider time with patients to develop the integrative aspects of care. We also needed individual follow-up time with each patient to zero-in on the unique aspects of the case as defined by our professional backgrounds. We settled on a schedule that allowed for two consecutive 30-minute family intakes with all three providers. While the first new family was being interviewed, the second new family was filling out our paperwork: the family information sheet, parent and child versions of our eating and activity questionnaire, and a self-perception profile. After 30 minutes, the families switched activities. Each family was subsequently seen for 40 minutes by each provider separately. The provider not seeing a new family was working with another family returning for a follow-up appointment. From noon to 1:30 the team met over lunch. This extended lunch hour was critical to the review and preview of patient care, communication of professional information, troubleshooting, planning for the program, and team cohesiveness. There was only one day of the week that all team providers were physically at the clinic at the same time, so opportunity for interaction had to be built in. The afternoon was divided into 30-minute follow-up appointments. Many patients wanted to see all three providers. Others were interested in following up with only one or two. The team could not have survived without the skillful help of the team receptionist who made this complex scheduling system work.

The 40-minute individual provider intake session was brief by professional standards for the psychologist. This was partially compensated by the 30-minute joint intake session. In fact, the joint intake created an opportunity for providers to observe each other's professional "moves." After hearing each other pursue their pet topics and questions, a general interdisciplinary format arose, and questions were professionally cross-pollinated, that is, the nutritionist might ask a psychologically oriented question while the psychologist might ask directly about exercise and nutrition habits. The physician might be quiet in order to listen carefully to the whole story that the patients and families were telling.

As the health psychologist began to get to know and influence the other members of the team, behavioral change became a central outcome of care rather than an assumed expectation of patients (Kaplan, 1990). Behavioral change precedes, indeed is a prerequisite for, medically de-

	High Resources for Coping	Low Resources for Coping
Simple Problems	Level 1: Coaching	Level 2: Counseling
Complex Problems	Level 2: Counseling	Level 3: Management

Figure 9.1. Levels of clinical intervention based on risk dimensions of problem complexity and family resources for coping.

sired physiological outcomes, such as decreased body fat or improved cholesterol or blood pressure. Simultaneously, there was an expanded focus for interventions from patient based care to family based care.

We developed a structure for understanding the problems of the patients we encountered. It is our belief that an individual patient has three fundamental factors that influence behavior: what they know, how they feel, and what they do. These factors are dynamically and reciprocally interconnected. An individual is also dynamically and reciprocally connected to situations and relationships. When families seek our help, their system may be unhealthy with respect to weight management, but it is balanced and stable in such a way to meet certain needs or to solve certain problems that are often covert. The context of care is this dynamic system.

C. J. Peek (personal communication, 1986) has observed another shared concept, which is illustrated in Figure 9.1. There are three levels of clinical intervention, which are based on two risk dimensions: complexity of the problem and availability of resources. Patients in the lowest risk group, level 1, have relatively straightforward problems and sufficient material and psychological resources to cope. They require more traditional "coaching," which includes information, feedback, and support. Level 2 patients have more, complex and/or diminished resources to cope. They require what might be called a "counseling" style of care. This care is highly individualized and is designed to facilitate problem solving and/or to enhance the patient and family coping resources so that relevant information, feedback, and support is effective. Level 3 patients have both complex problems and limited resources to cope. Problems are typically chronic and pervasive. Often these patients require a period of direct clinical management in order to offset feelings of hopelessness, helplessness, and demoralization. The immediate goal of intervention is to help these patients move to level 2 care.

The team used these shared concepts to analyze cases and plan care. We recognized that these clinical classifications were an internal common currency for discussion and comparison. Classification of a family was typically withheld until the second visit, giving them time to demonstrate their readiness and capacity to respond to initial plans. The team fortunately had the autonomy to define itself and its therapeutic approach. Our concepts and "voice" were shaped and consolidated when we made presentations to other providers inside and outside of the HMO—the quickest way to clarify one's thinking is to be faced with giving a public presentation.

We also recognized the need to look beyond ourselves as simply a unique set of professionals who worked as a team. We recognized that being effective and ultimately efficient would require measures of outcomes. For an obese adult population, one can simplistically use weight in pounds and percentage of body fat as direct measures of weight status. Successful weight control programs show improvement in weight status of their clients. In growing children and adolescents, lean body mass naturally increases with growth. Improved body composition, not total weight, is the better measure of success. A clinic database and flow sheet were developed to provide consolidated data for review, analysis, and follow-up. The nutritionist also developed a separate follow-up shingle that could be easily updated and followed by any nutritionist who might fill in when the team nutritionist might be off.

We made many other modifications in the program as a result of the cross-pollination of professional knowledge, skills, and values. For example, it was the custom of the physician to write an "exercise prescription" for each patient's exercise program. This was designed to improve compliance. If exercise were made analogous to medicine, it would surely be taken more seriously and followed more consistently. Unfortunately, compliance with traditional pharmaceutical prescriptions is much lower than physicians care to recall (Meichenbaum & Turk, 1987). Furthermore, parents considered the prescription more seriously than did the patient. Often the exercise prescription, which was ceremoniously handed to the patient in the office, became an acrimonious point of contention at home. In its place, the team developed an activity planner to be done as a collaborative effort between parent and child. Together they could identify different activities that could be done under each of four different circumstances: indoors alone or with others, and outdoors alone or with others. A guideline sheet was provided, if necessary, that gave examples of possible activities in each circumstance. Once activities were selected, the family was asked to identify resources necessary for these activities to occur. For example, bike riding requires a bike that works, a helmet, and a safe route. Swimming requires a pool and most likely transportation to the pool, membership or money for access, and a partner or supervision. And, each of these requires planned use of time.

Lionel Tripp is a 17-year-old who has been chronically ill with flu-like symptoms for about six months. He has been treated for Lyme disease recently, with about 50% improvement. He is able to do some activity before extreme fatigue and chest pain set in. Lionel also has delays in his intellectual, social, and emotional development. He receives special education at school. He is on amitriptyline for depression. His low self-esteem has worsened with his illness, which is compounded by a 25-pound weight gain in the last five to six months. Lionel skips breakfast and drinks about three to four cans of regular soda a day. His overall eating habits are erratic. He is unable to complete the initial treadmill test due to leg cramps. Mr. & Mrs. Tripp separated four years ago and are divorcing, but they still share a house; Mr. Tripp lives upstairs and has kitchen privileges.

Lionel appears to have many problems and no readily apparent strength on which to build our treatment. Although he is willing to attend our sessions, it is often difficult to know the degreee to which he benefits from our work together. Indeed, Lionel gains eight pounds without change in his height over the first six to seven weeks in our program. Despite this lack of progress, he continues to participate. We teach him some basics about weight management and offer him a few practical, small, concrete steps that he might take. We give him encouragement and celebrate progress in any area of his life—not just changes in his weight.

At the same time, Lionel's physical symptoms begin to improve and he is more able and willing to go for walks around the neighborhood without having to be nagged to do so. Over the next several months, several other changes occur independent of our efforts. We celebrate these improvements and work to make them relevant to his weight control. Lionel and his mother move into an apartment complex that has exercise equipment available to all tenants; Lionel gets a part-time job at a retail store; and a physical education teacher encourages Lionel to join a group of other students in a weight lifting class at school. His physical activitiy level becomes more consistent.

As Lionel feels more successful, he makes voluntary dietary changes. He now wants more information from the dietitian on healthy eating, and his intake of soft drinks decreases remarkably. Success is breeding success, and our earlier seeds of knowledge and encouragement are beginning to blossom in this richer environment at home and at school. His weight trend shifts back to levels he was at when we first met him, but his body composition now consists of much more muscle and much less fat. His performance on the treadmill is significantly better.

Vicky Newton is an only child whose mother has weight concerns for both Vicky and herself. Mother is more concerned than Vicky, and recalls her own lifelong problems with weight control. At ten years old, Vicky is a good eater, consuming larger portions than peers. She is well above the 99th percentile of weight for her age. She has many interests, including piano, art, swimming, and dance. She also likes to ride her bike and play video games with her friends. Her self-perception profile shows high scores on most subscales with median scores on the athletic competence and physical appearance subscales. Her heart rate response during the modified Balke treadmill walk suggests that she isn't consistently active. There is room for improvement in eating and activity habits, and her family appears motivated to change.

Our treatment strategy was to stabilize the larger system and identify the "drivers" of the system that can be modified or influenced to achieve therapeutic goals. With a greater appreciation for the system complexity and dynamics, the team has a more complete grasp of the global system than any individual provider could. The team also has the range of "moves" necessary to interact with and modify the global system.

During the intervention phase there is an immediate decrease in Vicky's weight trend. This is accomplished by an increased awareness of eating and snacking habits and an increase in physical activity. Exercise capacity and measure of body fat consistently show improvement. With the onset of summer, Vicky's daily patterns shift as she is often home alone. Her weight begins to rebound and between June and September, she gains 11 pounds. The nutritionist detects an increase in power struggles over limits that had previously been set on foods such as french fries and sugared soft drinks. Activity level is higher than baseline but not as active as during the during the period of decreasing weight.

We respond by reinforcing the positive changes that occurred, acknowledging the influence of puberty on weight control at this age, and setting tiny goals for reestablishing consistent choices in the new school year. We are also tempted to reestablish more parental control of diet and exercise, which appeared to work initially. However, this move would clearly increase parent-child conflicts, risk long-term cooperation, and jeopardize the likelihood of success. Instead, we reinforce the family's trust in Vicky's ability to balance her eating and activity habits. At her age, Vicky needs her parents to provide the macroenvironmental support for change to occur; she needs to do the daily work of managing the microenvironment.

Vicky's weight trend continues to rise until her weight returns to a point in the 98th percentile. This would be Vicky's last visit. A repeat treadmill test shows better exercise capacity than at the time when weight was at its lowest point. This confirms Vicky's consistent activity effort. It also reveals that fitness and fatness are not mutually exclusive states. There is hope. The goals are to become more fit, not simply to lose weight, and to stabilize eating and activity habits. If these behavior changes occur, the weight trend will follow.

The third and final phase of Vicky's story involves the follow-up of her progress which reveals the impact of the intervention. For two years, Vicky has stabilized her weight trend on a slope that is returning her toward the 95th percentile. Her weight trend has remained stable throughout the entire time. Basketball has become a special sport, and Vicky is reinforced by her athletic image and success. She and her mother both feel successful with this lifestyle change.

PRINCIPLES OF TEAM FORMATION

The experience of forming the CENT team has shown us many principles that will be useful to others in planning, evaluating, and troubleshooting team functioning. We define a multidisciplinary team as a community of professionals, some from different professional backgrounds, who are bound by common mission, goals, and expected outcomes. They work with a shared population of patients within the same physical space. Over time, they develop their own values, principles, practices, and history. At the core of this definition are the concepts of a shared population of patients and a community of professionals.

A population of patients may be defined by a common set of clinical conditions or problems. It is these people and the problems they experience that literally brings the team together and focuses the team's thinking and actions. Like the mythical blind men and the elephant, each team member may see each patient somewhat differently, but through the combined vision of the team, the picture is more complete and better integrated. Furthermore, it is their shared commitment to those patients — to *their* patients — that provides the foundation for team building, the bond of team identity, and the synergy of a well-functioning team. A team's shared population of patients will pace and lead the team, and if time for team communication is built in, it will teach the team and help it improve.

A professional community may be defined by a number of parameters, including:

- membership
- status, roles, and responsibilities
- knowledge base and decision-making principles
- common language, practices, and experiences

Membership

Each member of an interdisciplinary team is a member of at least two communities: his or her primary professional community and the shared community of the team. Membership is often defined by the status of the provider in his or her professional community, with the expectation that this knowledge, skill, judgment, and wisdom is necessary for the team to be successful with the population of patients they serve. But, simply being good at what you do professionally is not enough. To a large degree, it is actually the capacity of the provider to function in the "foreign culture" of the other professional communities while maintaining one's own professional identity that characterizes a member of an effective and well-functioning team.

Status, Roles, and Responsibilities

To gain and maintain status in the team, each provider must represent, interpret, and apply the knowledge, skills, judgment, and wisdom of his own profession to the common problems presented to the team. Although one team member, typically the physician in whose clinic the team practices, is the leader and "keeper" of the team, each member must "pull his own weight" and contribute his own expertise to make the team effective. It is critical that all key team members represent and deliver the knowledge, wisdom, and skills of their professions, and that conflicts in professional viewpoints, values, and intervention strategies be identified and resolved. Integrated primary care teams, like the well-functioning team in baseball, have players who play their position well while supporting and enhancing the performance of the team to get the job done.

Knowledge Base and Decision-Making Principles

Integrated care draws on the knowledge base and decision-making principles of the multiple disciplines represented on the team. This presents two challenges: first, to identify and communicate relevant knowledge, theory, and principles to others outside one's professional domain, and, second, to find ways to establish priorities and resolve conflicts among competing ideas.

Most of us have experience in communicating our professional knowledge to others who have not shared similar training and cultures: We reduce our use of professional jargon, we speak to issues that are relevant and "real" to our colleagues, and seek out "teachable moments" when our colleague's need to know is high. We speak neither condescendingly nor without sensitivity to the issue that an expert in one field may be a novice in another. We translate and interpret. We teach and we listen. We also seek common ground, common understandings, and common principles.

Early in the development of the team, areas of expertise are typically defined by professional backgrounds, and for some teams and some clinical problems this structure may be sufficient, such as when services by each provider are offered at different times and in different places rather than in a truly coordinated and integrated fashion. However, in our opinion, much greater effectiveness and efficiency is gained when each provider begins to learn the knowledge, skills, practices, and decision-making principles of the others, and each provider is able to identify and respond to clinical issues and teachable moments that are clinically significant to fellow team members. Based on the experience of quick hallway consults, more in-depth case conferences, and direct observation of the other's "craftsmanship" while interacting with patients, the integrated care provider gains appreciation of the multiple, overlapping aspects of clinical problems, and the variety of interventions required to treat the patient. Each team member is able to provide a response to patient concerns that is more on target and adds leverage to the interventions of other team members. This does not mean that physicians become psychologists, that physical therapists practice medicine, that psychologists become dietitians; as with all professional practice, this level of functioning requires knowledge of one's own professional limits and the ethical requirement not to practice outside of one's own competence. But, for the patient (and for the team), each provider is like a point on a hologram, in which each part of the picture contains information about the whole picture.

Common Language, Practices, and Experiences

Over time, common language, practices, and experiences become part of the team's culture, the team's shared voice. This voice flows from (1) the language, practices, and experiences of each provider in his or her primary professional community, (2) the shared experiences of observing, consulting, and criticizing case work together, and (3) deliberately developing new behaviors, knowledge, skills, judgments, values, and relationships within the team. Membership is no longer based solely on professional qualifications. Trust is established. Relationships are consolidated. The professional values of fellow team members are appreciated and supported. The array of provider approaches is broadened, resulting in less provider frustration, anxiety, or defensiveness when challenged by the complexities of clinical practice.

In sum, individual contributions in the service of a shared population and shared mission build effective multidisciplinary teams, enhance care, and produce better clinical outcomes.

REFERENCES

American College of Sports Medicine. (1978). Position statement on the recommended quantity and quality of exercise for developing and maintaining fitness in healthy adults. *Medicine and Science in Sports, 10*, vii.

Ford, D. E. (1994). Recognition and under-recognition of mental disorders in adult primary care. In J. Miranda, A. A. Hohmann, C. C. Attkisson, & D. B. Larson (Eds.), *Mental disorders in primary care* (pp. 186–205). San Francisco: Jossey-Bass.

Kaplan, R. (1990). Behavior as the central outcome in health care. *American Psycholoist, 45*(11), 1211–1230.

Lipchik, E. (1988). Purposeful sequences for beginning the solution-focused interview. In E. Lipchik (Ed.), *Interviewing*. Rockville, MD: Aspen.

Maine, M. (1991). *Father hunger: Fathers, daughters, and food*. Carlsbad, CA: Gruze.

Meinchenbaum, D., & Turk, D. (1987). *Facilitating treatment adherence: A practitioner's guidebook*. New York: Plenum.

Price, J., Desmond, S., Ruppert, E., & Stelzar, C. (1989). Pediatricians' perceptions and practices regarding childhood obesity. *American Journal of Preventive Medicine, 5*(2), 95–103.

Rosenbaum, M., & Leibel, R. (1989). Obesity in childhood. *American Journal of Family Therapy, 14*(3), 247–253.

Sheslow, D., Hassink, S., Wallace, W., & DeLancey, E. (1993). The relationship between self-esteem and depression in obese children. *Annals of the New York Academy of Sciences, 699,* 289–291.

Wagner, E. H., Austin, B. T., & Von Korff, M. (1996). Improving outcomes in chronic illness. *Managed Care Quarterly, 4*(2), 12–25.

10

Integrated Primary Health Care For Women

Margaret Heldring

Margaret Heldring's chapter is a call for integrated primary care for the population that makes up the largest group of patients in primary care: women. Women as a group are sometimes thought of by providers as better patients than men because they are more willing to seek health services for illness or injury and to comply with a treatment regimen. Women also seem to make up the group that is most likely to encounter the faults and inadequacies of the health care system. A majority of the overserviced and underserved patients that Peek and Heinrich describe (Chapter 7) are women. Women comprise the majority of patients who present with "undefined" disorders (Malterud, 1992), the painful and destructive disorders such as fibromyalgia and chronic fatigue syndrome in which there are few objective findings. The more providers are limited to the biomedical lens in approaching these conditions and are unable to understand psychosocial factors or to give credence to the experience of the patient separate from the findings, the more difficult and frustrating the treatment for patient and provider.

Integrated primary care provides one antidote for the problem of the single lens approach. It offers routine experience for providers in

247

polyocular vision, that is, looking at a phenomenon with two or more perspectives or lenses at the same time. As is true with the process of normal human visual perception, each perspective provides a slightly different angle on the phenomenon being viewed. If, however, one must choose between perspectives, if it is an either/or process in which the "right" perspective must be isolated, the depth perception given by simultaneously using both perspectives is lost. When providers are part of an integrated primary care setting, they are are likely to develop the depth of vision that is necessary to effectively approach the problems that their patients bring.

> "Women around the world share a common health problem, whether they are missing from U.S. clinical drug trials or are nowhere to be seen in a malaria clinic in Thailand. As chronicled in report after report, aspects of women's health — including nutrition and aging, responses to illnesses such as AIDS, the diseases that plague only women — have received only minimal attention or funding. Upgrading women's health entails, in part, reexamining sexuality and cultural mores. Securing women's health means social transformation." (Holloway, 1994, p. 77)

WORKING IN THE field of women's health care is essentially both a personal and a political act. To ignore the "social transformation" that is required for, and is brought about by, providing quality health care to women is to give up one of the most important resources in making this work possible: the commitment of women and men of good will to make better health care for women possible. This chapter is typical of work in this field, partly political, partly very personal. Initially, it will focus on the importance of the movement for women's health care and discuss the role of primary care, which is central to meeting the particular needs of women. It will make the case that an integrated or biopsychosocial approach is ideal and imperative to address the health needs women bring to primary care. The chapter ends with a story of one attempt to provide this kind of care.

THE STUDY OF WOMEN'S HEALTH

Consideration of women's health care necessarily involves attention to public policy and the sociocultural and political context in which it is constructed and implemented. Support for women's health care has been historically sparse (Schroeder, 1992). Until recently, women have not had nor assumed a sufficient political voice to call clear attention to the public policy neglect of women's health (Schroeder, 1993). They have not had sufficient numbers in the employment sector to lobby for good and meaningful benefits for themselves, their children, and families. Women's health was assumed to mean reproductive issues, some major cancers, and aging. Aging was generally understood as physical and psychological deterioration and loss of value to society.

Recent years have seen an increase in the theory, clinical study, and scholarship about women's health (Rodin & Ickovics, 1990). Health care delivery systems increasingly identify women's health as a specialty area. Architects of public policy now attend to women's health issues (Bass & Howes, 1992; Wood & Ransom, 1994). Gender as a critical variable in health and illness is now understood more broadly (Strickland, 1988). Elected and appointed government leaders like U.S. Secretary of Health and Human Services Donna Shalala and former Congresswoman Patricia Schroeder have spoken, written, and established programs and assistance for the study of women's health (Schroeder, 1992, 1993). Professional organizations like Planned Parenthood and associations like the AARP have called for a comprehensive women's health care agenda. The recent health care reforms on the federal and state levels have provided new opportunities for greater recognition of women's health issues and greater validation for women as leaders in health care policy. Women are increasingly involved in rule-making about health care benefits and reimbursement systems (Washington State Health Services Commission, 1993).

All this increased attention is not a policy fluke. Historically, women's health has received greater support and protection as women have achieved a greater political voice. The Maternity and Infant Act was the first national legislation to specifically address women's health. It was passed in 1921, one year after universal suffrage. In that same year, Margaret Sanger founded the Birth Control League. The Supreme Court handed down *Roe v. Wade* in 1973, a few years into the twentieth century's second wave of feminism. As women began to be elected to political office in increasing numbers, legislation and policies focused on women's concerns have correspondingly increased. In 1989, the Congressional Caucus for Women's Issues uncovered inequities in funding for women's health: only 13.5% of the NIH budget was allocated to women's health. In response came the passage of the 1990 Women's Health Equity Act and the NIH Reauthorization Act of 1992, providing greater support for women's health. The U.S. Public Health Service established the Office of Women's Health in 1991.

There is a clear rationale for the greater support and study of women's health. Women comprise 51% of the population of the United States, 59% of the population over age 65, and 69% of the population over age 85 (U.S. Census Bureau, 1997). The Medicare and Medicaid populations are dominated by women. Forty-six perecent of the workforce is women, 40% of whom have children under the age of 18 (U.S. Bureau of Labor Statistics, 1996). Women have poorer health outcomes than do men and suffer greater disability from disease (U.S. Public Health Service, 1995). The United States ranks thirteenth in life expectancy for women and fifteenth in maternal mortality (U.S. Public Health Service). In addition, W.H.E.R.E. (Women for Healthcare, Education, Reform, and Equity; 1995) reports the following: The lower a woman's income, the less likely she is to receive preventive care; women make the majority of the health care decisions for their families; and the most common reason women go on welfare is to obtain health care benefits for their children.

In response to these data, the U.S. Public Health Service (1995) identified the following clinical health issues for women:

1. *Cardiovascular disease.* Cardiovascular disease is the most frequent cause of death in American women. Women often experience a myocardial infarction in ways that are different from the classic chest and arm pain that are seen in men. There may also be less expectation that women will have heart attacks and therefore less urgency in the response. Forty-nine percent of women who have a heart attack die within the following year, compared to 31% of men.

2. *Cancer.* Lung cancer is the leading cancer death of women, followed by breast cancer. Breast cancer is recognized as a major public health problem and was responsible for 46,000 deaths in 1993 in the U.S. (U.S. Public Health Service, 1995). Women of color have higher mortality rates for breast and cervical cancer.

3. *Autoimmune diseases.* There is remarkably little known about why women would have higher rates of autoimmune disease than men. The beginnings of a literature on the relationship of life experience to autoimmune disease is emerging (Adams, 1994) and the relationship of traumatic events in women's lives, such as being physically or sexually abused, to later numbers of physical symptoms is being documented (McCauley et al., 1997). In this area, as in many areas of women's health care, the movement from a clinical knowledge base that is "unsubstantiated" to a researched knowledge base is painfully slow.

4. *Mental health.* Rates for depression and anxiety disorders are higher for women than men. Eating disorders, posttraumatic disorders, and

some personality disorders appear more frequently among women with each of these correlating in incidence or intensity with histories of abuse (Tice, Hall, Beresford, Quinones, & Hall, 1989).

5. *Substance abuse.* Substance abuse among women has been consistently underrecognized, yet may have significant implications for the incidence and prevalence of diseases like STDs, HIV/AIDS, tuberculosis, and blood cancers, as well as social and psychological functioning. Substance abuse by women has a major impact on family life and functioning.

6. *Violence.* Homicide is the leading killer of women in the workplace and in 1991 was the leading cause of death among African-American women aged 15 to 24. Estimates of the percent of emergency room visits that are the result of domestic violence have run as high as 30%. Recent studies have been lower saying that closer to 12% of visits are the result of domestic violence. However, of the population of women who come to emergency rooms for all causes, over 50% have experienced domestic violence at some point in their lives (Abbott, Johnson, Koziol-McLain, & Lowenstein, 1995; Vivian & Langhinrichsen-Rohling, 1994).

7. *Reproductive health.* Three major issues are adolescent pregnancy, contraception, and reproductive technology. Each of these issues bears on women's autonomy, on their ability to exercise options. Adolescent pregnancy in particular is an expression of what young women judge the future to hold for them. Pregnancy is often seen as a way for an adolescent to gain a brief period of autonomy in a life where few options are available. When young women perceive a value to their life and options for their future, postponing pregnancy is much more likely.

8. *Other issues.* Further critical issues specified by federal policy are maternal-infant death; STDs; environmental health; chronic illness conditions; and disease prevention and health promotion. The Public Health Service has noted that chronic illness, more than 50% of which is caused by behavioral and lifestyle factors (U.S. Public Health, 1995), places the greatest demand on health care systems.

SOCIAL IMPACT OF WOMEN'S HEALTH ISSUES

Statistics about the numbers of women diagnosed or at risk for any of these health care issues do not reveal the whole story. Many women are part of a larger system, such as a significant relationship, family, employment, and community. Many women have social roles of caretaking that require high levels of responsibility for and attention to others.

Many women, as single parents, are the primary wage earner for their family. The health status of an *individual* woman has a potentially major impact on others who are around her and dependent on her, and, because of her high levels of connection and responsibility, the problems of those around her are more likely to be a cause of stress and to impact her health. The health status of the *population* of women has comparable implications for the health and well-being of communities and many social structures. National policy is obligated to attend to women's health.

The health status of women is highly related to the position of women in power relationships. The health problems women have that correlate with histories of abuse are clearly related to unequal and exploitive power relationships. The problems that correlate with high levels of stress are possibly related to unequal power relationships. The risk factors and illness trajectories of these health care issues reveal opportunities for prevention, early intervention, and rehabilitation. Substantial sociocultural, behavioral, and psychological factors are involved. In order to improve care for the health problems of women, an integrated, biopsychosocial approach is imperative. Attention both to psychological and physical factors in health and the interactions between the two is a strategy consistent with the World Health Organization's revised definition of health. This new definition focuses on the positive condition of physical, mental, and social well-being rather than the absence of disease (Jones & Meleis, 1993). Psychological interventions contribute positively to both quality of care and economic factors in health care (Katon & Gonzales, 1994; Rinaldi, 1985).

Primary health care for women must therefore be multidimensional, a complex configuration of physical, psychological, sociocultural, economic, and even political factors. Primary health care services for women should include prevention and education, early intervention by routine screening for psychological and physical indices of normal and abnormal development, treatment and rehabilitation for women's common and critical health care needs, and coordination with community-based resources and personnel, the public health system, and subspecialties like cardiology, psychiatry, and surgery.

To dichotomize the emotional and physical health of women is to ignore the obvious connections between the two. Such a dichotomy, as still persists throughout most of the health care system, is reductionist and discriminatory. Where such a dichotomy exists, there is almost always a greater nod given to physical health than mental and emotional. Many women today are still left with subtle or sometimes not-so-subtle messages, that "it's all in your head." While this literally may be largely true (biochemically-based disorders, distorted and depressive cognitions, diminished self-esteem, notions of dread and fear), the context in which this message is delivered is dismissive. Too many women are left unheard and isolated from the healing powers of credibility, support, and psychosocial interventions.

Candib (1995), who offers a feminist analysis of health care delivery, argues that inequalities in power relationships between women patients and medical service providers, in addition to the American medical tendency to honor patients' striving for autonomy over their ability to achieve relatedness, greatly lowers the ability of medical services to effectively treat women. To effectively serve women, physicians need to work in understanding partnership with their patients rather than as fast-acting directors of treatment. Malterud (1992), describing the "undefined" disorders that women commonly bring to primary care says, "Perhaps the doctor [or other health care provider] will need to revise the image of an intervening, organizing actor towards a more patiently caring and listening professional role in order to satisfy the medical needs presented by her female patients. Such a professional role is challenging the traditional omnipotency of the doctor, but is perhaps more efficatious and satisfying for the patient with "undefined" disorders—as well as for the doctor" (p. 302).

Optimally, every health care encounter with women should be framed by an integrated approach that gives equal recognition and value to the diverse, interactive, and systemic emotional, physical, and social factors influencing health and illness. A health care provider, initiating a health care encounter with a woman, with the assumption that she has to distinguish whether the problem brought is *either* a physical problem entirely *or* an emotional problem is practicing medicine that is swiftly becoming dated and highly divergent from both the science of health and the art of health care.

MULTIDISCIPLINARY HEALTH CARE

Primary health care settings provide the best opportunity to apply these principles of health to the many women who utilize established primary care services like family practice, general internal medicine, obstetrics/gynecology, and pediatrics. Health care services for women are a set of multidisciplinary services particularly suitable for collaboration between behavioral health and primary care providers. The behavioral sciences are an essential part of all aspects of primary health care for women. Therefore behavioral health providers should be essential members of a primary health care team.

Two theoretical models blended together provide the foundation for conceptualizing primary health care for women as multidisciplinary. These are the biopsychosocial model (Engel, 1977) and the collaborative model of health care (Blount & Bayona, 1994; Doherty & Baird, 1983; Dym & Berman, 1986; Mauksch & Leahy, 1993; McDaniel, Campbell, & Seaburn, 1995). Engel's all-encompassing theoretical system and the collaborative model of practice taken together can integrate approaches to women's health care needs across the life span. The biopsychosocial model widens the aperture on factors contributing to health and illness by including psychosocial ones. The collaborative model recognizes the unique perspective of mental and physical health providers and proposes that quality, cost-effective care is best provided when each joins together in a manner that preserves the integrity of each, but recognizes the complementarity of the other. The routines of collaboration that develop between mental health and medical providers in these approaches parallel and foster the kind of collaborative work with patients that Candib and Malterud espouse.

Making the Practice Work: Greenside Primary Care

Collaborative practice for women's health care is growing nationally. One such partnership has existed in Seattle, Washington. At Greenside Primary Care I had the experience of being the psychologist in a partnership of seven Board-certified women family physicians. We worked together for nearly ten years to provide care that reflected the multidimensionality of patients' visits to primary care providers. Although I was not located at the same physical site with the physicians, we sought to act consistently within a multidisciplinary framework. We met regularly to discuss patient care issues and our collaborative process. All patients were fully informed and gave signed consent for this communication between their health care providers.

The most common psychological and psychosocial issues encountered by this primary health care team included affective and anxiety disorders, grief and loss, substance abuse, trauma and physical/sexual abuse, reproductive disorders, aging, adaptation to chronic illness, and the behavioral complexities of managing personality disorders and somatization in their primary care patients. Psychologist-physician clinical collaboration included any or all of the following modalities: brief case consultation in person or by telephone; psychoeducational groups like "coping with infertility" or "parenting the difficult child"; short-term individual or family psychotherapy; long-term individual or family psychotherapy; and facilitating referrals to other mental health providers like psychiatrists. Consultation, education, diagnosis and treatment, and coordination with community-based resources were all regular collaborative clinical activities.

The psychologist-physician team developed, as well, a set of nonclinical activities designed to support their collaborative process. Our common goal was to provide quality, accessible, effective, satisfying, and cost-efficient care to our mutual patients. Two activities particularly useful to the promotion of collaboration were behavioral rounds and Balint groups. Both of these activities were part of the culture of the family medicine residency in which most of the physicians in the practice trained. I was the behavioral science faculty member in this residency for many of the years in which these physicians were residents, so the relationship of collaborative work and mutual respect carried over into the culture of the practice quite easily.

Behavioral Rounds

Behavioral rounds occured every four to six weeks and included discussion of clinical, theoretical, ethical, pragmatic (reimbursement systems, working with managed and capitated care), and political/public policy issues. The psychologist led behavioral rounds. These rounds often focused on a particular patient who presented a challenging diagnostic or treatment issue. These rounds also focused on such general topics as recognizing depression and when to utilize psychopharmacology, understanding lesbian health care, teaching prevention to sexually active adolescent females, finding strategies to enhance compliance with breast self-examination or other health promotion activities, and building good relationships with nursing staffs and office managers.

The range was considerable. Flexibility on the part of the psychologist, who was often simultaneously facilitator, partner, educator, and consultant, was essential. I respected the limited time availability of the physicians and their occasional ambivalence about integrating the psychological dimensions of their patients' health status and functioning. It takes time to listen to patients' stories. It uses emotional energy. It is a role not generally well-understood or respected by a psychologist's physician colleagues from other specialities. Psychological treatment remains somewhat mysterious to many primary health care providers.

Often behavioral rounds focused on identifying personality disorders in primary care settings. One family physician arrived at these rounds and expressed her uncertainty about a patient's diagnosis. Her question, a common one from primary health care providers to their collaborative partners, was, "What's going on with this patient and how do I help her?"

After listening to a summary of the patient's history and care-seeking behavior, the psychologist talked about identifying personality disorders by looking for well-established behavior patterns, the manner in which help from a physician is received and utilized, and the affective responses providers feel in attempting to care for such patients. The providers talked together about coordinating their efforts with these patients and relinquishing some of their expectations that they should be able to "cure" these patients. Facilitating communication, providing information, and modeling empathy were the major contributions the psychologist made to the behavioral rounds.

Balint Groups

Balint groups are a second strategy to promote collaboration. Balint groups are a well-known experience in many family practice residency programs. Michael Balint (1957) was a British psychoanalyst intrigued by the dynamics and complexities of the doctor-patient relationship in general medical practice. He instituted a program for general medical physicians to meet regularly to reflect on their relationships with patients. Particular emphasis was placed on transference and countertransference issues.

Today, Balint groups typically address issues like empathy, boundaries, context, and the confluence of personal and professional development. Recently, many Balint meetings have been opportunities to commiserate jointly about the loss of medical practice as it was known before managed care. Balint meetings became an important mechanism of adaptation to the new world of health care.

Meetings followed a predictable format. The primary objective was to heighten awareness of the provider-patient relationship and understand this relationship as a key instrument in patient health. Secondary gains included greater cohesion among providers, increased psychological mindedness in the primary care practice, increased tolerance for those factors influencing health and illness that cannot be controlled, reduction of provider stress, greater professional satisfaction, and a willingness to trust the art of medicine as well as the science. One family physician provider commented at the end of a Balint group, "I think good psychology *is* the art of medicine."

A Case Illustration

Balint groups and behavioral rounds are ways of attending to the emotional/behavioral dimension of both the patients and the providers in the practice as a regular part of the routine, not something that occurs only in crisis. They are a way of modeling and maintaining a biopsychosocial approach. Such a routine contributes to medical providers' being able to involve a behavioral health provider who is a regular part of the health care team without conveying any sense of failure or stigma to patients. It gives physicians a way of obtaining consultation and support in caring for patients, often heading off problems in the doctor-patient relationship, which might otherwise compromise the quality of care. The process helps physicians engage in a broader range of their patients' experience and contextual stressors than they otherwise might attempt, knowing there is help if the physician "gets in over her head."

Jane was a 25-year-old single woman when she was referred to the psychologist by a resident in the family medicine residency in which the psychologist was a faculty member. Jane was referred for help with depression and obesity. Her mother, who had adopted her as an infant, had died six months before, and Jane's grieving had begun to look more and more like depression.

Jane had been adopted by a couple who were in their mid forties. Within a few years of her adoption, they adopted a second little girl. Jane was overweight in early childhood. Although she was gregarious and had many friends, as a teenager her weight was experienced as physical unattractiveness to boys, which became an important issue for her. Jane's sister grew up thin and pretty. She was very popular with her peers and in her teen years had lots of male admirers. The roles of Jane as the "unattractive one" and her sister as the "attractive one" were a painful part of the everyday expectations of her family. As an adult, Jane had a work history of steadily increasing responsibility in her jobs. She was very bright and very organized.

Over the course of her care, the psychologist and all of the physicians in the practice had numerous contacts with Jane. She came to see her physicians for her hypertension and for pains in her knees and back, pain aggravated significantly by her obesity. She told the physicians and the psychologist, "I am depressed because I am never going to find anyone who loves me until I lose weight, and I can't seem to lose weight because I am depressed." During her episodes of intense involvement with the practice, a number of approaches were tried. Behavioral approaches for weight loss, cognitive approaches for increased self-esteem, counseling for depression, medication for depression, feminist discussions and readings, an eating disorders program, and a highly managed liquid diet for weight loss were all tried without lasting success. Each time she came back, there would be a period of intense involvement with both her primary care physician and the psychologist, who spoke to each other often and occasionally met with Jane together. This tended to last three or four months, after which she would give up and cease active treatment for six months to a year.

All of the providers knew Jane well and liked her a great deal; however all of them were also very frustrated with her. Finally this frustration lead to her being the focus of the Balint group.

The discussion was typical in many ways. It moved from the particulars of Jane's situation and people's frustration with trying to help her to the larger issues of how to work with women who internalize cultural norms about what they should look like and what women's lives should be like, on the other. Group members wrestled with the question, "Should we help women adjust to what their life is, or should we help them change their views and their lives?" Jane, like many of the practice's patients, wanted only to meet the demands she had been raised to understand about how women should look in order to be worthy of love.

As with many conversations in the Balint group, the providers came to no resolution and yet the process somehow seemed to be helpful. After the meeting, we all felt less frustration. We sensed that she was doing the best she could under her life circumstances. Whether our greater acceptance of Jane was related to her moving forward can never be known. It is certainly true that this pattern is commonly experienced by practitioners who use the Balint process.

It was not long after the Balint group that a story caught Jane's eye about adults who had been adopted finding their birth parents. She reinitiated counseling sessions and spent several visits talking over the idea with both the psychologist and her physician. At the same time, she considered having a child. She said that she did not want her life to be on hold, waiting to find a partner. Ultimately, it was the desire to find her birth mother that was the most immediate to her.

During this time she seemed more animated, more upbeat. She lost 20 to 30 pounds, not nearly what she had to lose, but it was the first weight she had ever lost and kept off. Finally she hired a person who was a professional in finding birth parents for adoptees. She got the name and telephone number of a woman along with very convincing evidence that this was her biological mother. When she finally made the call, everyone in the practice knew it was coming and was anxious to know the outcome.

The woman who answered the phone listened to Jane's explanation of who she was and why she was calling and then was silent for a long time. Finally she said, "No one can ever know that this happened and you are never to call me again." Jane was devastated and at the same time emancipated. She spent several counseling sessions grieving the loss. This was the first crisis since the providers had known her in which she did not gain weight. At the present time she is back on a slow weight-loss regimen and has broadened her circle of friends and the types of activities that engage her. Her utilization of outpatient medical services is lower. Her doctors feel that they are working in partnership with her as she continues her journey.

SUMMARY

Women's health care needs are best met within the biopsychosocial or integrated care model. Given the complexity and constantly changing physiology, psychology, and social roles of women across their life span, an integrated approach to their health is both sensible and necessary. In fact, the growing attention to women's health care creates an opportunity to move toward an integrated approach to primary care.

Behavioral health providers and primary care physicians can form effective partnerships and work as respectful, mutually beneficial teams in health care. Women of all ages will benefit as their health care needs are better recognized and addressed. Healthier women may actually mean healthier families and communities, a universal social policy goal, and a promising means to reduce overall health care costs.

REFERENCES

Abbott, J., Johnson, R., Koziol-McLain, J., & Lowenstein, S. R. (1995). Domestic violence against women: Incidence and prevalence in an emergency department population (and subsequent commentary). *JAMA, 273*, 1763–1767.

Adams, D. O. (1994). Molecular biology of macrophage activation: A pathway whereby psychosocial factors can potentially affect health. *Psychosomatic Medicine, 56*, 316–327.

Balint, M. (1957). *The doctor, his patient and the illness.* New York: International.

Bass, M., & Howes, J. (1992). Women's health: The making of a powerful new public issue. *Womens Health Issues, 2*, 3–5.

Blount, A., & Bayona, J. (1994). Toward a system of integrated primary care. *Family Systems Medicine, 12*, 171–182.

Candib, L. (1995). *Medicine and the family: A feminist perspective.* New York: Basic.

Doherty, W. J., & Baird, M. A. (1983). *Family therapy and family medicine: Toward the primary care of families.* New York: Guilford.

Dym, B., & Berman, S. (1986). The primary health care team: Family physician and family therapist in joint practice. *Family Systems Medicine, 4*, 9–21.

Engel, G. L. (1977). The need for a new medical model: A challenge to biomedicine. *Science, 196*, 129–136.

Holloway, M. (1994). A global view. *Scientific American, 271*, 77–83.

Jones, P. S., & Meleis, A. I. (1993). Health is empowerment. *Advances in Nursing Science, 15*, 1014.

Katon, W. J., & Gonzalez, J. (1994). A review of randomized trials of psychiatric consultation-liaison studies in primary care. *Psychosomatics, 35*, 268–278.

Malterud, K. (1992). Women's undefined disorders—a challenge for clinical communication. *Family Practice, 9*, 299–303.

Mauksch, L., & Leahy, D. (1993). Collaboration between primary care medicine and mental health in an HMO. *Family Systems Medicine, 11*, 121–135.

McCauley, J., Kern, D. E., Kolodner, K., Dill, L., Schroeder, A. F., DeChant, H. K., Ryden, J., Derogatis, J. R., & Bass, E. B. (1997). Clinical characteristics of women with history of childhood abuse: Unhealed wounds. *JAMA, 227*, 1362–1368.

McDaniel, S. H., Campbell, T. L., & Seaburn, D. B. (1995). Principles for collaboration between health and mental health providers in primary care. *Family Systems Medicine, 13*, 283–298.

Rinaldi, R. C. (1985). Positive effects of psychosocial interventions on total health care: A review of the literature. *Family Systems Medicine, 3*, 417–426.

Rodin, J., & Ickovics, J. R. (1990). Women's health: Review and research agend as we approach the 21st century. *American Psychologist, 45*, 1018–1034.

Schroeder, P. (1992). Women's Health: A focus for the 1990s. *Womens Health Issues, 2*, 1–2.

Schroeder, P. (1993). We've come a long way, maybe: Women's health reseach in the 103rd Congress. *Nursing & Health Care, 14*, 292–293.

Strickland, B. R. (1988). Sex-related differences in health and illness. *Psychology of Women Quarterly, 12*, 381–399.

Tice, L., Hall, R. C., Beresford, T. P., Quinones, J., & Hall, A. K. (1989). Sexual abuse in patients with eating disorders. *Psychiatric Medicine, 7*, 257–267.

U.S. Public Health Service, Office on Women's Health. (1995). *Report on women's health.* Washington, DC: Author.

Vivian, D., & Langhinrichsen-Rohling, J. (1994). Are bi-directionally violent couples mutually victimized? A gender-sensitive comparison. *Violence and Victims, 9*, 107–124.

Washington State Health Services Commission. (1993). *Women in health care policy.* Olympia, WA: Author.

Wood, S. H., & Ransom, V. J. (1994). The 1990s: A decade for change in women's health care policy. *Journal of Obstetric, Gynecologic, and Neonatal Nursing, 23*, 139–143.

11

Training Issues in Integrated Care

JoEllen Patterson   Richard J. Bischoff
Leita McIntosh-Koontz

Training is a way of ensuring the future. If integrated primary care is to be a regular feature of the future health care landscape, physicians and behavioral health professionals in training must gain experience in integrated settings. The program described by Patterson, Bishoff, and McIntosh-Koontz is one of very few programs in the country where the regular training experiences that lead to a basic credential are carried out in an integrated setting. It took a great deal of commitment and creativity to pull this overlapping of training experiences together.

Currently, the more common approach to training is to train people who already have their credential. Postdoctoral fellowships in primary care psychology are beginning to be developed around the country. Summer courses for physicians and mental health practitioners in working collaboratively are available in several settings. A few graduate schools in mental health disciplines train practitioners to practice collaboratively in medical settings.*

---

*The Collaborative Family Health Care Coalition attempts to keep an up-to-date list of training programs in this area. They can be reached via e-mail at cfhcc@ sprynet.com.

Peek and Heinrich's discussion of training in Chapter 7 demonstrates how important this function is for large health systems that are trying to implement integrated primary care. The fact that large capitated health systems are often the most evolved settings in terms of primary care integration means that training in the routines and practices of integrated care is developing faster outside rather than inside of academia. This creates a new situation for teachers in academic medicine and behavioral science who are used to seeing innovations develop in the training centers and gradually be exported to the "masses" of providers in the field. In the area of integrated care, faculty would do well to keep an eye out for practices in the most advanced health systems in their area. The more training faculty are aware of these practices and utilize the best of them, the more trainees will be ready for the health care world they will be facing.

D R. KNOLLS, a medical resident at a primary care clinic, peruses the brief chart notes on his new patient. Mrs. Stimpson, a 71-year-old woman, has a six-month history of frequent presentations to the local hospital's ER for shortness of breath and chest pain. Despite some 50 years as a smoker, Mrs. Stimpson's chest x-rays are clear, and EKGs and other work-ups are negative. Dr. Knolls glances quickly through notes on the patient's recent visits and sees that Mrs. Stimpson's husband, a retired military commander, died one year ago from an unidentified pulmonary infection. He thinks about what role this might play in Mrs. Stimpson's complaints, and picks up the phone to call Dr. Nelson, a fellow intern—a psychotherapy student who's on board the clinic's behavioral health program. After a quick phone conversation, Dr. Nelson makes room in her schedule to join Dr. Knolls for his afternoon appointment with Mrs. Stimpson. Later that day, the patient and therapist explore the psychosocial issues that might underlie Mrs. Stimpson's somatic problems. Three weeks later, Mrs. Stimpson is doing well on a carefully coordinated treatment plan that includes close monitoring of her physical health, antidepressant medication, and weekly therapy for bereavement problems. Dr. Nelson is grateful for her colleague physician's input and medication management, and Dr. Knolls is equally thankful that his patient is getting supportive psychotherapy. This integrated approach has resulted in a decrease in the patient's symptoms. Most of all, Mrs. Stimpson is feeling better.

The trainees in the vignette above are part of a movement among many health care organizations to integrate medical and mental health care. The medical resident and psychotherapy intern demonstrate the kind of relationship trainers seek as they prepare clinicians to work in integrated, primary care settings. Aiming one's sights on an integrated model of practice is a goal that reflects a realistic "read" on the future of health care delivery, as well as an ethical, even noble, desire to treat the whole patient. Whether integration occurs within the context of a large health maintenance organization or by a collaborative group of private practitioners, the trend to combine primary care with mental health services is still in its infancy. And as is so often true in science and business, we usually know where we want to go before we know how to get there. The road map for training in an integrated model is a "work in progress" with partially constructed streets and avenues and yet-to-be-planned highways and bridges.

Our ideas about important issues in training spring from our experiences in a family medicine residency program that is embedded in a large health maintenance organization (Patterson, Bischoff, Scherger, & Grauf-Grounds, 1996). Four years after launching an integrated approach, we find ourselves developing training models while concurrently examining, changing, and evaluating integrated care models. In these early stages, and without preestablished "maps," flexibility has allowed us to experiment with different ways of doing things. Today, physicians, nurse practitioners, family therapists, psychiatrists, midwives, other health care providers, and myriad office staff work together as essential members of an interdisciplinary team. Training occurs for family practice residents and family therapists at two residency clinics. Interns in family therapy are connected with one of the country's few family therapy graduate programs to provide curriculum on managed care practices in addition to biomedical and biopsychosocial models (Patterson, Baron, Bischoff, & McIntosh-Koontz, 1996).

Although new issues emerge daily in this interdisciplinary endeavor, a primary assumption underlying our work is that the practice and training models a clinician experiences during training strongly influence his or her later practice strategies. It follows then that if primary care is ever going to be truly integrated in a universal manner, changes must be made in how physicians and therapists are trained. It is our belief that if physicians and psychosocial providers are trained together by a faculty demonstrating mutual respect, they are likely to emulate this same model when they establish their own clinical practices after graduating.

As we interact with other established professionals in our community who are trying to adjust to the changing health care environment, we often see—even in those who consider their work collaborative— attempts to carve out areas of practice and to protect professional expertise. Our conclusion is that even when faced with external pressures to adopt new models for providing care, most professionals will resist changing their practice strategies from the way in which they were trained. This makes sense when we consider that people attempt to preserve what is familiar to them in the face of change. If someone is trained to work independently, he or she will probably practice independently or find the transition to collaborative models rather difficult. Integrated primary care requires a different way of thinking than the traditional independent practice models commonly taught five to ten years ago. Emphasizing collaborative models in training programs will enable practitioners to walk right into the practice world of today and tomorrow without the loss of time that it takes for people to learn to function effectively in an integrated primary care environment.

RELATIONSHIPS, RELATIONSHIPS, RELATIONSHIPS

In order for training to be effective, a comfortable, efficient working relationship must be established at the trainer level. Medical residents and psychosocial provider trainees need to see a model of collaboration in action—"showing" enhances "telling." In a study of medical student education in managed care settings, students experienced the "unique characteristics of these sites . . . through observing the practice of physicians and other health care providers, not through formal lectures or other didactic sessions" (Veloski, Barzansky, Nash, Bastacky, & Stevens, 1996, p. 669).

Modeling for residents/interns drives home the importance of the skills and relationships we teach. Consequently, before an effective teaching program can be established, a working relationship needs to exist between members of the clinical faculty, across disciplines. Faculty physicians need to have successful experiences working with the behavioral science faculty as clinicians and vice versa. Without this relationship in place, neither residents nor psychotherapy interns are likely to see behavioral science providers as integrated within the treatment program. This situation may be particularly challenging for seasoned physician-trainers who find themselves teaching practices that are contrary to long held habits and views about other disciplines.

Outcome data on the effectiveness of psychotherapy have lessons to teach professionals who are implementing an integrated model. These data suggest that it is not the theory or even the treatment that predicts achieving treatment goals. Instead, the two major predictors are the relationship between the therapist and the client or, more specifically, the client's perception of the therapeutic alliance, and the client's motivation or readiness for change. This is true even when the only treatment is pharmacotherapy.

In a similar manner, we assume that the strength of the relationship between the therapist and physician is probably one of the strongest predictors of the effectiveness of a collaborative, integrated model. While communication between providers is critical, especially when training future clinicians, real interest in a new way of working significantly enhances the model's success. Practitioners from individual disciplines have to be somewhat dissatisfied with the way care is currently provided. Training is more effective and meaningful when faculty/trainers believe that an integrated model offers a better way of working. The costs of the model (e.g., time needed for communication and consultation, less autonomy) should not outweigh the benefits (e.g., more satisfying work, cost savings, sense of providing optimal patient care). Simply announcing that a clinic is going to create a new, improved (integrated) model and then place different professionals next door to each other will not work.

In our model, physician and behavioral science faculty were able to work together before the first class of residents and therapists arrived. During this time, we collaborated on cases, watched each other work, and developed a mutual respect for one another. This further increased the likelihood of referral and consultation. A foundation was laid for us to continue building relationships and for trainees to learn and ultimately elaborate on our earlier work.

While many aspects of a true interdisciplinary approach will become apparent to residents/therapists during training in integrated settings, we believe it's helpful to sometimes articulate why the relational model works. First, a natural tendency exists for professionals to refer their patients to other providers whom they know and respect. Second, this sense of mutuality of referrals and care can create an accountability for individual patients' needs and, ideally, a sense of professional community that can be felt by patients. This is in marked contrast to many HMO models in which patients frequently must "call an anonymous number and get three provider names." Market research on HMOs suggests that patients want to pick their providers and want a relationship with them. Clearly, relationships among practitioners underlie collaborative work. Seeing this kind of connection is important for trainees because it grounds the practical in the philosophical — a factor that always enhances learning.

Along the way, trainees can also discover and utilize the unique personal traits and experiences of their colleagues from other disciplines. In our experience, areas of subspecialty that may not be part of a professional's title or formal education often lead to valuable consultations — for example, a therapist who comes with experience from a child protective service is recognized by a primary care physician as a good resource for families that present with trauma-related medical concerns. The mutual respect between professionals soon extends to flexibility around exchanging information, using e-mail or voice mail when face-to-face meetings are difficult to coordinate, and otherwise considering both patient needs and colleagues' time pressures. The office or clinic becomes a community of professionals who share a common vision of optimizing patient care, while keeping lines of communication up and running.

CLOSE QUARTERS: A MUST FOR INTEGRATED CARE AND TRAINING

Proximity is essential for integration to work. We believe that multidisciplinary professionals should ideally be located within the same office — with patients sharing the same waiting room and practitioners passing each other in the hall. All too often, professionals are housed according to their discipline, with different disciplines assigned space that prohibits frequent contact with those with whom they should be collaborating. Housing medical and mental health professionals according to discipline in different buildings, on different floors, and sometimes even on the same floor but at opposite ends of the hall, can prohibit collaboration. Frequently, mental health carve-out models in managed care usually mean the patient is seen by a physician in one part of town, and a therapist in another — and the two professionals may never know each other or communicate about the patient. It follows then, that training occurring within these environments would place trainees in positions where they do not have contact with the professionals with whom they are learning to collaborate.

Proximity makes integration possible by facilitating five-minute hallway conversations and rapidly planned consultations between doctors, therapists, and other providers. Increased face-to-face contact also helps the therapist trainee come to understand the pragmatic, problem-solving focus of the primary care physician, while the physician trainee comes to understand the therapist's focus on process, not just content. Any training clinic or group setting out to integrate care should assign office and work space so that regular contact between professionals at both the faculty and trainee level becomes a fact of daily practice.

Proximity refers not only to space but also to time. Time is one of the most precious commodities to most professionals. A 15-minute lunch together or an impromptu 10-minute conversation at the end of the day allows professionals the chance to have an ongoing awareness of each other and of the progress of their mutual patients. Every practitioner has experienced the frustration of playing "telephone tag," a game that requires unproductive time and can delay conversations about mutual clients for days, and sometimes longer. We are convinced that practitioners who share the same space communicate about patients more frequently and with less frustration. Because of this, practitioners are more likely to access the expertise of other professionals and collaborate care. Practitioners trained in this environment develop habits of collaboration based on ease of communication. This helps trainees come to value the care provided by others and, we believe, increases the likelihood that they will coordinate care in similar ways in other practice settings in which they may work.

Taking time to socialize is also important. In our office, the staff does an excellent job planning pot-luck lunches, birthday celebrations, and holiday events. Practitioners across disciplines have the opportunity to work together on mutual patients and socialize even in the midst of hectic and demanding schedules. Physician and therapist trainees are also involved in these activities and are able to see the collegiality that exists between professionals.

THE REALITY OF HIERARCHY

Hierarchy refers to the often unstated, but quite powerful, understanding of status and rankings among different professionals. Hierarchical issues here frequently refer to responsibility and authority. In the managed care environment in which we work, the primary care physician always has the final say about treatment decisions. Although behavioral health care providers, such as therapists, may be treated as peers in some medical environments, this usually happens because roles are made clear and are respected. In the context of training, we emphasize that integration does not necessarily reduce or otherwise change certain hierarchies that exist between different disciplines. It does, however, demand that professionals in multidisciplinary settings become familiar with each other's role in patient care, and respect the validity of each other's opinions and ideas about common cases. So, while an integrated clinic may place the physician "at the top" in decision-making power, the therapist should feel free to offer the physician his or her own diagnostic observations or inquire about medications without fear of disrespecting the hierarchy. For example, a physician referred a patient to the in-office family therapist intern after prescribing an antianxiety drug. During a session later in the week, the therapist noticed that the patient's depressive symptoms were as prominent as the anxiety symptoms. The therapist wondered about using a medication that would address both. She consulted with the physician, and the medication was changed. Again, optimal patient care unites disciplines, while maintaining necessary differences in power. Trainees gaining clinical experiences within this environment learn first-hand how hierarchies can be respected while collaborating patient care.

BRIDGING DIFFERENCES: SPECIFIC TRAINING NEEDS

While the assumptions discussed above cut across disciplines, important differences between primary care and mental health professionals need to be addressed in any training model. This includes understanding and making room for the other professional's unique education, view of problems, and ideas about treatment.

Medical Professionals' Training Needs

Medical residents in our integrated clinic need hands-on experience with psychosocial treatment in order to appreciate the complexity involved in considering psychosocial issues, and to understand how therapy works. During residents' month-long behavioral science training (rotation), we make every effort to get the physician in the therapy room as a cotherapist with the behavioral science provider. For example, during a recent behavioral science rotation, one of the therapist-trainers scheduled most of his patients to coincide with one of the resident's schedule. The resident was brought in as a cotherapist with all these cases, and she became a behavioral science treatment provider during that month-long rotation. The experience gave her a greater appreciation for what occurs in psychotherapy. It also provided her an opportunity to sharpen her skills of assessing for mental health concerns and providing time-limited mental health interventions.

Time is an important consideration in ensuring that residents get adequate exposure to psychosocial work and training. Because residents struggle with so many time demands, they tend to make decisions based on a priority system of what they need to devote time to, and what they can give minimal attention to or let slide altogether. When faced with a difficult patient or one with whom psychosocial issues are prevalent, the easiest thing to do is to make a referral to the psychosocial provider. This is the least favorable option from a training perspective. It is far better for the psychosocial provider to counsel, supervise, and instruct the medical resident on providing mental health care. For example, a decision was made at our facility to always consult about patients with residents before accepting a psychosocial referral. During this consultation, the behavioral science faculty member's priority is to instruct the resident on how to manage the behavioral science concern within the medical interview. As a result, decisions are often made for the resident physician to continue working with the patient using the behavioral science provider as a consultant. In these cases, the behavioral science faculty member may even view the physician's interview with the patient through closed circuit television so that the resident can receive immediate instruction about his or her work with the patient. When a decision is made to schedule the patient with the psychosocial provider, efforts are made to bring the resident in as a cotherapist. These strategies allow the resident to become intimately involved in the psychosocial care of his or her patient and allows him or her to receive experiential instruction on how psychosocial care is provided. Merely making a referral to a therapist contributes to the separation of medical and psychosocial concerns. The same problem can occur if therapists merely accept referrals at convenient times rather than try to coordinate the timetables of patient, patient's family, physician, and therapist.

Psychotherapists' Training Needs

Just as medical residents need training in psychosocial assessment and intervention, therapist interns require information and experience with the medical model and its practitioners. In our experience, in order to function effectively in primary care a mental health clinician must have a basic understanding of pharmacology and general medical terminology (e.g., anatomy, disease, treatment). The mental health provider must also be able to diagnose and treat psychopathology and understand how chronic illness and medical conditions impact and are impacted by patient emotional and mental conditions. The therapist must understand the role of preventive care and patient education and be familiar and comfortable with the conceptual underpinnings of managed care, namely, the symptom focus and pragmatic problem-solving perspective of primary care medicine. For example, physicians often consider the worst case scenario a symptom might represent, and then rule it out (e.g., ruling out a brain tumor when a patient complains of headaches). Finally, the mental health professional must understand that medical care and mental health care providers are trained differently and they must be taught to respect these differences in training. For example, physicians are trained to make rapid judgments while psychosocial professionals prefer a more tentative stance.

One way to address these issues is through exposure to other disciplines in training. At the residency clinics, different disciplines offer continuing education lectures about clinical issues. And in the family therapy program associated with the clinics, we have moved outside our discipline to find capable teachers who not only impart information but also serve as role models for students who are just beginning to form opinions about working with other disciplines — a psychiatrist teaches a course about pharmacology, a psychologist teaches a class in psychopathology, and a family physician teaches a course on such family health issues as preventive care, chronic illness, and death and dying. Indeed, most of the course work for trainee therapists takes a biopsychosocial approach, thus enhancing their "fit" within a medical environment.

Bringing mental health professionals into a primary care environment means training must address requirements regarding assessment, diagnosis, and treatment planning that are congruent with an integrated, medical environment. To address this need, our family therapy program recently initiated a course that covers essential skills for working in a managed care setting (Patterson, Baron, et al., 1996). For example, therapist interns learn about "medical necessity" and the need to address and document certain diagnostic and functional criteria before treatment is authorized. While medical practitioners will be familiar with set treatment protocols, therapists frequently are not. Training also includes instruction on identifying and rationalizing treatment modality. Therapist interns are oriented toward using limited sessions creatively and effectively, using preset treatment guidelines for certain disorders, and for being familiar with and responsive to utilization review methodologies that also impact medical practice.

COMMON TRAINING ISSUES IN TODAY'S INTEGRATED SETTINGS

Other challenges need to be addressed in training and education of professionals who will work in integrated settings. In an editorial on medical education and managed care, editors from the *Journal of the American Medical Association* stated:

> Physicians practicing in managed care settings provide more ambulatory care and less inpatient care, face new pressures to practice cost-effectively and to work in interdisciplinary teams, must deal with new forms of payment and administrative controls, and are required to think about maintaining the health of populations rather than just individual patients. Education of young physicians should . . . display two attributes: flexibility as to the institutional arrangements in which education takes place, and a sure sense for the skills that, regardless of organizational setting, will prove essential to effective practice. (Blumenthal & Thier, 1996, pp. 726–727)

The *JAMA* editors called for educators to define those necessary skills while simultaneously recognizing that health care providers must be trained in a way that scientific, organizational, social, and financial change is the rule rather than the exception. Similarly, diverse groups within mental health struggle with these issues. Psychotherapists are confronted with using mandated treatment guidelines, choosing the "least-extensive intervention that has proven efficacy," or denying longer-term treatments which, though they may help, lack empirical data to support them (Sanderson, 1995, p. 97). These are some of the concerns leaders in medical and therapy education must address.

While individual differences between disciplines will result in specific training for each group, all players in an integrated setting must address the relatively new issues that arise with managed care, including patient advocacy, protecting confidentiality, population-based interventions, and treating chronic illness.

Patient Advocacy

Helping trainees understand potential pitfalls of managed care can build a sense of patient advocacy across disciplines. For example, patient rights advocates have identified physician gag rules as a tremendous threat to both the doctor-patient relationship and optimal care. These rules, set by certain HMOs, forbid physicians from giving patients information on different treatment options. To emphasize the importance of their patient advocacy role and to instruct them in how to act within this role, we share and discuss with the trainees patient experiences such as was cited in the *New England Journal of Medicine* (Weston & Lauria,

1996). In this paper the authors tell of a family enrolled in an HMO whose infant was diagnosed with leukemia. The child needed a costly bone marrow transplant that was authorized by the HMO in an out-of-state facility. This meant the family would be separated and the mother would lose her job in order to accompany the infant. The caregivers asked for an exception to allow the treatment to occur in a nearby medical center with which the HMO had no cost-saving agreement. The request was denied. The transplant was done at the HMO-authorized, out-of-state hospital and the baby responded well. However, the mother was demoted at work, the father lost his job, and the older sibling was sent to live with relatives in another state. After the infant relapsed, a second transplant was set up at yet another site that had obtained the HMO's latest contract before the oncology social worker and oncologists had decided what course of treatment she needed. In the end, the mother lost her job, the family lost its home and savings, and the older sibling had increasingly severe behavior problems. Examples such as these facilitate discussions with physician and therapist trainees about their roles as patient advocates and allow them to see the consequences on their patients' lives of the treatment decisions that are made.

Confidentiality

Training programs must integrate issues of law and ethics into their curriculum, and confidentiality is a central issue. Medical records are seen by more institutions and individuals than any other personal records, so trainees must learn protocols to protect patients' confidentiality. The issue of segregating mental health issues from physical data must be addressed. We use articles like one that appeared in the *New York Times Magazine* by M. Scarf (1996) highlighting the confidentiality issue. This article tells of a woman who went to see her HMO internist for a routine treatment of a urinary tract infection. The doctor she saw that day (not her regular physician) said, "I can help you with your medical problems, but I can't help you with your mental problems." To her dismay, she discovered that a detailed note on her psychiatric sessions had been stored in a computerized medical record that was accessible to anyone, including clerks and nurses, within her large HMO. Discussing experiences such as these help trainees recognize the importance of maintaining confidentiality of information and encourages discussions of how information contained within the medical record should be used. Trainers need to ensure that therapist-interns and residents are aware of relevant laws affecting confidentiality (such as the Health Insurance Portability and Accountability Act of 1996, which directs Congress to address the need for confidentiality) (Chase, 1996).

In addition, mental health and medical providers must be alerted to common failures in protecting confidentiality. These include sending patient information by fax to the wrong number or to the wrong e-mail address, leaving information about patients in a fax machine, and leaving information on a telephone answering machine when you are not sure who might listen at the other end. Other risks that should be addressed during training include inappropriate use of pagers, passwords for voice-mail, e-mail, or computer programs that put case notes, billing, and scheduling all on the same program, and requiring patients to describe to receptionists some medically sensitive information — in front of a filled waiting room — in order to get the type of appointment they need.

Population-Based Treatment

Members of integrated, multidisciplinary teams will increasingly be required to focus on treating populations, not just individuals. The goal is to provide broader resources and group approaches to address common problems (e.g., obesity, smoking, and diabetes). At the training level, residents and therapist-interns will benefit from some knowledge of epidemiology to ascertain different patient-population needs. Trainees can be an integral part of the process to further identify groups of patients with common problems, and to design group interventions. For example, in one of our clinics, within a matter of weeks the therapists received a large number of referrals and requests for consultation of patients with chronic pain. In meeting with the physicians, the psychosocial providers developed a psychoeducational group for these patients. This group allowed both therapists and physicians to educate patients about chronic pain, and allowed the patients to receive support from individuals suffering from similar conditions.

Any type of chronic illness or chronic condition appears to be a good target for these groups. The groups balance education with a space for troubled patients to share their feelings and experiences. Current research should be emphasized in these groups, giving residents, therapist-interns, and patients a greater appreciation for how illness can be managed and quality of life increased, without creating expectations of miracle cures. Therapist-interns are in an ideal position to spearhead these endeavors, while using resident physicians' knowledge of specific medical problems.

Ideally, these groups have coleaders — a therapist and resident physician. Residents are thus able to sharpen their educational and psychosocial skills while gaining an appreciation for psychosocial care. Because of time demands, there may be a tendency to include the physician for the educational portion only, and leave the supportive/psychosocial portion to the therapist. In our estimation, this is a mistake because it further emphasizes the separation between disciplines in the eyes of the resident physician, the therapist trainees, and the patients.

Chronic Illness

One of the foremost issues perfectly suited to integrated care is that of chronic illness, but cotreatment models are few and far between. Thus, our development of training models around cotreatment runs parallel to treatment model development itself.

Chronic illness is a common problem in primary care. Physicians and therapists can become frustrated and defensive when they see little change with chronic patients, especially when they consider the myriad providers often involved in the care of chronic patients. The balance of responsibility over time between different providers can become confusing. Cost-containment issues also become increasingly important as multiple, costly treatments are tried for numerous problems, with few successes.

Coordinating treatment planning and relational issues between providers clearly needs to be addressed in training so that physicians and therapists are prepared for chronic patients. At the same time, trainees from different disciplines can provide important insights that might be missed when treatment (and training) is provided piecemeal. Both therapists and physicians should be involved in some in-service and training meetings together where protocols, strategies, and other issues related to the treatment of chronic illness are discussed. For example, residents and therapists in our integrated clinic were discussing a treatment technique commonly used by the therapists at the facility when working with chronic pain patients. The technique is called the "miracle question" and is a hallmark of solution-focused therapy (de Shazer, 1985). The therapist using this technique says something like, "Suppose one night, while you were asleep, there was a miracle, and you no longer had your problem. How would you know? What would be different?" Although the therapists felt this question accesses hidden resources that even chronically ill patients have, the residents felt it would be inappropriate to use a question suggesting the possibility of cure for patients with longstanding, debilitating illnesses. As a result of this discussion, a variation on the miracle question was developed that would apply to the medical setting and the treatment of chronic illness. The technique became one in which both therapists and physicians felt comfortable using with their chronically ill patients. In the process, both residents and therapist-interns learned from one another and increased their awareness of the special needs of this population.

OBSTACLES AND ANSWERS: PAST AND FUTURE
CONSIDERATIONS FOR TRAINING

"Start small and build." This could be the motto for our practice and training program during the last four years. In this final section of the chapter, we take a look at the practical considerations and steps that helped us get started. We also offer suggestions for monitoring progress. And finally, we consider some important points that, discovered in retrospect, might get in the way of effectively integrating primary care and mental health services — grist for the mill of future practitioners and trainers.

Resources, Funding, and Other Bumps in the Road

Our initial steps toward interdisciplinary training and model building started with existing resources that we redirected toward our goals. We knew that the survival of any ideas or models we implemented depended on a low-cost/high-satisfaction ratio. We initially exchanged faculty between an academic family training program and the family medicine residency using traditional positions that were already funded. A family physician began teaching a family therapy course. A part-time family therapy faculty member became the "behavioral scientist" for the residency. Family therapy faculty members gave guest lectures in the residency, and family physician residents participated in some of the family therapy classes during their mental health rotations.

These initial exchanges incurred no new costs and allowed the faculty to get to know each other. Based on a few small successes, we expanded. The residency behavioral scientist was funded for more time, and part of this time was then allocated for supervision of family therapy interns. This allowed the residency to add three nonsalaried family therapy interns. They saw patients with the residents and received supervision from the behavioral science faculty.

As mentioned earlier, the residency program has three locations and each site has been somewhat autonomous. Over time, the number of faculty, residents, and interns grew at each site, but the responsibilities and tasks performed varied from clinic to clinic. A site with more residents emphasized education and teaching, while other locations emphasized patient care and collaborative model building. Many problems arose. Providers were not on some panels, or strict regulations regarding faculty seeing patients alongside residents had to be followed for reimbursement. These meta-issues were addressed on an individual basis.

Solutions to financial and structural meta-issues are still being created and tried.

External funding was sought for some projects. For example, money was obtained to start a research project examining the interface between family functioning, mental health, and physical illness. One residency site is located near the Mexican border, and funding is being sought to hire more bilingual therapists who can do more community outreach. At the same time, curriculum revisions were made within the family therapy training program. These included the aforementioned addition of courses in families and health, pharmacology, and professional issues in managed care (Patterson, Baron, et al., 1996; Patterson & Magulac, 1993; Patterson & Scherger, 1995). The program continued to emphasize a biopsychosocial model, preparing therapy students for a place in integrated medical settings. At the residency sites, the behavioral science curriculum guideline from the Society of Teachers of Family Medicine and the American Academy of Family Physicians were streamlined to make them applicable and practical for our settings. Instead of trying to cover every topic, we identified those that faculty thought were most important, and focused our energy on teaching these.

A common goal among medical and therapy faculty was to create a model of exemplary patient care and training within an integrated, managed care setting. At times, this goal took precedence over individual gain. The most practical example of this is that work was sometimes done despite lack of remuneration. In addition, there was often uncertainty about the future of the collaborative relationship, and even of the viability of the residency, as rapid change in health care provision pressed on. The residency program was one part of a larger-scale negotiation addressing for-profit versus nonprofit issues. Faculty had no idea how these issues would be resolved, but kept focusing on individual work responsibilities. In the midst of dramatic health care changes, and in the early phases of integrating care, people simply kept working!

Evaluating Progress

As efforts to integrate medical and mental health services continue, and training issues become more apparent, a significant question arises: How do we know if this model of care is working, if these are the right training protocols for the job at hand? At the beginning of this chapter, we talked about a common dilemma in so many fields of endeavor — being clear about the destination before being certain about the means to get there. Answering the question asked above relies on our ability to measure our progress, without the benefit of reliable instruments. In the beginning phases of model development, we often depend on anecdotal or ad hoc data and forge ahead. While this remains a natural and sometimes beneficial process (in the serendipitous sense), we begin to attempt to measure training effectiveness, and integration itself, by looking at process and outcome research in distinct fields (e.g., biomedical, psychosocial, health care quality).

We assume that training will ultimately improve patient care, increase patient satisfaction, and boost provider morale. One could argue that measures of patient and provider satisfaction, remission rates, and rates of improvement are indirect measures of success in training within an integrated model of care. Measures such as these should be easily administered within a training environment. Indeed, integrated primary care training programs can establish habits of collecting ongoing outcome data, and can expose students to evidence-based medicine and cost-effective analysis (Clancy & Kamerow, 1996). We can train physicians and psychosocial providers to think about micro and macro measurements of quality and expose them to meta-analysis and decision sciences. Therapy interns and medical residents can also be trained in the use of common pencil and paper measures of outcome, and computer-scoring software that can be used on personal computers. Frequently, residents and therapy interns begin their clinical training having received considerable exposure to statistics, research design, and program evaluation during the didactic portion of their education. These skills can and should be utilized in integrated settings.

Finally, in evaluating the training program in integrated care, it's important to recognize our goal at this early stage of developing models of training in integrated primary care, namely, to promote a model of integrated care. Promote does not mean force residents and therapists to accept a new way of doing things. Although there is much self-selection within our training program—most residents and therapists choose to receive clinical training with us because of their interest in psychosocial concerns and in integrating medical and psychosocial treatments—we also acknowledge that physicians and therapists can choose to accept this way of working, or reject it. So, although we may be able to evaluate the degree to which the training program changes treatment protocols, physicians become more aware of psychosocial issues, therapists become more aware of medical concerns, and physicians and therapists attempt to seek collaborative relationships, the best determination of success at this early stage of model development may just be the degree to which training programs expose residents and therapists to this way of working.

Stumbling Blocks to Integration

We began this chapter by presenting our assumptions about integrative care and the issues we felt must be addressed in order to train both therapists and medical providers in integrated primary care. Equally important is the following collection of common assumptions — false ones in our experience — that can impede both training and the development of an integrated care model. It is our hope that this retrospective can serve others as they prepare to combine medical and psychosocial clinicians' efforts.

1. *Everyone wants to integrate services.* One of the biggest mistakes to be made in training is to assume that all the players want to join forces. Typically, decisions to include behavioral science in a primary care setting are made at the administrative level, and are handed down to clinicians who are expected to carry them out. When we were exploring the joint training model described in this chapter, we first formed alliances with the directors of the medical residency program. The decision to integrate was made without much consultation with the physicians about the particulars of integration or the degree to which the integration would occur. Once the behavioral science providers were on the scene, it quickly became clear that medical and support staff were not aware of the new clinicians' role in either treatment provision or training. After much consternation, we adopted a strategy of scheduling patients around physicians' timetables and giving medical staff maximum flexibility to access our services and interact with us. These efforts helped increase the likelihood that physicians and residents would ask for consultations, make referrals, become involved in psychosocial treatment, and request a therapist's involvement during medical interviews.

Over time, some medical providers and behavioral science faculty have developed close working relationships built on a model of integrated care. Others are still skeptical, but there exists a mutual respect for the talents and knowledge each clinician brings to patient care, even when time demands or differential conceptualizations of illness prevent true integration. With some others, a great separation still keeps the different disciplines apart. Clearly, not all faculty and residents/trainees will "buy" the integrated approach we teach. Many physician faculty members don't have the time or interest to invest in the model. Some prefer sending the patient off for mental health treatment without expecting that psychosocial care will be coordinated with them. Many residents come to training with little interest in mental health issues and limited impetus to be involved with the behavioral science portion of the program. Forcing the integrated model onto these people could result in resentments that might sabotage integrative treatment.

We believe, however, that by responding to individual and group skepticism about integrated care we indirectly enabled the model, and training, to progress. Taking a nonassuming, one-down position and making ourselves available for consultation has been most beneficial. Indeed, some of the medical providers who were initially most resistant to the integrative model are beginning to involve psychosocial providers in treatment, and when referrals to therapists are made, we are careful to keep physicians updated on treatment progress.

2. *Hierarchies don't matter.* One of the most serious mistakes a clinician can make is to disregard the hierarchy that exists within the training program. Physicians generally carry greater authority in terms of clinical work and training. When residents enter the training program they look to physician faculty for direction about who they should listen to, what they should attend to, and how seriously they should regard the behavioral science faculty. Expecting across-the-board equality in decision-making about training issues is not a realistic stance for behavioral science providers to take, and in fact could sabotage the formative stages of integrating care. By modeling a mutual respect for multidisciplinary team members, the input provided by behavioral scientists gradually carries more weight. Residents and therapy interns who "grow up" within an integrated model demonstrate true collaboration in a way that seasoned veterans might find difficult, if only because it is unfamiliar territory—essential hierarchies are respected and maintained, while consultation and collaboration become a part of everyday life.

3. *Nursing and ancillary staff can be disregarded in training.* The behavioral science faculty initially underestimated the importance of nursing and administrative staff in providing collaborative care. Frankly, the faculty were so focused on establishing a working relationship between the physicians and nurse practitioners and psychosocial providers that they didn't focus sufficient attention on informing nursing and support staff of their roles and how they were attempting to work together. As a result, therapists were not seen by these groups as integrated members of the provider team. Other problems emerged. For example, the names of behavioral science staff were inadvertently not included on office publications and their business cards were not ordered. To rectify this problem, residency faculty provided an in-service training for the entire office staff. A behavioral science faculty member led the training, which emphasized the importance of collaborative care to a patient's total well-being—the influence of biological, psychological, relational, and environmental factors on health was described. The presenter was careful to discuss the value of collaborative efforts not only among medical and psychosocial providers, but between office staff as well.

4. *In integrated care, a common language will bridge differences between disciplines.* Medical and psychosocial clinicians are trained differently, practice differently, and use different languages to conceptualize problems and discuss treatment issues. So far, our efforts to devise a common language to bridge communication problems between disciplines have not borne much success. For example, in one of our colleague's clinical settings, administrators are attempting to design a multidisciplinary assessment form. The initial draft was presented in a meeting of physicians, family therapists, psychologists, and social workers. Under a section that assessed for family functioning, the physicians and psychologists balked at such phrases as "boundaries poorly differentiated" and "engulfment of member," some stating they had no idea what these phrases meant or how they might be used. Similarly, a physician noting "no significant family history" is saying something quite different from what a therapist might read into the phrase.

Attempts made at developing a common language invariably result in compromising various assumptions underlying the practice of either the behavioral science or medical provider. Compromising these assumptions can result in confusion in developing and implementing treatment plans, as well as sacrifices to professional identity. Because of the realities of hierarchy discussed above, these sacrifices are often made by the behavioral science provider. This is especially true in the early part of model development when professional roles are still taking shape. We believe these sacrifices are too great.

Perhaps the best that can be achieved is for behavioral scientists to understand the language of the physician, and for the physician to understand the language of the behavioral scientist. Clearly, in situations where people are frequently informing decisions by reading reports and chart notes that other disciplines design and use, we need to make sure each understands what the other is saying. Any common language that might grow out of integrated care would be superficial, and could detract from the richness, descriptiveness, and therapeutic meaning of each discipline's theory and practice. An awareness and understanding of diverse languages (medical and behavioral) will enhance an integrated model immensely. While didactic courses, though limited in scope, can help professionals within the various disciplines understand each other, the best supplement is exposure and collaboration throughout training—the immersion model of learning any new language.

5. *Across-discipline training schedules always support integrated care.* In order to encourage and teach integrative care, a substantial amount of the behavioral science rotation needs to take place within the facility where the resident is seeing patients. Because our program is located

at three distinct sites, we initially had one individual at the main site coordinating rotation schedules. We soon discovered that schedules varied from site to site, and that limited communication between residents and behavioral science faculty meant that sometimes the rotation actually supported a separation between disciplines! The behavioral science faculty members who work with the residents need to have input into the rotation schedule, and the schedule needs to be coordinated with these teachers so that residents can have regular, hands-on experiences with behavioral science faculty.

6. *Behavioral science automatically gets equal time in integrated training programs.* In order for integration to be emphasized, the behavioral science component needs to be treated as an important part of the curriculum by faculty and administrators. Traditional residency programs often appear to treat behavioral science as an unwanted requirement that can be taken care of through the behavioral science rotation and an occasional in-service training. The importance and value of integrative care can only be communicated to trainees when psychosocial concerns are a prominent part of all aspects of training. In our program behavioral science faculty regularly give in-service presentations of psychosocial issues affecting patient medical care. They are also available for consultation, live supervision of cases, and cotherapy, outside the behavioral science rotation. We have found that as the psychosocial component of care has gained equal time in regularly scheduled in-service meetings and other training forums, residents are more likely to engage in integrative care.

FUTURE DIRECTIONS

As integrated care models become more widespread in health care delivery, we can expect a growing demand for specific training protocols. Those who plan to implement integrated care will be looking for a standardized method to train clinicians, as well as an overall model of integrated care itself. While some groundwork has been done, three issues must be addressed in the future.

First, specific training models with curriculum guidelines and steps for implementation must be developed. As previously mentioned, we usually know where we want to go before we know precisely how to get there. This is certainly true for training in integrated primary care. As trainers experiment with and adjust training programs, they learn what works and what doesn't. Models of training, complete with curriculum guidelines, training strategies, and achievable competencies need to be written in training manuals that are accessible to others. Professionals from different programs need to meet to share ideas and develop training models based on what is most successful across training programs. Because training in integrated primary care is still in its infancy, it may be premature to expect that these models currently exist. However, the future of training depends on this standardization.

Second, training programs need to develop methods of self-evaluation. It will be important for programs emphasizing models of integrated primary care to evaluate trainees on both a short-term and long-term basis. These evaluations can take the form of assessments of attitudes about working with other professionals, actual practice strategies, and treatment success. This information will provide feedback to the program about areas of deficit and competence. Then programs can make the necessary curriculum and other adjustments to effectively instruct trainees in the workings of integrated primary care.

Third, models of integrated care must begin to address the truly multidisciplinary nature of the primary care environment. For example, models of integrated care (ours included) frequently overlook the important contribution made by nursing and other medical staff personnel. In our setting, we have found that the nursing staff is really the backbone to patient care. Considering the prominent and important role the nursing staff plays in patient care, it is a mistake to not consider nursing in models of integrated care and integrated training. Including these medical professionals in the models of integrated care being advocated in training programs will improve patient care and increase provider communication and morale.

SUMMARY

Much has been written, debated, and discussed about a biopsychosocial model of treatment — usually from the unique perspective of individual disciplines. Perhaps no model of care is better suited to providing this kind of comprehensive attention than an integrated one in which multidisciplinary teams treat the whole patient. As yet, we have no clear map to show us the best way to reach this wonderful destination. This has sometimes hampered, but never stopped, our efforts to train a new group of physicians and therapists who will provide better care. In this chapter we have explored some of the most important assumptions that drive our training, and have outlined some of the pitfalls and how they can be avoided. We especially encourage other pioneers in integrated care to create signposts and markers along the way — evaluations, perhaps, of our own and others' assumptions and methods—so that future maps to guide training will clearly point the way.

REFERENCES

Blumenthal, D., & Thier, S. (1996). Managed care and medical education. *Journal of the American Medical Association, 276*(9), 725-727.

Chase, M. (1996, December 11). Medical records may be private but they're hardly confidential. *San Diego Union Tribune*, p. 27.

Clancy, C., & Kamerow, D. (1996). Evidence-based medicine meets cost-effectiveness analysis. *Journal of the American Medical Association, 276*(4), 329-330.

de Shazer, S. (1985). *Keys to solution in brief therapy*. New York: Norton.

Patterson, J., Baron, M., Bischoff, R., & McIntosh-Koontz, L. (1996). *Responding to health care reform: Implications for education and training of marriage and family therapists*. Manuscript submitted for publication.

Patterson, J., Bischoff, R., Scherger, J., & Grauf-Grounds, C. (1996). University family therapy training and a family medicine residency in a managed-care setting. *Family Systems & Health, 14*(1), 5-16.

Patterson, J., & Magulac, M. (1993). The family therapist's guide to psychopharmacology: A graduate level course. *Journal of Marital and Family Therapy, 20*, 151-174.

Patterson, J., & Scherger, J. (1995). A critique of health care reform in the United States: Implications for the training and practice of marriage and family therapy. *Journal of Marital and Family Therapy, 21*(2), 127-135.

Sanderson, W. (1995). Can psychological interventions meet the new demands of health care? *The American Journal of Managed Care, 1*(1), 93-98.

Scarf, M. (1996, June 16). Keeping secrets. *New York Times Magazine*, pp. 38-40.

Veloski, J., Barzansky, B., Nash, D., Bastacky, S., & Stevens, D. (1996). Medical student education in managed care settings. *Journal of the American Medical Association, 276*(9), 667-674.

Weston, B., & Lauria, M. (1996). Patient advocacy in the 1990s. *New England Journal of Medicine, 334*(8), 543-544.

Index